Pomegranate, Broccoli (sulforaphane) & Turmeric (Curcumin):

FROM THE FOOD CART TO THE MEDICINE CART

BY

Prof Randolph M. Howes MD, PhD
Physician, Surgeon, Scientist (Biochemist)
Author and Scholar

A CRITIQUE & SELECTIVE REVIEW

Pomegranate, Broccoli (sulforaphane) & Turmeric (Curcumin):

FROM THE FOOD CART TO THE MEDICINE CART

BY

Prof Randolph M. Howes MD, PhD

Physician, Surgeon, Scientist (Biochemist), Author and Scholar

**Adjunct Assistant Professor of Plastic Surgery, (RET.)
The Johns Hopkins Hospital, Baltimore, MD USA**

**Espaldon Professor of Plastic and Reconstructive Surgery,
University of Santo Tomas, Manila, Philippines**

**Adjunct Professor of Biological Sciences,
Southeastern Louisiana University**

**Founder, Director and Chairman of the Scientific Advisory
Board;
U.S. Medical Scientific Research Foundation, Inc.**

Copyright © 2015
Free Radical Publishing Co.
ISBN-13: 9781517475406
ISBN-10: 1517475406

By Dr. Randolph "HealR" Howes
Copyright © 2015
Free Radical Publishing Co.
27439 Hwy 441
Kentwood, Louisiana 70444

DISCLOSURE AND DISCLAIMER

drug therapy are required. The author and the publisher of this work have checked with sources believed to be reliable in their efforts to provide information that is complete and generally in accord with the standards accepted at the time of publication. However, in view of the possibility of human error or changes in the medical sciences, neither the authors nor the publisher nor any other party who has been involved in the preparation of publication of this work warrants that the information contained herein is in every respect accurate or complete, and they disclaim all responsibility to any errors or omissions or for the results obtained from use of the information contained in the work. Readers should confirm the information contained herein with other sources. For example and in particular, readers are advised to check the product information sheets (or labels) included in the package of each drug they plan to administer to be certain that the information contained in this work is accurate and that changes have not been made in the recommended dose or in the contraindications for administration. This recommendation is of particular importance in connection with new or infrequently used drugs, additives or supplements.

Disclaimers: Please note: only your personal physician or other health professional you consult can best advise you on matters of your health based on your medical history, your family medical history, your medication history, and how information from any of these databases may apply to you. Neither Dr. Howes nor any party involved in creating, producing or delivering this web site shall be liable for any damages arising out of access to or use of this material or web site, or any errors or omissions in the content thereof.

The information given herein is not intended as medical advice. Always consult with your doctor for underlying illness. Before beginning dietary investigation, consult a dietician or a physician with an interest in nutrition. Information is drawn from the scientific literature, web research, and personal enquiry; while all care is taken, information is not warranted as accurate and the author cannot be held liable for any errors and omissions.

The information contained herein is not intended to replace a one-on-one relationship with a qualified health care professional and is not intended as medical advice. It is intended as a sharing of knowledge and information from the research of Dr. Howes. Dr. Howes encourages you to make your own health care decisions based upon your research and the advice of a qualified health care professional.

Financial disclosure: **Dr. Howes has no financial conflicts of interest and is not involved in the sale of dietary supplements or fitness equipment. The author holds no stocks or interests in companies in the food additive or antioxidant supplement business.**

ACKNOWLEDGEMENTS

Special thanks Don Neale Piatt, Sr. for proof reading. Also, special thanks to Michael R. Root, M.S. for his unwavering encouragement.

DEDICATION

To the Nobel Prize Winners I have known:
George Wald, Andrew V. Schally,
Louis J. Ignarro, Fritz Albert Lipmann,
Linus Pauling, Joseph E. Murray,
and James Dewey Watson.
Thanks for the inspiration.

Pomegranate, Broccoli (sulforaphane) & Turmeric (Curcumin):

FROM THE FOOD CART TO THE MEDICINE CART

TABLE OF CONTENTS:

SECTION FOUR

ABBREVIATIONS

reactive oxygen species (ROS); electronically modified oxygen derivatives (EMODs); Free Radical theory (FRT); electron transport chain (ETC); catalase, (CAT, CT); superoxide dismutase, (SOD); glutathione peroxidase (GPx, GSH-Px); antioxidant (AOX, AO); lipid peroxidation (LIPOX); encapsulated antioxidant concentrate (EAC); FRTA (free radical theory of aging); MFRTA (mitochondrial free radical theory of aging); deoxyribonucleic acid (DNA); mtDNA (mitochondrial DNA); nDNA (nuclear DNA); methionine sulfoxide reductase (MsrA); basal metabolic rate (BMR); prostate-specific antigen (PSA); ORAC, Oxygen Radical Absorbance Capacity; Trolox equivalents (TE); USDA's Nutrient Data Laboratory (NDL); TEAC, Trolox Equivalent Antioxidant Capacity; FRAP, ferric reducing ability of plasma assay; TRAP, total radical trapping antioxidant parameter; FOX, refers to ferrous oxidation of xylenol orange; CAP-e refers to cell-based antioxidant protection in erythrocytes; thiobarbituric acid reactive substances (TBARS); ornithine decarboxylase (ODC); low density lipoprotein (LDL); triglycerides (TG); High density lipoprotein (HDL); serum total cholesterol (TC); high fat diet (HFD); Methicillin-resistant *staphylococcus aureus* (MRSA) and methicillin-sensitive *staphylococcus aureus* (MSSA); myosin light chain kinase (MLCK); *vascular cell adhesion molecule-1* (VCAM-1); sulforaphane (SF); complementary and alternative medicine (CAM); N-acetylcysteine (NAC); xeroderma pigmentosum A (XPA) protein; isothiocyanate (ITC); mitochondrial membrane potential (MMP); antioxidant response element (ARE); cancer stem cells (CSCs); chronic atrophic gastritis (CAG); Phenethyl isothiocyanate (PEITC); oxidative phosphorylation (OXPHOS); Beta-Phenylethyl isothiocyanate (PEITC); Ascorbigen (ABG); Cytochrome P450 (CYP); Indole-3-carbinol (I3C); tumor necrosis factor-related apoptosis-inducing ligand (TRAIL); heme-oxygenase 1 (HMOX1); thioredoxin (TXN); á-tocopherylquinone (TQ); Tetrahydrocurcumin (THC); (diferuloylmethane, CUR); rheumatoid arthritis (RA); non-steroidal anti-inflammatory drug (NSAID); Food and Drug Administration (FDA); colorectal cancer (CRC); aberrant crypt foci (ACF); monoclonal gammopathy of undetermined signifi cance (MGUS); cervical intraepithelial neoplasm (CIN); Head and neck squamous cell carcinoma (HNSCC); Irritable bowel syndrome (IrBS); type 2 diabetes (T2DM); acute renal failure ARF; 5 Fluoruracil (5FU); "Generally Recognized as Safe" (GRAS); cyclooxygenase-2 (COX2); 5-lipoxygenase (5-LOX); visible light (VL); Dinitrophenol, DNP; human papillomavirus (HPV).

SECTION ONE

PROLOGUE

Many foods, such as pomegranate, broccoli and turmeric, have claimed to possess magical antioxidant properties and capabilities which claim to heal a wide spectrum of human diseases and increase one's lifespan. Yet, I have collected well over 500 studies showing the ineffectiveness and the potential harm of these very same supplemental antioxidants.

Many of the articles concerning antioxidants are "awash with adjustments, nonsignificant results and unfamiliar statistical methods," and convincing conclusions or "plausibility" are hard to come by, particularly as it relates to cause and effect or provability.

I do not "shoot from the hip," based on my pre-conceived ideas, but I look at the relevant papers and give a thoughtful critique on the peer-reviewed literature.

Contrary the erroneous claims of antioxidants, in article after article, which I have read, and in book after book that I have written, I have been impressed with the fact that many of the beneficial effects of antioxidants can be attributed to their prooxidant activity, including cancer cell kill which is primarily an EMOD-induced (ROS, prooxidant) apoptotic event.

This has proven to be the case with pomegranate, broccoli and curcumin.

When researched, antioxidants which claim to have tumoricidal activity have been found to trigger apoptosis primarily prooxidatively, not antioxidatively.

Curiously, antioxidant zealots deny any prooxidant role in these mechanisms and continue to preach the wonders of antioxidants and the pernicious character of oxidants or EMODs.

For the sake of scientific accuracy and truth, this must stop.

This most recent article by Janet Helm exemplifies the fact that the free radical theory has fallen and that "antioxidant mania" is over. I have been promoting this approach for over 15 years and it is now coming to fruition.

It has been a long and arduous path for me but it has been worth it to set the scientific record straight as regards antioxidants and reactive oxygen species (ROS), which are more accurately called electronically modified oxygen derivatives (EMODs).

In spite of spurious claims, there are no "super foods." So, Helm's article will serve as a starting point for this book.

The Antioxidant Era Is Over -- and What's Next

U.S. News and World Report
By Janet Helm

9-14-15 I have adapted Helm's article as follows:

RMH Note: refers to insertions by Prof. Randolph M. Howes MD, PhD (**RMH**).

The public was once enamored by antioxidants. This technical-sounding term used to be plastered on food and beverage labels -- from cereal, snack bars, chips and chocolate to juices, tea and even soft drinks.

RMH Note: I found that in the past, if one wanted a boost in product sales, all they had to do was to plaster "Loaded With Antioxidants" on their product and it would sell like snake oil, which it was.

You'll still find some products touting the antioxidants inside, but **the number of such claims has plummeted. Only 2 percent of new products in the U.S. boasted about antioxidants last year, according to Mintel's Global New Products Database, which tracks food and beverage launches.**

RMH Note: Companies still pushing antioxidants should be part of a class action law suit, because of the well established harmful potential associated with excessive levels of antioxidants.

Much of the decline resulted from the Food and Drug Administration clamping down on companies making claims about antioxidants. Some manufacturers even faced lawsuits. The biggest nail in the antioxidant coffin was the decision by the Department of Agriculture to yank the ORAC Database for Selected Foods from its website in 2012. ORAC, which stands for oxygen radical absorbance capacity, is a test to esti-mate the antioxidant activity of foods.

Antioxidants are substances that inhibit oxidation -- or the potential damaging effects of oxygen. They **supposedly** help protect the body from rogue molecules called free radicals that have been implicated in everything from heart disease to cancer.

RMH Note: Please remember that there are at least seven es-sential oxidative pathways that are crucial to our well being and survival: cancer protection, wound healing, detoxification, pathogen protection, immunity, energy production, and intercellular cross talk, all of which can be interfered with or blocked by excess levels of antioxidants.

The ORAC test was once widely used by food and supplement makers; ORAC scores were flashed on package labels, cited on charts compar-ing different antioxidants and featured in ads touting antioxidant super powers. Trouble is, **the ORAC test looked only at what goes on in a test tube, which turns out to have little to do with what actually happens in the body**.

On its website, the USDA explains: "**There is no evidence that the beneficial effects of polyphenol-rich foods can be attrib-uted to the antioxidant properties of these foods. The data for antioxidant capacity of foods generated by in vitro (test-tube) methods cannot be extrapolated to in vivo (human) effects and the clinical trials to test benefits of dietary an-tioxidants have produced mixed results. We know now that antioxidant molecules in food have a wide range of func-tions, many of which are unrelated to the ability to absorb free radicals.**"

Around the same time the USDA removed the ORAC data-base from its website, research was underway that showed

antioxidant supplements -- including beta-carotene, vitamin E and selenium -- did not offer protection against cancer and cardiovascular disease. In fact, some studies showed the supplements could even be harmful at high levels.

RMH Note: Please refer to my companion books at the end of this tome.

This doesn't mean that antioxidants found naturally in foods, such as fruits, vegetables and whole grains, are not a good thing. They certainly are. But now scientists are discovering the reasons plant-derived foods are so beneficial go far beyond their antioxidant properties or ability to fight free radicals.

Rather than worrying about a food's ORAC score, you're better off knowing about the phytonutrients inside. Also called phytochemicals, these naturally-occurring compounds are the real workhorses in fruits, vegetables and other plant foods, protecting our health in many wondrous ways.

Phytonutrients help fight inflammation, influence blood vessel function, affect certain hormones and signaling systems that regulate cell growth, and even influence whether genes that protect health are turned on or temporarily silenced, says registered dietitian Karen Collins, a nutrition advisor to the American Institute for Cancer Research.

RMH Note: Please keep in mind that **many of the phytonutrients have very low bioavailability** and those that do, have beneficial properties are have significant prooxidant character.

So my wish is that people will stop referring to all the good stuff in fruits, vegetables and other plant-based foods and beverages -- even chocolate and wine -- as antioxidants. It's almost insulting to their multi-tasking abilities.

It's time to learn a new lexicon. Now it's all about polyphenols, flavonoids, flavanols, carotenoids, resveratrol, anthocyanins, proanthocyanidins and other phytonutrients. Maybe these words don't roll off your tongue quite the same way as antioxidants easily do, but these are the terms that will soon be breaking through as we learn more about the disease-protecting attributes of phytonutrients.

RMH Note: I have written about each of the **polyphenols, flavonoids, flavanols, carotenoids, resveratrol, anthocyanins,**

proanthocyanidins and other phytonutrients in my various books discussing chocolate, tomatoes, blueberries, wine, etc. Please refer to my companion books.

From fruits and vegetables to grains, beans, nuts and seeds -- if it's a plant, it contains phytonutrients. Often these mighty phytonutrients provide the pigment in plants, so take a cue from the color. Orange-tinted beta carotene gives carrots, pumpkin and other winter squashes their distinctive hue. Bright red cherries are packed with anthocyanins and purple grapes are rich in resveratrol. Typically, the darker the color, the more phytonutrients inside.

However, don't lose sight of the big picture. Focusing only on antioxidants or single phytonutrients is like "zeroing in on a section of an impressionist painting and seeing only the dots," says Collins. "Step back and you see the big picture: that making nutrient-rich plant foods the focus of your meals protects your health through a whole range of pathways."

RMH Note: It appears that current studies indicate that it is the microbiome breakdown products of the phytonutrients that may be having a beneficial effect on human health - not so-called antioxidant activity or the effect of the primary phytochemical.

Once again, this is an important reminder to emphasize whole foods, instead of individual nutrients. It's about looking at your overall diet, not a single component. And, as always, **your health is better protected by what you put on your plate than what you can buy in a pill**.

RMH Note: I agree with Helm's conclusion that none of the chemically concocted supplements are equivalent to the nutrition provided by fresh fruits and vegetables.

**Truth be told,
I can scarcely begin to explain
the overwhelming, biochemical complexity
of a singular living, breathing critter.
In truth, it approximates
being utterly ineffable,
all the while, reflecting the
stunning beauty of Creation.**
R. M. Howes, M.D., Ph.D.
2/2/15

**The free radical theory
has more holes in it than
a warehouse full of Swiss cheese.**
R. M. Howes, M.D., Ph.D.
1/2/15

**In life, opposites may attract opposites
and likes interact with likes.
The latter is assuredly the case with
ground state triplet oxygen,
a magically unique elemental entity.**
R. M. Howes, M.D., Ph.D.
2/2/15

**If one were to pull the thread
of a singular biochemical pathway,
you would inadvertently tug on
the totality of the living cellular fabric.**
R. M. Howes, M.D., Ph.D.
9/21/06

**A state of health is only maintained
by a continuously vigilant oxidative defensive system,
without which we quickly succumb to
bugs, drugs and thugs called cancer cells.
Debilities and anomalies of our somatic condition are
pounced upon by pathogens and mutagens
but they are quickly
"rebuffed by radicals."
Oxidative "radical outbursts" of EMODs
are proven tireless workers.
So it is in the world of
homeostasis.**
R. M. Howes, M.D., Ph.D.
6/11/06

**Oxygen is not optional.
It is essential for creating and
perpetuating aerobic life and for
sustaining homeostatic health,
especially in man.**
R. M. Howes, M.D., Ph.D.
4/2/15

Radically increase your chances
for establishing long term homeostatic health
by increasing your oxidative capacity,
- your oxidative bliss.
R. M. Howes, M.D., Ph.D.
4/3/15

The voracious vortex of the free radical theory
has sucked up the common sense of medical biochemistry.
This anomaly of logic posits the artifice that
oxygen is the primary instrument of the Grim Reaper and
that it is the root system from which sprouts nigh all
pathophysiologies.
Author after author acquiesces to this cheap parlor trick and
appears blind to this scientific sleight of hand.
I beg you to look around at the beauty of aerobic nature,
take a deep breath, relax and reconsider.
Oxygen is the indispensable energy ingredient,
sustaining the magic and mystery
of all human experiences.
It is self evident.
R. M. Howes, M.D., Ph.D.
5/21/06

EMODs are not as harmful as you might've imagined,
not as destructive as you might've thought
and not the "inner enemy" you might've feared.
In fact, your life depends on them.
R. M. Howes, M.D., Ph.D.
5/28/10

INTRODUCTION

My new readers must have a basic background in redox chemistry and on the flawed history of antioxidants. Antioxidants are not the saviors they have been made out to be. In fact, in excessive levels, they can be quite harmful.

The first section of this book will be for an introduction to scientific facts, as they relate to antioxidants and EMODs.

So, let's go back to 2010. This is from an interview that I did with WWL TV.

Doctor says extra vitamins aren't just unnecessary -- they may be harmful

WWL Staff, WWLTV.com December 10, 2010

NEW ORLEANS -- Vitamins are essential to good health. But now a local doctor is questioning conventional thinking.

Do we already get enough vitamins from our diets and is taking extra vitamins potentially harmful?

For years we've been told to load up on the antioxidant vitamins, that they would mop up the byproduct or waste of using oxygen in our bodies. We were told those byproducts were bad for us and made us age faster or get sick.

Well now a local doctor and scientist is challenging that theory that's been around for years.

'Back in the earlier days in the late '60s, early '70s, these things were glamorized. It's a vitamin so it's got to be good for you, right?' said Dr. Randolph Howes of Kentwood. LA.

RMH: 'And in fact, I personally took them myself for many years, until I started researching it and I saw the harmful potential was incredibly there. It was shockingly there.'

Howes got his M.D. and Ph.D. from Tulane. He has professor appointments at Johns Hopkins, Southeastern Louisiana University and the University of Santo Tomas in the Philippines. He is a surgeon and Biochemist.

For years he practiced plastic surgery, but retired after he invented a type of catheter that saves critically ill people. It's used in ER's and OR's in 100 countries around the world and has been credited with helping save the lives of over 20 million critically ill people worldwide.

Now he is privately funding his own research. He thinks we need to change our thinking about antioxidant vitamins.

RMH: 'No one worldwide has ever assembled the number of studies that I have, showing that these antioxidants vitamins, in particular Vitamins A, Vitamin C and Vitamin E, are basically frequently ineffective and then on the other hand they are frequently causing harm,' he said.

Howes said he started noticing that the studies, beginning around 2000, starting shifting away from the free radical theory, and the notion that the waste from oxidation was bad and we needed antioxidants to mop them up. He now believes oxygen free radicals do good things in the body, like turn on and off over 200 genes.

RMH: 'Everything from fertilization of an egg, to almost the thought process. See, the brain is interesting. It only weighs 2 percent of the body, but it uses 20 percent of the oxygen we take in. It's an oxygen sponge and it forms these free radicals at an amazing rate. So why isn't it sitting there rancid in our head all of the time? It isn't,' Howes said.

RMH: 'I'm saying that they are the most important molecules in the body, in that they protect us from pathogens, such as bacteria for infections, fungi for infections, for even agents such as malaria, even agents such as HIV/AIDS, the virus,' he said. 'Then it protects us against new cancerous growths.'

And he now believes the science is showing that by mopping up these free radicals in the body, we are causing illness or harm.

RMH: 'What diseases: cancer, heart disease, strokes, diabetes, arthritis, cataracts. There are now quite a few studies starting to show with multivitamins that there are problems, problems such as increased risk of the aggressive form of prostate cancer with multivitamins, increased risk of problems in children with multivitamins, allergies, asthma,' he said.

Prof Randolph M. Howes MD, PhD

Are there doctors who think he is controversial?

RMH: 'Yes, yes, in fact, last night just before coming down, I went on the internet on Amazon, pulled up on the book section, just typed in anti-oxidants, 3,300 list showed of that. There might be four or five leaning toward what I am saying here,' Howes said.

When he gives lectures to medical students and faculty, there are doctors who disagree with his information.

RMH: 'Once you point out to them there is no war between the good, being antioxidants, and the bad, oxygen free radicals, they understand it a lot better,' he said.

He's put all the science in his book, 'Death in Small Doses,' and says we don't need to mega-dose on vitamins. Americans get enough in their diets, he believes. More research over time will unveil if he is a pioneer in his thinking or on the wrong track.

Howes said exercise, which increases oxygen consumption, and getting vitamins from fruits and vegetables is proven in the medical literature to decrease the risk of disease.

Go here for more information: http://www.iwillfindthecure.org

The following is another interview and this is with Gambit magazine in New Orleans.

Gambit - Nov 2, 2010

Do synthetic antioxidant supplements do more harm than good ?

By Missy Wilkinson @missy_wilkinson

Vitamin A, C and E supplements are touted as a panacea for everything from crow's feet to the common cold. However, **Dr. Randolph M. Howes**, who earned his doctorate in medicine and biochemistry from Tulane School of Medicine and serves as adjunct associate professor of plastic surgery at Johns Hopkins Hospital, argues that synthetic antioxidant supplements do more harm than good. His book, *Death In*

Small Doses?: Antioxidant Vitamins A, C & E in the 21st Century (Trafford Publishing), debunks the free radical theory.

Q: What is the free radical theory?

A: The free radical theory was proposed by Dr. Denham Harman in 1954. He erroneously concluded that oxygen free radicals were responsible for most of the diseases in man. So if oxygen free radicals were causing diseases like cancer, heart disease and stroke, then antioxidants would reverse, cure or prevent these diseases. This theory has been around for more than half a century, and it became accepted as being true.

Q: Is the free radical theory a sound one?

A: The free radical theory lacks predictability, ergo it fails to be validated by the scientific method. So many studies that show the nullification of the free radical theory have either been ignored or denied. One of the most accepted theories for aging is the oxygen free radical theory of aging, but these over-exuberant claims for antioxidants have been wrong. No theory of aging has been proven. Today, with the antioxidant vitamins, it is not about scientific evidence. It is about clever marketing.

Q: Are synthetic vitamin A, C and E supplements good for you or even necessary?

A: Unless you have a known deficiency of a vitamin, all you need is a well-balanced, nutritious diet. You need to consume nuts and five servings a day of fresh fruit and vegetables. Fresh fruits and vegetables are very complex biochemically, with tens of thousands of compounds in them. We can't determine or define what they are doing on their own or synergistically with all these other compounds. So taking a supplement is not even close to the same thing as eating fruits or vegetables.

Q: Can these antioxidant supplements hurt you?

A: Everywhere from Johns Hopkins Hospital and Harvard (Medical School) to Tufts (University School of Medicine) have found that antioxidants can increase total or overall mortality. They increase risks of prostate and lung cancer, the risk of various forms of heart disease, the rates of bone fractures, the risk of gestational (or pregnancy-induced) hypertension ... and the list goes on and on.

Q: What should we do to stay healthy?

A: If there is one thing that is consistent in medical literature, it is the fact that exercise decreases the risk of disease. When you exercise, you increase your oxygen consumption, and we want to increase our oxidative capacity. The second best way is with vitamin D3. A substance in the skin is converted into vitamin D3, a pro-oxidant, when exposed to sunlight. Fifteen minutes of sun a day is enough, but it is also available as a supplement, and it appears to be very effective in that form, unlike other supplements. And you need to consume fresh vegetables, fruits and nuts. Even fast food places are offering salads and fresh fruits, so it is a matter of choice.

Frequently, I have been asked for my opinion regarding various products that have created a marketing craze amongst the people, such as Plexus Slim, Protandem and Cuties.

Invariably, these products are the result of clever marketing campaigns of persuasion. These products may have some nutritional value but lack the magical preventative or curative properties attributed to them.

They are classic examples of con games, schemes and scams. This type of crime has been around since the days of the "medicine man", who sold snake oil from out of the back of a covered wagon.

This is exactly the case with the foods containing antioxidants and which have erroneously been dubbed as "super foods."

Studies on the naked mole rat have lifted the curtain and allowed us to see that even with the accumulation of high levels of oxidative products, this unique critter has the longest healthspan and lifespan of all rodents.

Please refer to my book: **Cancer and Longevity Answers: Naked mole rats, Exercise & EMODs (ROS).** CreateSpace and Free Radical Publishing, © **2015.** (Howes, 2015, Cancer)

I have come to recognize and point out the fact that a state of "oxidative bliss" is necessary to maintain homeostasis and provide pathogen and neoplasia protection.

Also, please refer to my book: **Hyperbaric oxygen, Hypoxia, Hyperoxia & EMODs (ROS): Separating Fact From Factitious.** CreateSpace and Free Radical Publishing, © **2015.** (Howes, 2015, HBOT)

For over six decennia, we have been misled by the lamentable free radical theory, which dragged a huge red herring across the trail of scientific oxidative truth. My friend, the late Dr. Denham Harman, was truly a nice guy but his erroneously concocted theory, based on radiation studies, held us at a nigh standstill for over half a century and still holds back scientific progress.

Please refer to my book: **Antioxidant Failures and Dangers, The fall of the free radical theory.** CreateSpace and Free Radical Publishing, © **2011.** (Howes, 2011)

We have only been able to move forward by opening our cumulative minds to the beneficence of ground state, di-radical oxygen.

Please refer to my book: **Exercise and Reactive Oxygen Species. Likely the only health miracle out there.** CreateSpace and Free Radical Publishing, © **2015.** (Howes, 2015, Exercise)

My research has established that antioxidants have failed to block, reverse or prevent diseases, such as cancer, strokes and cardiovascular disease, in randomized clinical trials with over 16 million participants and clearly show that the free radical theory lacks predictability and fails to fulfill the requirements of the scientific method.

Please refer to my book: **Antioxidants Linked To Deadly Unintended Consequences,** CreateSpace and Free Radical Publishing, © **2012.** (Howes, 2012)

I have researched this extensively and my results can be found at amazon.com or www.iwillfindthecure.org.

Please refer to my books: **Death In Small Doses? Book One:** Antioxidant Vitamins A, C & E in the 21st Century *A Health Impact Statement For The Layman.* Trafford Publishing, © **2010.** (Howes, Book 1, 2010)

- Death In Small Doses? Book Two: Antioxidant Vitamins A, C & E in the 21st Century *A Health Impact Statement For The Medical Scientist.* Trafford Publishing, © **2010.** (Howes, Book 2, 2011)

Basically, oxygen free radicals are of low toxicity and are crucial metabolic agents for pathogen and neoplasia protection. The studies showing the failure of antioxidants to prevent or reverse diseases were based on the nullified free radical theory.

Please refer to my book: **Reactive Oxygen Species vs. Antioxidants: The Oxypocalypse or The War That Never Was,** CreateSpace and Free Radical Publishing, © **2014.** (Howes, 2014, ROS)

**There is no consistent evidence
that the foods we eat
have a health benefit
due solely to their
so-called antioxidant content.
Many of the foods recommended
for a healthy diet,
are, indeed, nutritious,
but for other
biochemically complex reasons
apart from
the antioxidants contained therein.**
R. M. Howes, M.D., Ph.D.
2/8/15

The late Dr. Denham Harman was responsible for the introduction and popularity of the currently invalidated free radical theory.

**The free radical theory
is more than just a theory.
Undeniably,
it is a scientifically invalidated
and an indubitably nullified theory.
Cleanse this misleading paradigm
from your thoughts and your studies.**
R. M. Howes, M.D., Ph.D.
2/8/15

Antioxidant overview

Antioxidants are (man-made or natural) substances that inhibit the oxidation of other molecules and may therefore protect cells from the alleged damage caused by free radicals. Antioxidants are found in many foods, especially fruits and vegetables.

There are literally thousands of different substances that can act as antioxidants.

Some of the most popular antioxidants are, beta-carotene, selenium, vitamin A, ascorbic acid (vitamin C), tocopherol (vitamin E), ubiquinol (coenzyme Q).

Since 1990's, antioxidants have gained in popularity as scientist theorized that free radical or oxidative damage was involved in the early stages of artery-clogging atherosclerosis and allegedly contributes to cancer, vision loss, and some chronic conditions.

Unfortunately, antioxidants have erroneously become a synonym for good health.

Due to their profitability, high popularity and demand supplemental antioxidants also found their way to supermarket shelves, where sales have been brisk.

However, <u>more and more well-designed studies show that antioxidants, in supplement form, do not deliver promised health benefits.</u> In fact, my research has shown that excessive ingestion of supplemental antioxidants is harmful and it increases the risk of cancer, heart disease, strokes and overall mortality.

Therefore, I decided to dig into the scientific literature to bring you the facts about these very popular supplements.

What are Antioxidants, Free Radicals, and What is Oxidative Stress?

Free radicals (reactive oxygen species) are relatively unstable molecules that are naturally formed during exercise, sun exposure, cigarette smoking, and when your body converts food into energy.

Theoretically, they may cause cellular damage via a process cleverly called oxidative stress.

Oxidative stress is described as increased production of oxidants or a significant decrease in the effectiveness of antioxidants, which may potentially lead to damage. (Sies, 1997)

Betteridge defined oxidative stress as "disturbance in the balance between the production of reactive oxygen species (free radicals, EMODs) and antioxidant defenses". (Betteridge, 2000)

Allegedly, severity of damage caused by oxidative stress depends upon the size of changes. It may cause anything from small deviations in the cell to cellular death. (Choi et al, 2009)

According to the nullified free radical theory, to prevent free radical damage the body has a defense system of **antioxidants.**

Many believe that they are produced by our bodies to fight off the free radicals formed by normal body processes. They can also be ingested by eating a healthy diet or as a supplement.

However, I believe that so-called antioxidants serve as co-oxidants or pre-oxidants, because they provide an electron source for essential oxidants and the formation of EMODs.

Exercise and Oxidative Damage

Strenuous physical exercise can increase oxygen consumption from 10 to 20 times over the resting, which leads to oxidative stress via increased production of free radicals (EMODs) and in vitro lipid peroxidation. (Clarkson, 1995)

Skeletal muscle, which makes up about 42% of body weight, uses about 30% of oxygen consumed at rest, and over 86% of oxygen consumed during heavy work.

The abdominal organs use 25% and the brain uses 20% of the oxygen consumed at rest. Their relative contributions proportionately decrease during heavy work.

The human brain and heart can survive for only brief intervals of O_2 deprivation without sustaining irreversible damage or cell death.

This fact raised a few questions: does this increased oxidative stress enhance damage to muscles and other tissues and do athletes need to supplement with antioxidants?

Well, some scientists weasel their way out of this paradox by stating, "luckily our bodies can adapt to regular physical exercise via improved antioxidant defense system." (Clarkson, 1995)

Please refer to my book, **Exercise and Reactive Oxygen Species. Likely the only health miracle out there.** CreateSpace and Free Radical Publishing, © **2015.** (Howes, 2015, Exercise)

Whether athletes should ingest extra antioxidants remains controversial. However, a diet rich in fruits and vegetables is suggested.

Please refer to my book, **Sex, Performance, Reproduction, Naked Radicals And Antioxidants,** CreateSpace and Free Radical Publishing, © **2012.** (Howes, 2012, Sex)

Please refer to my other books as follows:

- **Death In Small Doses? Book One: Antioxidant Vitamins A, C & E in the 21st Century. A Health Impact Statement For The Layman.** Trafford Publishing, © **2010.** (Howes, Book 1, 2010)

- **Death In Small Doses? Book Two: Antioxidant Vitamins A, C & E in the 21st Century. A Health Impact Statement For The Medical Scientist.** Trafford Publishing, © **2010.** (Howes, Book 2, 2011)

- **Antioxidant Overkill,** CreateSpace and Free Radical Publishing, © **2011.** (Howes, 2011, Overkill)

- **Dangers of Excessive Antioxidants in Cancer Patients;** The Consequent Downfall of the Free Radical Theory, CreateSpace and Free Radical Publishing, © **2011.** (Howes, 2011, Dangers)

- **Heart Disease and Antioxidant Failures,** CreateSpace and Free Radical Publishing, © **2011.** (Howes, 2011, Heart Disease)

- **Antioxidant Failures and Dangers,** CreateSpace and Free Radical Publishing, © **2011.** (Howes, 2011, AOX Failures)

- **Anti-Aging Anti-oxidant Scams,** CreateSpace and Free Radical Publishing, © **2011.** (Howes, 2011, AOX Scams)

- **Alzheimer's Disease: Forget Antioxidants and Supplements,** CreateSpace and Free Radical Publishing, © **2012.** (Howes, 2012, Alzheimer's)

- **Sex, Performance, Reproduction, Naked Radicals And Antioxidants,** CreateSpace and Free Radical Publishing, © **2012.** (Howes, 2012, Sex)

- **Antioxidants Linked To Deadly Unintended Consequences,** CreateSpace and Free Radical Publishing, © **2012.** (Howes, 2012)

- **U.T.O.P.I.A.: Unified Theory of Oxygen Participation In Aerobiosis,** CreateSpace and Free Radical Publishing, © **2014, revised.** (Howes, 2014, UTOPIA)

- **Hydrogen Peroxide: A Health, Homeostatic and Protective Essentiality,** CreateSpace and Free Radical Publishing, © **2014.** (Howes, 2014, H2O2)

- **Reactive Oxygen Species vs. Antioxidants: The Oxypocalypse or The War That Never Was,** CreateSpace and Free Radical Publishing, © **2014.** (Howes, 2014, ROS)

- **Diabetes and Oxygen Free Radical Sophistry,** CreateSpace and Free Radical Publishing, © **2014, revised.** (Howes, 2014, Diabetes)

- **FISH OIL (Omega3 fatty acids): Facts, Fantasies & Failures.** CreateSpace and Free Radical Publishing, © **2014.** (Howes, 2014, Fish oil)

-**Vitamin D: Benefits & False claims.** CreateSpace and Free Radical Publishing, © **2014.** (Howes, 2014, Vit D)

- **Chocolate & Red Wine Antioxidants (Polyphenols, Flavonoids & Resveratrol): Facts vs. Falsehoods.** CreateSpace and Free Radical Publishing, © **2015.** (Howes, 2015, Chocolate)

- **Blueberry, Tomato & CoQ10 Antioxidants (Anthocyanin, Lycopene & Ubiquinone): Claims vs. Facts.** CreateSpace and Free Radical Publishing, © **2015.** (Howes, 2015, Blueberry)

- **Cancer and Longevity Answers: Naked mole rats, Exercise & EMODs (ROS).** CreateSpace and Free Radical Publishing, © **2015.** (Howes, 2015, Cancer)

- **Hyperbaric oxygen, Hypoxia, Hyperoxia & EMODs (ROS): Separating Fact From Factitious.** CreateSpace and Free Radical Publishing, © **2015.** (Howes, 2015, HBOT)

Let me summarize a bit.

Why Antioxidant Supplements Do Not Work as Marketed?

Widespread use of antioxidants has failed to put an end to the current pandemic of cancer, diabetes, and cardiovascular disease and it also failed to reverse the aging process.

Furthermore, **most clinical randomized, double-blind, controlled trials in humans using supplemental antioxidants have failed to provide substantial health benefits**. (Howes, 2006, Fantasy)

The Women's Antioxidant Cardiovascular Study failed to show any effects of ascorbic acid (500 mg/d), vitamin E (600 IU every other day), or beta carotene (50 mg every other day) on cardiovascular events among women at high risk for cardiovascular disease. (Cook et al, 2007)

Same was reported in a large-scale study in men where neither vitamin E (400 IU every other day) nor C (500 mg/d) supplementation reduced the risk of major cardiovascular events. (Sesso et al, 2008)

Meta-analysis of randomized trials discouraged the use of vitamin supplements containing beta-carotene and vitamin A, beta-carotene's biologically active metabolite, because this family of agents is associated with a small but significant excess of all-cause mortality and cardiovascular death. (Vivekananthan et al, 2003)

Furthermore, beta-carotene and vitamins C and E had no effect on the age-related lens opacities or visual acuity loss in 4,757 participants (who were followed for 6.3 years). (AREDS report no. 9, 2001)

Findings of the Hercberg et al. study advised against supplementing with vitamins and trace element antioxidants as they may not always provide beneficial effects. (Hercberg et al, 2007)

In 13,017 men and women, **rates of skin cancer were higher in women (but not in men) who were assigned to take vitamin C, vitamin E, beta-carotene, selenium, and zinc**.

According to National Center for Complementary and Alternative Medicine several reasons may contribute to these findings, including:

(http://nccam.nih.gov/health/antioxidants/introduction.htm Retrieved 4. May 2014)

— Relationship between free radicals and health is more complex than previously thought as in some (many) cases free radicals may actually be beneficial. Some recent data shows that cells use reactive oxygen species as part of the signaling process responsible for activating an important mechanism for eliminating cancer cells. (Lopaczynski et al, 2001)

— Health benefits from a diet rich in vegetables and fruits may be caused by other substances present in such food rather than antioxidants.

— High doses of supplemental antioxidants used in studies may have different effect on the body than small amounts found naturally in foods. Differences in the chemical composition of antioxidants in foods versus those in supplements may also influence their effects.

— For some diseases, specific antioxidants may be more suitable than others and act as cooxidants.

Potential Hazards of Antioxidants

Not only that most studies failed to show health benefits of antioxidants, a few raised the possibility that taking antioxidant supplements, alone or combinations, could interfere with health and longevity.

For example, **a study in Finnish male smokers found an 18% excess of lung cancer in participants receiving beta-carotene compared to placebo after 6 years and increased the incidence of cardiac death and the risk for major coronary events**. (Heinonen et al, 1994)

The trial was stopped early due to increase in lung cancer among those taking the supplement. Excess in lung cancer (28%) was also reported in another trial where 18,314 smokers, former smokers and workers exposed to asbestos were given beta-carotene and vitamin A for 4 years. The trial was stopped 21 months early.

Conclusion

It is well established that a diet rich in vegetables and fruits is desirable. **However, how much of this benefits can be credited to their antioxidant content remains unclear.**

Just because so-called oxidative stress contributes to some chronic diseases and vision loss that doesn't mean that antioxidant supplements will fix the problem. The studies thus far are controversial and in general don't provide strong evidence that antioxidant supplements have a considerable impact on disease. Also, they may be quite harmful.

If you decide to take dietary antioxidants keep in mind that they may interact with some medications as their combination may cause serious problems like kidney damage, bleeding problems, nerve damage and may interfere with absorption of medications used. (http://www.drugs.com/drug-interactions/multivitamin-with-minerals, antioxidant-formula.html Retrieved 4. May 2014)

The best overall advice is not to use antioxidant supplements to replace a healthy diet or conventional medical care. (http://nccam.nih.gov/health/antioxidants/introduction.htm Retrieved 4. May 2014)

Also, try to get as much information as you can from reliable sources.

Basics On Oxygen Metabolism

Cellular respiration and the electron transport chain are crucial for aerobic life, as we know it, and oxygen and oxidation are at the center of these processes.

Oxidation equals aerobic life and excessive antioxidants can threaten, jeopardize, endanger or terminate this vital process and its attendant EMOD formation and EMOD reactions.

Oxygen and EMODs are not the demons they have been made out to be.

Still, the free radical theory remains one of the most popular theories relating to disease and aging causation. Calculated lies and scientific myths can be very hard to overcome, especially when they have been repeated for over six decennia. Such is the case with Harman's free radical theory.

The PERMANENT gases in the atmosphere by percent are:

Nitrogen 78.1%
Oxygen 20.9%
these two permanent gases together comprise 99% of the atmosphere.....Other permanent gases:

Argon 0.9%
Neon 0.002%
Helium 0.0005%
Krypton 0.0001%
Hydrogen 0.00005%

VARIABLE gases in the atmosphere and typical percentage values are:

Water vapor 0 to 4%
Carbon Dioxide 0.035%
Methane 0.0002%
Ozone 0.000004%

Thus, we are surrounded by di-radical oxygen, which enters our bodies on a continual basis at the rate of each breath, which totals approximately 21,600 times a day, at rest.

Please remember that we are radical beings in a radical universe.

I believe that, in general, we fail to appreciate the fact that we swim beneath and within a sea of di-radical oxygen molecules, which constantly bathes all external and most internal parts of our being.

One in every five atmospheric molecules is an oxygen molecule, a di-radical. We are continually immersed in this ocean of di-radical ground state, triplet oxygen.

Thus, I do not accept and emphatically reject the customary hoopla concerning the killer-toxicity of oxygen radicals (EMODs).

Consider the free radical, hydrogen

Hydrogen is, by definition, a free radical, in that it has only one unpaired outer orbital electron.

The sun is a big ball of hot gases. The gases are converted into energy in the sun's core. The energy moves outward through the interior layers, into the sun's atmosphere, and is released into the solar system as heat and light.

Most of the gas — about 72 percent — is hydrogen. Nuclear fusion converts hydrogen into other elements. The sun is also composed of about 26 percent helium and trace amounts of other elements — oxygen, carbon, neon, nitrogen, magnesium, iron and silicon.

These elements are created in the sun's core, which makes up 25 percent of the sun. Gravitational forces create tremendous pressure and temperatures in the core. The temperature of the sun in this layer is about 27 million degrees F (15 million degrees C). Hydrogen atoms are compressed and fuse together, creating helium and a lot of energy.

This process is called nuclear fusion.

The energy, mostly in the form of gamma-ray photons and neutrinos, is carried into the radiative zone. Photons can bounce around in this zone for about a million years before passing through the interface layer, or tachocline. Scientists think the sun's magnetic field is generated by a magnetic dynamo in this layer.

The convection zone is the outermost layer of the sun's interior. It extends from about 125,000 miles (200,000 km) deep up to the visible surface or the sun's atmosphere. Temperatures cool in this zone, enough for heavier ions — such as carbon, nitrogen, oxygen, calcium and iron — to hold onto their electrons. This makes the material more opaque and traps heat, causing the plasma to boil or "convect."

The convective motions carry heat quite rapidly to the surface, which is the bottom layer of the sun's atmosphere, or photosphere. This is the layer where the energy is released as sunlight. The light passes through the outer layers of the sun's atmosphere — the chromosphere and the corona — before reaching Earth about eight minutes later.

Astronomers who have studied the composition of the sun have catalogued 67 chemical elements in the sun. There may be more, but in amounts too small for instruments to detect.

Hydrogen, a radical, is 91.2% in abundance of the total number of atoms on the sun and it is 71% of the total mass of the sun.

Thus, our source of life on earth is from a radical star.

The sun's light is captured in the process of plant photosynthesis, which is again an EMOD generating photochemical pathway. The earth is a huge photon-collector, which takes the sun's photons and converts them into foodstuffs, such as sugar (glucose).

The chain of electrons is the chain of life

The glucose then passes into Krebs cycle (or the citric acid cycle) and is a part of cellular respiration. Named after Hans Krebs, it is a series of chemical reactions used by all aerobic organisms to generate energy.

Krebs cycle basically produces electrons and hydrogen from our foodstuffs and these electrons are utilized in our mitochondria to produce energy in the form of adenosine triphosphate (ATP) and gives off CO_2 and water.

Cellular respiration, which is essential to our very existence, is an oxidative process, which can be interfered with or blocked by excessive amounts of antioxidants. This is a key observation, which is primarily overlooked by scientists, who push antioxidants.

ATP is a molecule which carries energy in chemical form (a high energy phosphate bond) to be used in other cell processes. To summarize energy production:

- Two molecules of carbon dioxide are given off
- One molecule of ATP is formed
- Three molecules of NAD+ are combined with hydrogen (NAD+ $\rightarrow$ NADH)
- One molecule of FAD combines with hydrogen (FAD $\rightarrow$ FADH$_2$)

Because two acetyl-CoA molecules are produced from each glucose molecule, *two cycles are required per glucose molecule*. Therefore, at the end of two cycles, the products are: two ATP, six $NADH_2$, two $FADH_2$ two QH_2 (ubiquinol) and four CO_2.

Kreb's cycle thus provides a source of electrons because of the production of $NADH_2$, $NADPH_2$ and $FADH_2$. Those electrons are then directed to the electron transfer chain, where they participate in oxidative phosphorylation and the production of ATP.

What is glycolysis (anaerobic metabolism)?

a) 6 carbon glucose is split into two 3 carbon pyruvates
b) anaerobic - proceeds whether or not O_2 is present ; O_2 is not required
d) net yield of 2 ATP per glucose molecule
e) net yield of 2 NADH per glucose ---> sent to the electron transport chain (ETC) in mitochondria

The pyruvic acid diffuses into the inner compartment of the mitochondrion where a **transition reaction** occurs that serves to prepare pyruvic acid for entry into the next stage of respiration, this converts them an acetyl CoA which enters the Kreb's cycle.

If oxygen is not present, pyruvate is converted to lactic acid in the cytoplasm -- **anaerobic respiration**

What is the citric acid or Krebs cycle?

a) it occurs in the inner mitochondrial matrix
b) it is an aerobic process; it will proceed only in the presence of O_2
c) net yield of 2 ATP per glucose molecule
d) net yield of 6 NADH and 2 $FADH_2$ (NAD+ is reduced to NADH, FAD+ is reduced to FADH)
e) in this stage of cellular respiration, the oxidation of glucose to CO_2 is completed.

What is the electron transport chain (ETC)?

a) it consists of a series of enzymes on the inner mitochondrial membrane
b) electrons are released from NADH and from $FADH_2$ and as they are passed along the series of enzymes, they give up energy which is used to fuel a process called **chemiosmosis**, which drives the process of ATP synthesis using an enzyme called ATPase.
c) net yield of 32 ATP per glucose molecule

d) 6 H_2O are formed when the electrons unite with O_2* at the end of electron transport chain.

* Note: This is the function of oxygen in living organisms!

Dr. Hekimi of McGill University interprets the cellular redox situation as follows:

- Dr. Hekimi has been refuting the free radical theory of aging for many years [Cellular Molecular Life Science, Jan 2010]

- Dr. Hekimi specifically notes that "reactive oxygen species" or so-called oxygen free radicals (EMODs) are needed to activate the immune system in cell energy compartments called mitochondria [Oncoimmunology, April 2013]

- Dr. Hekimi says "our finding indicate that maintaining normal stress resistance is not crucial to the rate of aging [Proceedings National Academy Science, April 2012]

- In 2011 Dr. Hekimi said increased free radicals are "necessary and sufficient to increase longevity, "an effect that "is abolished by vitamin C or N-acetyl cysteine (NAC) antioxidants." He identifies a particular oxidizing agent called superoxide as the trigger to produce a longevity effect. [PLoS Biology, Dec 2010]

- In a press release issued by Dr. Hekimi, he said, "when stimulated in the right way by free radicals, this actually reinforces the cell's defenses and increases its lifespan [Science Daily, May 8, 2014]

Until the majority of investigators change their view (interpretations of the data), they are going to continue to demonize oxidation and oxidative products. Even if oxidative products are of low levels or concentrations, they will be seen as harmful. Only when the current bias against oxidation and oxidative products is eliminated, will this situation change. However, more and more scientists are adopting the view that EMODs are crucial to normal homeostasis and that antioxidants have harmful potential.

The following was adapted from: Diabetes and Oxygen Free Radical Sophistry. Copyright © 2006, by Prof. R.M. Howes MD, PhD (Howes, 2006, Diabetes)

Oxygen at work. Do not disturb

Inscribed on the aerobic cell wall hangs a sign which reads, "Oxygen at work. Do not disturb." Yet, we repeatedly attempt to interfere with the intracellular nano-biochemical factory, which operates nearly flawlessly without our so called medical or nutritional meddling.

Yes, oxygen and its derivatives are continually at work to provide us with prooxidant protection from pathogens and to provide for oxidative healing.

I am amazed that investigators assume that any harmful result must be due to oxidants and can not be due to antioxidants. Thus, when they see bad results from the use of antioxidants, it must be due to the fact that the antioxidants are changing or converted into prooxidants.

Following decades of brain washing, they fail to see the harmful potential of antioxidants whatsoever.

Even more astounding, to me, is the fact that they can not see the incredible salutary effects of prooxidants.

A major stumbling block to our progress in the understanding of diseases has been the obfuscation introduced by the erroneous free radical theory.

This theory has prevailed for over sixty years, without the perspicacity and intellectual integrity necessary to remove it from the hodgepodge of confusing and conflicting scientific data de jour.

Without logic, there is only mayhem.

Logic tells us that oxygen is an essential agent for aerobic life. Logic tells us, that in times of medical emergencies, we must establish an airway and administer oxygen.

Instead, specious reasoning would tell us to administer antioxidants, which would sound the death knell for the patient.

Nonetheless, there are many who presently press for forced widespread supplementation of antioxidant vitamins in our food supply and who insist on the beneficence of these questionable and potentially harmful agents. Perchance, this is related to the surprising increases that are seen in the incidence of diseases such as cancer, diabetes and atherosclerosis.

Since so called oxidative stress is seemingly increased in so many disease states and since antioxidants fail to prevent or curtail these same diseases, I believe that the increased oxidative state may be or is a natural reaction to disease.

We build a state of "oxidative bliss." We need a state of oxidative bliss.

The increased oxidative state is the body's attempt to control or cure the disease. It appears to me that oxidation is the primary process that the body has to deal with pathogens and neoplasia.

The presence of the increased EMODs has little or nothing to do with disease causation but has everything to do with disease control, progression or cure.

Even though many feel that we are now firmly entrenched in the 'information age,' the knowledge we so desperately need to maintain health and meet the challenges of disease is still outside of our grasp.

Our dependence upon a system in which standards of care are dictated by pharmaceutical advertising is evolving into a self-devouring monster yielding unprecedented increases in the adverse consequences of polypharmacy.

A new standard of care, which recognizes that half of our current scientific papers will ultimately prove to be false, must attempt to adhere to a wide spectrum of well-studied, scientifically validated interventions not solely disseminated by the prescription pad or by dogged adherence to flawed theories.

My mission is to see oxidative therapy, utilizing EMODs, at the patient's bedside in my life time. Based on the results seen with photodynamic therapy and with my singlet oxygen generating system, I know that good things await us in the near future.

My general observations on antioxidants

A major observation of the pancreatic ß-cell is its unusually low complement of the antioxidant enzymes, SOD, catalase, and GPx. This situation is also found in the critically important organs of the heart and the brain.

After decades of study, I believe this is telling us that these organs have normal requirements for high levels of EMODs and consequently, they have evolved correspondingly low antioxidant enzyme levels.

This is especially curious in the brain, because of its high concentration of lipids and free iron. According to the teachings of the free radical theory, this is a mistake of Nature and thus, the brain, heart and pancreas should undergo the effects of chain reactions of lipid peroxidation with impending cellular death, summarily.

However, that does not happen. Nature must have created this situation by Darwinian design and we must have the intellectual acuity to discern its meaning. I have diligently attempted to do so.

The free radical theory has been falsified on the basis of its lack of predictability. It fails to conform to the standards of the scientific method.

I have asked myself recurring questions concerning disease clustering and what I term an "EMOD insufficiency syndrome" as follows:

- Why do we see clustering of cancer, atherosclerosis, diabetes, obesity and cataracts?

- Why do diabetics get recurring infections and have trouble healing wounds?

- Why do patients get gestational diabetes?

- Why can patients have spontaneous regression of gestational diabetes, cancer, atherosclerosis and arthritis?

- Why do obese patients have more difficulty in healing wounds and have increased risk of developing cancer, diabetes and atherosclerosis?

- Why does it appear that one good EMOD deficiency disease deserves another?

- Why does exercise reduce diabetic tendencies and improve overall health?

- Why can diabetic ulcers, delayed wound healing and neuropathy be successfully treated with hyperbaric oxygen?

Diabetes appears to be inextricably related to other disease conditions, such as atherosclerosis, CVD, cancer, hypertension, cataracts, strokes, infections and obesity. This has made the research into this complex of diseases very difficult and arduous.

It has been an investigative maze of open and dead ended passageways and has been rife with conflicting and confusing data. This is especially true as it relates to the questionable involvement or the role of oxygen free radicals or as I have named them, "electronically modified oxygen derivatives (EMODs)" in diabetogenesis.

The data has been so abundant that I have had to divide the material into another book on this disease clustering phenomenon, which I have entitled the "**Howes' EMOD insufficiency syndrome.**"

With cancer and atherosclerosis I am convinced that oxygen is definitely not causative of these conditions and I further believe that oxidants can be used in their control or cure.

With most diseases I am also convinced that EMODs are not causative but I can not say that raising the body's oxidative capacity will be capable of controlling or curing the diseased condition.

Again, diabetes is a most complex disease. That is not to say that cancer and CVD are not complex diseases but diabetes has so many facets of other diseases within it.

Failures of the Big Three Antioxidant Enzymes: Catalase, Superoxide Dismutase & Glutathione Peroxidase

Without oxygen, we die. Further, without electronically modified oxygen derivatives (EMODs), we die.

The big three antioxidant enzymes (i.e., catalase, CAT, superoxide dismutase, SOD and glutathione peroxidase, GPx) fail to support the invalidated free radical theory and may have negligible effects or harmful potential. These endogenous (internally generated) antioxidant enzymes are more potent in preventing free radical damage than are dietary antioxidant vitamins, such as vitamins A, C and E.

Any agent which interferes with fundamental bodily biochemical processes must be taken seriously and substances, such as dietary antioxidants and antioxidant enzymes, which indiscriminately attack essential cellular signaling agents (i.e., electronically modified oxygen derivatives, EMODs) must be viewed with considerable caution. Such is the case for protecting essential EMODs and preventing their annihilation by antioxidant vitamins, low molecular weight antioxidants and antioxidant enzymes.

The antioxidant enzymes, which also attack EMODs, have more specificity but they also more vigorously attack these same vital EMOD signaling molecules.

Various isoforms of CAT, SOD and GPx are dispensable (expendable, nonessential, unessential, unneeded, unnecessary, superfluous) and not needed for normal growth and survival.

CAT, with **hydrogen peroxide is its only substrate,** is believed to be one of the fastest and most perfect catalysts and is believed to be the predominant H_2O_2-removing enzyme in human erythrocytes. Yet, we can live normally without it. GPx is the powerful scavenger of oxygen free radicals. CAT is the unsurpassed, highly efficient scavenger of hydrogen peroxide and SOD is the scavenger of superoxide anion. **Humans with genetic deficiency of catalase ("acatalasemia") or mice genetically engineered to lack catalase completely, suffer few ill effects.**

My conclusions on the big three, CAT, SOD and GPx are that CAT and GPx are both dispensable (expendable, superfluous, unessential, unnecessary, replaceable, surplus to requirements, etc.), since **both can be eliminated and the animal can live a normal life**; whereas, **SOD is not an antioxidant enzyme at all, since it generates hydrogen peroxide from superoxide**.

Even ecSOD is somewhat expendable since mice without the extracellular SOD have minimal defects (only being sensitive to hyperoxia). **This is in contrast to species which lack NOX, NADPH oxidase, which generate superoxide (an EMOD). They are prone to repeated infections, granulomas and die an early death.**

There are at least four different glutathione peroxidase isozymes in animals. **Glutathione peroxidase 1 is the most abundant and is a very efficient scavenger of hydrogen peroxide, while glutathione peroxidase 4 is most active with lipid hydroperoxides. Surprisingly, glutathione peroxidase 1 is dispensable, as mice lacking this enzyme have normal lifespans**, but they are hypersensitive to induced oxidative stress.

SOD enzymes will lead to an increase in the local concentration of H_2O_2. This also means that it can be viewed as a prooxidant enzyme and not an antioxidant enzyme.

I believe that it is of utmost importance to consider the fact that animals null for CAT and Gpx1 and Gpx2 appear to develop normally and live normal lives. This must weaken the argument that EMODs are extremely toxic and causative of up to 200 pathophysiologies.

Gpx1 reduces the fatty acid hydroperoxide to alcohol and water.

SOD, CAT and GPx, generate H_2O_2, O_2 and organic alcohols, respectively. I find it extremely interesting that the 3 big antioxidant enzymes, i.e., SOD, CAT and GPx, generate H_2O_2, O_2 and organic peroxides.

Thus, I ask, "Does that sound like ANTI-oxidants?" **I believe that an argument could be made that they are producing conditions favorable for oxidation or they are acting as "cooxidants."**

Apoptosis and Cell Death

Cell death is an essential phenomenon in normal development and homeostasis, but also plays a crucial role in various pathologies. **This means that generation of EMODs is essential also.** Our understanding of the molecular mechanisms involved has increased exponentially, although it is still far from complete.

The morphological features of a cell dying either by apoptosis or by necrosis are remarkably conserved for quite different cell types derived from lower or higher organisms.

At the molecular level, several gene products play a similar, crucial role in a major cell death pathway in a worm and in man. However, one should not oversimplify. It is now evident that there are multiple pathways leading to cell death, and some cells may have the required components for one pathway, but not for another, or contain endogenous inhibitors which preclude a particular pathway.

Furthermore, different pathways can co-exist in the same cell and are switched on by specific stimuli. Apoptotic cell death, reported to be non-inflammatory, and necrotic cell death, which may be inflammatory, are two extremes, while the real situation is usually more complex. The distinguishing features of the various cell death pathways are: caspases (cysteine proteases cleaving after particular aspartate residues), **mitochondria and/or electronically modified oxygen derivatives are often, but not always, key components**.

As these various caspase-dependent and caspase-independent cell death pathways are becoming better characterized, we may learn to differentiate them and perhaps exploit the knowledge acquired for clinical benefit. (Fiers et al, 1999)

Innate immunity is the primary host defense against invading microorganisms. Pathogen recognition, mediated through an elaborate 'microbial sensing' system comprising the Toll-like and Nod-like receptor families results in the activation of caspase-1, which is a prerequisite for pathogen clearance.

Tight regulation of caspase-1 is necessary to control the magnitude of the innate immune response and protect the organism from possible damaging effects such as sepsis. EMODs are integral to the innate immune system.

Apoptosis Eliminates Cancerous and Precancerous Cells

One of the important functions of apoptosis is the elimination of preneoplastic and neoplastic cells. (Thompson, 1995)

Apoptosis Utilizes EMODs

In most forms of cell suicide, the signaling cascade utilizes electronically modified oxygen derivatives as essential intermediate messenger molecules. (Albright et al, 2003)

Antioxidant Depleted Diet Causes Reduction in Brain Tumor Size

Salganik et al. observed a reduction in brain tumor size in the TgT transgenic mouse model, which spontaneously develops brain cancer, when these mice were fed diets depleted of antioxidants. (Slater et al, 1995)

There was enhanced apoptosis within tumors of antioxidant depleted mice. (Salganik et al, 2000)

Breast Cancer Showed Increased Apoptosis with Antioxidant Depleted Diet

Recently, colleagues extended this observation to another cancer type, breast cancer. (Albright et al, 2004)

Antioxidant Depleted Diet Led to Decreased Metastasis and Increased EMODs

Using a transgenic mouse model of mammary tumorigenesis with defined rates of tumor growth and lung-targeted metastasis, they determined that **dietary antioxidant depletion inhibited tumor growth and diminished metastasis**. Compared with control mice fed a standard diet, **mice fed an antioxidant-depleted diet exhibited tumor-targeted generation of electronically modified oxygen derivatives; the number of apoptotic cells in tumors increased 5-fold, and the percentage of tumor cells undergoing mitosis decreased by half.** The mice fed the antioxidant-depleted diet had more small primary tumors and fewer large primary tumors than did controls, and they also had <30% of the number of lung metastatic tumor foci compared with mice fed the control diet.

Antioxidants may exert a cancer-promoting effect in cancer patients and in individuals with precancerous DNA changes. Inhibition of apoptosis by antioxidants may explain why, in several studies in heavy smokers, vitamin E and β-carotene enhanced carcinogenesis in the lung, where, presumably, precancerous lesions caused by smoking predated antioxidant treatment. (De Luca, Ross, 1996)

I believe that the fact that ß-carotene is a singlet oxygen scavenger is also of prime importance in the increased rate of cancer seen in this study.

Administration of antioxidants subsequent to a mutagenic event may effectively intercept free radicals that are critical in promoting apoptosis. This imbalance may allow the rate of proliferation in tumors to exceed the capacity for apoptosis. It seems reasonable to suggest that **the potential risks and benefits of high-dose antioxidants need to be considered on a case-to-case basis, and indiscriminate use of antioxidant dietary supplements should be avoided. I wholeheartedly agree.**

Antioxidant Vitamin and Supplement Failures

For years, I have written about the rise and fall of the free radical theory. **Antioxidant vitamins and supplements have repeatedly failed to reverse, nullify or cure** what have been believed to be oxidation-caused diseases. **Antioxidant vitamins do not work.** This can best be summed up by the following results of a most recent evaluation of antioxidants relative to cancer.

A recent study that found calcium and vitamin D supplements don't reduce the odds of developing breast cancer is the latest to deflate the cancer-prevention claims of some vitamin proponents. **A federal science panel in May 2006 had concluded there is no evidence for recommending certain vitamin supplements for cancer prevention. Even the Council for Responsible Nutrition, a supplement trade association, won't say that vitamins prevent cancer.**

"There is no vitamin or mineral supplement proven to reduce the risk of cancer," said **Eric Jacobs, a senior epidemiologist and vitamin specialist with the American Cancer Society**. However, many doctors continue to recommend daily multivitamins for general health. And some experts say certain supplements may yet prove to be a help in the fight against cancer — once scientists can work out the right amounts and better ways to study their effects.

I believe that there is total denial of the failures of vitamins by the followers of the Free Radi-Crap theory.

"More than half of Americans are taking dietary supplements — mostly multivitamins — but scientists aren't certain about their benefit," said Dr. J. Michael McGinnis, who chaired the National Institutes of Health panel that critiqued supplemental vitamins.

"For something used so widely, at such expense, among Americans, there is simply a need for much better information," he said. Scientists once suspected vitamin E and beta-carotene prevented lung cancer after a study showed people who took supplements appeared to have lower cancer incidence.

But a larger, more scientifically rigorous study found 50 milligrams a day of alpha-tocopherol, a form of vitamin E, had no effect on lung cancer incidence. And **20 milligrams of beta-carotene, a precursor of vitamin A, actually increased lung cancer incidence in smokers by 18 percent.**

Health officials now warn smokers not to take beta-carotene supplements.

Studies also have found that **beta-carotene has no impact on the incidence of lung cancer in non-smokers, or prostate or breast cancer.** And research has found **vitamin B2 and niacin had no impact on the occurrence of cancers, and selenium did not decrease skin cancer** in people with a history of that disease.

More recently, a study published in April 2006 in the Journal of the National Cancer Institute concluded that a **low-dose vitamin A derivative did not prevent head and neck tumors.**

Earlier research had suggested that higher doses of the derivative cut occurrence of subsequent tumors. **But those higher doses caused severe cracking of the lips, eyelid inflammation and other problems,** researchers said.

A study of about **36,000 post-menopausal women** released this month found **calcium and vitamin D supplements didn't cut the odds of developing breast cancer.**

Willett, the Harvard expert, faulted the study led by Dr. Rowan Chlebowski of Harbor-UCLA Medical Center in Los Angeles and said a different dose of vitamin D may be needed to show an effect. He also said it is possible vitamins and supplements reduce cancer risk at one stage of life, but not another, as a previous Canadian study suggested.

Much of the research into potential cancer-fighting powers of vitamins and other supplements have been **observational studies**, said Andrew Shao, the Council for Responsible Nutrition's vice president for scientific and regulatory affairs.

But **the gold standard is large, case-controlled trials** involving elaborate precautions to isolate cause and effect and prevent biased results. Such studies are expensive and take many years to complete. Meanwhile, patients are making their own decisions.

Emphasis has been placed on high antioxidant ability, which allegedly can protect cells against the adverse effects of **electronically modified oxygen derivatives** (**EMODs**).

Lester Packer (Department of Molecular Pharmacology and Toxicology, School of Pharmacy, Health Sciences Campus, University of Southern California, Los Angeles, CA) has highlighted his view of the crucial role antioxidants play in theoretically preventing so called oxidative stress and maintaining the physiological redox status of cellular constituents.

Antioxidants may:

-quench free radicals,

-change their redox state,

-be targeted for destruction,

-regulate oxidative processes involved in signal transduction,

-affect gene expression and pathways of cell proliferation, differentiation and death.

Yet, repeatedly antioxidants have failed to prevent cancer, heart disease, strokes and diabetes. Scientific study results have shown that Packer has a history of being wrong.

Some believe that this is being achieved at various subcellular and molecular levels including antioxidants that interact with the redox antioxidant network such as ascorbic acid (vitamin C) and a-tocopherol (vitamin E), thiols (glutathione, thioredoxin, lipoic acid), bioflavonoids,

Prof Randolph M. Howes MD, PhD

carotenoids and induction of phase 2 enzymes and immune cell stimulation. (Higdon, Frei, 2003) (Packer et al, 2004)

Dr. Packer **acknowledges the conditions under which redox-active substances can exert antioxidant as well as prooxidant action** in different organ systems and in various cell types.

I believe that it is extremely difficult to differentiate between the prooxidant and the antioxidant contributions of many of the supplements and antioxidants commonly used.

There is no doubt that many nutraceuticals, functional foods and naturally occurring polyphenols have other physiological and pharmacological activities in addition to their well-characterized antioxidant actions. (Mandel, 2005)

I believe that, in addition to their prooxidant activity, the other pharmacological activities (such as being a prooxidant) of these antioxidants are responsible for their cited salutary effects.

Even if the free radical theory was correct, antioxidants would still have to reach the intended cells (or the inner cellular parts) to produce their desired effect.

Yet, bioavailability is a major problem for many antioxidants, such as polyphenols, flavonoids and curcumin.

It is difficult to envision the effectiveness of these antioxidants if they are not readily bioavailable.

I have found that beta carotene, lycopene and omega-3 fatty acids all increase the risk of the aggressive form of prostate cancer.

I believe that these antioxidants result in cancer formation because they reduce EMOD levels to a level of insufficiency, which "allows" the development of neoplasia.

Also, I found that vitamin C, glutathione and lactate are all concentrated in cancer cells.

I believe that the concentration of antioxidants by cancer cells is for self protection from EMOD induced apoptosis (cellular suicide).

Some of the following was excerpted, adapted or modified from: (Fusco et al, 2007)

Effects of antioxidant supplementation on the aging process

Abstract

The free radical theory of aging

More than 300 theories have been proposed to explain the aging process, but none has yet been generally accepted by gerontologists. (Medvedev, 1990)

But, the initial proposal by Denham Harman that free radicals are causally related to the basic aging process is receiving growing acceptance as a possible explanation of the chemical reactions at the basis of ageing. (Harman, 1956) (De La Fuente 2002)

Theoretically, the accumulation of endogenous oxygen radicals generated in cells and the consequent oxidative modification of biological molecules (lipids, proteins and nucleic acid) have been indicated as being singularly responsible for the aging and death of all living beings. (Finkel and Holbrook, 2000) (Harman, 1956)

The free radical theory was revised in 1972, when mitochondria were identified as responsible for the initiation of most of the free radical reactions occurring in the cells. (Harman, 1972)

Allegedly, cells which use oxygen, and consequently produce reactive oxygen species, had to evolve complex antioxidant defense systems to neutralize reactive oxygen species and protect themselves against free radical damage.

In a normal situation, it is believed that a balanced-equilibrium exists but, **allegedly**, excess generation of free radicals may overwhelm natural cellular antioxidant defenses leading to oxidation and further contributing to cellular functional impairment. (Bowles et al, 1991) (Meydani et al, 1993)

According to Harman's flawed theory, the identification of free radical reactions as promoters of the aging process implies that interventions aimed at limiting or inhibiting them should be able to reduce the rate of formation of aging changes with a consequent reduction of the aging rate and disease pathogenesis. (Harman 2003)

RMH Note: Harman's approach has been tested and repeatedly it failed to have predictive value.

In fact, the free radical theory of aging fostered a **conflicted and confusing** body of research investigating the potential role of antioxidant nutrients in therapeutic or preventive strategies. (Mayne, 2003)

Surprisingly, even though antioxidant supplementation is receiving growing attention and is increasingly adopted in Western countries, **supporting evidence is still lacking and equivocal**.

SUMMARY OF 26 STUDIES IN CHAPTER FIFTEEN

Taken from my book: Sports, Athletes, Exercise Facts and Antioxidant Myths. CreateSpace and Free Radical Publishing, © 2011. (Howes, 2011, Sports) Please refer to this book for references.

- **Supplementation of diet with either single or multivitamin preparations containing B-complex vitamins, vitamin C or E does not improve physical performance in athletes with a normal biochemical vitamin balance resulting from a well-balanced diet.** (van der Beek, 1985)

- **3 mo of multivitamin and mineral supplementation was without any measurable ergogenic effect.** (Weight et al, 1998)

- **Supplementation** (with a high potency multivitamin-mineral supplement) **did not affect physical performance in well-nourished men who maintained their physical activity.** (Singh et al, 1992)

- **This study provided little evidence of any effect of** (vitamin and mineral supplementation) **supplementation to athletic performance for athletes consuming the dietary RDIs.** (Telford et al, 1992)

- **There is currently a lack of conclusive evidence that exercise performance or recovery would benefit in any significant way from dietary vitamin E supplementation. Most evidence suggests that there is no discernible effect of vitamin**

E supplementation on performance, training effect or rate of postexercise recovery in either recreational or elite athletes. There appears to be little reason for vitamin E supplementation among athlete. (Tiidus, Houston, 1995)

- To date, limited evidence shows that dietary supplementation with antioxidants improves human performance. This is an important area for future research. (Powers, Hamilton, 1999)

- Vitamin E and C supplementation was found to be ineffective in preventing muscle damage following an ultra marathon (50 km) run in healthy participants, although the supplements did decrease markers of lipid peroxidation and DNA damage. (Mastaloudis et al, 2004)

- The dogs ran, on average, 0.2 s slower when supplemented with 1 g of vitamin C, equivalent to a lead of 3 m at the finish of a 500-m race. Supplementation with vitamin C, therefore, appeared to slow racing greyhounds. (Marshall et al, 2002)

- Supplementation with high (1000 IU) but not moderate (100 IU) daily doses of vitamin E appears to slow racing greyhounds. (Hill et al, 2001)

- Seven trained male cyclists participated in 4 separate supplementation phases. They ingested 2 capsules per day containing vitamin C and Vitamin E treatments. However neither of these vitamins, either alone or in combination, will enhance exercise performance. (Bryant et al, 2003)

- Vitamin E supplementation had no effect on exercise performance or capacity in athletic students. (Gaeini et al, 2006)

- Horses supplemented with vitamin E, at nearly 10-times the 1989 NRC recommended level, did not experience lower oxidative stress compared to control horses. Additionally, lower plasma BC levels observed in the HI group, which may indicate that vitamin E has an inhibitory effect on BC metabolism. (Williams, Carlucci, 2006)

- There appears to be no independent or combined effect of a prior bout of eccentric exercise or antioxidant supplementation as used here on markers of muscle injury in resistance trained men. Moreover, eccentric exercise as used in the present study results in minimal blood oxidative stress in resistance trained men. Hence, antioxidant supplementation for the purpose of minimizing blood oxidative stress in relation to eccentric exercise appears un-necessary in this population. (Bloomer, Falvo et al, 2007)

- Vitamin C supplementation prevented endurance exercise-induced lipid peroxidation and muscle damage but had no ef-fect on inflammatory markers. (Nakhostin-Roohi et al, 2008)

- CVD is largely a disease associated with physical inactivity. A rapidly advancing body of human and animal data confirms an important beneficial role for exercise in the prevention and treatment of CVD. (Leung et al, 2008)

- Athletes (ultra-endurance runners) with a regular intake of vi-tamin and mineral supplements in the four weeks before the race finished the competition no faster than athletes without an intake of vitamins and minerals. (Knechtle et al, 2008)

- Recent meta-analyses have shown that large risk reductions for both ischemic and hemorrhagic stroke can be achieved by moderate or intense physical activity. Physical inactivity and obesity/overweight are not only associated with a number of health-related risk factors, but are considered to be indepen-dent risk factors for CVD, type 2 diabetes mellitus and hyper-tension. (Yung et al, 2009)

- Vitamin and mineral supplements are not needed if adequate energy to maintain body weight is consumed from a variety of foods. American College of Sports Medicine position stand. Nutrition and athletic performance. (Rodriguez et al, 2009)

- This work suggests that despite the enhanced levels of antioxi-dants, athletes undergoing regular strenuous exercise exhib-ited more oxidative stress than sedentary controls. (Teixeira et al, 2009, SNEM)

- Exercise-induced oxidative stress ameliorates insulin re-sistance and causes an adaptive response promoting endog-enous antioxidant defense capacity. Supplementation with antioxidants may preclude these health-promoting effects of exercise in humans. (Ristow et al, 2009)

- To the contrary, results indicate that administration of antioxidants during strenuous endurance training has no effect on the training-induced increase in insulin sensitivity in healthy individuals. (Yfanti et al, 2011)

- To assess the effects of an encapsulated **antioxidant concentrate (EAC)** and exercise on lipid peroxidation (LIPOX) and the plasma antioxidant enzyme glutathione peroxidase (Pl-GPx). **The EAC induced an increase of LIPOX as indicated by MDA and decreased pl-GPx concentrations pre- and postexercise.** (Lamprecht et al, 2009) **In this case, the antioxidants vitamins acted to stimulate prooxidant effects.**

- **AOX** (AOX; 272 mg of alpha-tocopherol, 400 mg of vitamin C, 30 mg of beta-carotene, 2 mg of lutein, 400 mug of selenium, 30 mg of zinc, and 600 mg of magnesium) **supplementation does not offer protection against exercise-induced lipid peroxidation and inflammation** and *may hinder the recovery of muscle damage*. (Teixeira et al, 2009)

- **Over 60% of the athletes reported using vitamin supplements, of which vitamin C (97.5%), vitamin E (78.3%), and multivitamins (52.2%) were the most commonly used supplements. Vitamin C and E supplementation was common in ultra endurance triathletes, despite no evidence of dietary deficiency in these 2 vitamins.** (Knez, Peake, 2010)

- **The consumption of an n-3 LC PUFA supplement increased oxidative stress at rest and did not attenuate the exercise-induced oxidative stress.** The addition of antioxidants did not prevent the formation of oxidation products at rest. (Flaire et al, 2011)

Please refer to the following book for references:

- **Cancer and Longevity Answers: Naked mole rats, Exercise & EMODs (ROS).** CreateSpace and Free Radical Publishing, © **2015.** (Howes, 2015, Cancer)

Summary: 100 fact nullifying versions of the Free Radical theory (FRT)

Selective summary of 100 fact and reasons that nullify the <u>FRT</u> (free radical theory), the <u>FRTA</u> (free radical theory of aging), the <u>MFRTA</u> (mitochondrial free radical theory of aging) and/

or the __MTA__ (mitochondrial theory of aging): (Whatever you call it, the FRTA has been negated, rebuffed and anulled!)

Since references are multiple on some items, chronology is only approximated. **As with the parent FRT, all of the decendant aging theories lack predictability and reproducibility. Thus, they fail to meet the requirements of the scientific method and are therefore invalidated.**

FRT (free radical theory); **FRTA** (free radical theory of aging); **MFRTA** (mitochondrial free radical theory of aging); **MTA** (mitochondrial theory of aging)

1) - **There is no clear evidence that EMOD (ROS) inhibitors delay mammalian aging.** (Hayflick, 1994)

2) - **Correlations between rate of aging and antioxidant levels in mammals are, if they exist, very weak.** (Finch et al, 1990) (Sohal, Weindruch, 1996) (Weindruch, 1996)

3) - **Genetic manipulations that increase CuZn-SOD activity and, thus, resistance to oxidative stress, have only a slight, if any, effect on maximum lifespan in several species.** (Warner, 1994)

4) - **Mice deficient for the antioxidant enzyme, glutathione peroxidase, do not age faster.** (Ho et al, 1997)

5) - Linus Pauling claimed that megadoses of vitamin C had antiaging effects because of its involvement in multiple redox reactions. Yet, **neither epidemiological nor vitamin intervention trials have demonstrated any major degree of protection from cancer, heart disease, stroke or aging.** (Hercberg et al, 1998)

6) - **Instead, vitamin C has been associated with increased oxidative damage to DNA, as levels of 8-oxoadenine are increased in persons taking vitamin C.** (Podmore et al, 1998)

7) - **A series of carefully designed studies established that the endogenous oxidative damage of mtDNA** (mitochondrial DNA) **is not greater than that of nDNA** (nuclear DNA). (Anson et al, 1999)

8) - **Transgenic mice that constitutively over express the human antioxidant enzyme, CuZnSOD, did not live longer than control animals.** (Huang et al, 2000)

9) - **A basal level of mitochondrial EMOD production is essential for the attainment of a normal length lifespan.** In support of this view, **the level of H_2O_2 affects the expression of at least 80 different genes or proteins,** including numerous components of the mitogen-activated protein kinase and nuclear factor κB signalling pathways. (Allen, Tresini, 2000)

10) - **In general, trials with vitamin E have been failures. Likewise, beta carotene trials have also been losers.** (Willett, Stampfer, 2001)

11) - **In most cases there is little or no scientific basis for these (antiaging) claims.** (Workshop Report, *Is There an Antiaging Medicine?* International Longevity Center, Canyon Ranch Series; New York, 2001)

12) - **The public is spending vast sums of money on these (antiaging) products and lifestyle changes, some of which may be harmful.** (U.S. General Accounting Office, 2001)

13) - **So far there is no scientific evidence to justify the claim that they (antioxidants) have any effect on human aging.** (Morley, Trainor, 2001) (de Grey, 2000)

14) - **Ubiquitous overexpression of SOD1** (Huang et al, 2000), **overexpression of glutathione peroxidase** (McClung et al, 2004), **and overexpression of catalase in the nucleus** (Schriner et al, 2000) **all failed to increase longevity.**

15) - In 2002, Hayflick et al stated, **"There are no lifestyle changes, surgical procedures, vitamins, antioxidants, hormones or techniques of genetic engineering available today that have been demonstrated to influence the processes of aging."** (Perls, 1999) (Kirkwood, 1999)

16) - This quote (15) was repeated in Scientific American. **"There are no lifestyle changes, surgical procedures, vitamins, antioxidants, hormones or techniques of genetic engineering available today that have been demonstrated to influence the processes of aging."** (Scientific American, 2002)

17) - Also, **mice without methionine sulfoxide reductase (MsrA) have a decreased longevity.** (Moskovitz et al, 2001)

18) - **Scientists are unwittingly contributing to the prolifera-tion of these pseudoscientific antiaging products.** (Scientific American, 2002)

19) - **The claim that ingesting supplements containing antioxi-dants can influence aging is often used to sell antiaging formu-lations.** (Hayflick et al, 2002)

20) - **"Nobody has ever shown that taking antioxidant vitamin pills helps prolong life."** (Mirkin, 2002)

21) - **Alfred Fisher and John E. Morely concluded in 2002, "Overall, at present, there is little evidence that free radical scavengers have positive antiaging effects."** (Fisher, Morely, 2002)

22) - **While the concept of antiaging therapies is intriguing, there is clearly little evidence-based medicine to support most of the generally touted approaches.** (Fisher, Morely, 2002)

23) - **Amazingly, the best antiaging medicine is exercise** (which increased oxygen consumption and EMOD production)! (Fiatarone-Singh, 2002)

24) - **"Currently, there is no proven way to reliably and safely de-lay, even ever so slightly, the aging of man."** (Olshansky et al, 2002)

25) - **The Women's Angiographic Vitamin and Estrogen (WAVE) Trial: All-cause mortality was higher in the antioxi-dant group + HRT** (hormone replacement therapy) **vs (hazard ra-tio) vitamin placebo group.** (Waters et al, 2002)

26) - **By feeding antioxidants to rodents it is possible to de-crease oxidative damage and sometimes even slightly increase longevity, but aging is not delayed.** (Hagen et al, 2002)

27) - **Short-term exposure to high oxygen concentration length-ens the life span in the nematode Caenorhabditis elegans. This is considered to be the result of an increase in antioxidant de-fense induced by short-term oxidative stress.** Mutations in genes such as age-1 and daf-2 that compose the insulin-like signaling network conferred oxidative stress resistance and an increase in Mn-SOD gene expression as well as life span extension. (Honda, Honda, 2002). **RMH Note: Some folks refuse to state that prooxidants can be ben-eficial under any circumstances.**

28) - **Manipulating components of antioxidant systems does not appear to affect aging in mammals.** (Sohal et al, 2002) (de Magalhaes, 2005)

29) - The Medical Research Council/British Heart Foundation **Heart Protection Study**, which is **the study cited by Dr. Gibbons, randomized 10,269 patients to 660 IU/day of vitamin E and 10,267 to placebo control. The vitamin E group was associated with about a 10% increase in mortality**. (Gibbons quote, 2002) (MRC/BHF, 2002)

30) - **In 2003,** eight years ago **Jacobs pointed out that the 'mitochondrial theory of aging has been neither proven nor disproven**. (Jacobs, 2003)

31) - **While heterozygous mice with reduced MnSOD** (an antioxidant enzyme) **activity have a life expectancy that is similar to wild-type mice, although these animals have increased oxidative damage to DNA**. (Van Remmen et al, 2003)

32) - **A causative effect of ROS (EMOD)-promoted oxidation in limiting life span has been hard to establish because of the inconsistent and/or nonexistent effects of antioxidants**. (Koubova, Guarente, 2003)

33) - **Ectopic expression of catalase** (an antioxidant enzyme) **in Drosophila mitochondria increases stress resistance but not longevity.** There was no impact on the life span of the flies at 25 degrees C, even in an exceptional line with a 149% increase in total catalase activity, and there was a **small decrease in longevity at 29 degrees C. There were no compensatory changes in the rate of metabolism or physical activity, or in the levels of other major antioxidants, suggesting that the aging process was largely unaffected**. (Mockett et al, 2003)

34) - **Mice heterozygous for SOD2** (an antioxidant enzyme) **showed increased oxidative damage at various levels, including DNA oxidative damage, but did not show significant changes in longevity or rate of aging, clearly arguing that oxidative damage alone does not drive aging in mammals.** (Van Remmen et al, 2003)

35) - **"No intervention will slow, stop, or reverse the aging process in humans."** (Hayflick, 2004)

36) - "**The overexpression of the antioxidant enzyme, GPx1** (an antioxidant enzyme), **which is better suited for the detoxification of low levels of H_2O_2, not only failed to extend the life span in mice, but resulted in the development of insulin resistance and obesity, metabolic problems often linked to aging."** (McClung et al, 2004)

37) - **Early attempts at antioxidant intervention as a means to delay aging were initiated soon after the free radical theory of aging was proposed, but these pursuits failed to extend life span in most cases.** (Blackett, Hall, 1980) (Thomas, 2004)

38) - **Two groups who attempted to test this theory (MTA) directly by generating knock-in mice with an elevated rate of mtDNA mutagenesis reported mixed results.** (Kujoth et al, 2005) (Trifunovic et al, 2004) (Trifunovic et al, 2005)

39) - **The pattern of aging-related changes in antioxidants in many tissues and species has been inconsistent. Substantial data exist indicating that there is no generalized decrease in antioxidant enzyme function.** (Matsuo et al, 1992) (Keaney et al, 2004) (Kevin et al, 2007)

40) - **Women with diabetes consuming at least 300 milligrams of vitamin C per day faced 2.3 times the risk of death from stroke and 2 times the risk of dying from coronary artery disease as did diabetic women who took in less of the vitamin C.** (Duk-Hee Lee et al, 2004)

41) - A 2004 article (Kris-Etherton et al., 2004) for the Nutrition Committee of the American Heart Association Council on Nutrition, Physical Activity, and Metabolism states that **the ATBC study showed:**

- **Increase in overall mortality (vitamin E)**

- **Increase in hemorrhagic stroke (β-carotene) with more deaths due to: ischemic heart disease, hemorrhagic stroke and ischemic stroke.**

42) - **Miller's Meta-analysis:** Johns Hopkins' investigator, Miller et al. performed a meta-analysis, including more than 135,000 subjects, and concluded that **high doses of vitamin E increased mortality by about 5%.** (Miller et al, 2005)

43) - The hypothesis that a specific enhancement of mitochondrial $O_2^{\cdot-}/H_2O_2$ catabolism would delay age-associated physiological changes and extend the lifespan was tested by simultaneous overexpression of MnSOD (manganese superoxide dismutase) and catalase, ectopically targeted to the mitochondrial matrix of transgenic *Drosophila melanogaster*. **The lifespan of the flies (***Drosophila melanogaster***) was decreased (shortened), by up to 43%, and this effect coincided with (i) an overall decrease in physical fitness, as measured by the speed of walking, and (ii) an age-related decrease in mitochondrial state 3 (ADP-stimulated) respiration. <u>These findings support the notion that mitochondrial $O_2^{\cdot-}/H_2O_2$ production at physiological levels is essential for normal biological processes leading to the attainment of a normal lifespan.</u>** (Bayne et al, 2005) **Again, this emphasizes the obvious. The use of MnSOD and catalase, which decreased hydrogen peroxide and superoxide, led to decreased life spans and physical fitness.**

44) - **Enhancement of the capacity for mitochondrial $O_2^{\cdot-}/H_2O_2$ catabolism** (breakdown) **leads to progressive decreases in the longevity of flies. This finding is at odds with the oxidative stress hypothesis of aging and with recent results obtained using transgenic mice.** (Schriner et al, 2005)

45) **One problem is that the lifespan extension, originally evaluated after 2–4 backcrosses to C57B6 mice, became less evident after further backcrosses. This is a problem as reduced oxidative stress should always increase lifespan if the core statement of the MFRTA is correct** (but it isn't). (Schriner et al, 2005)

46) - "**Traditional categorization of theories of aging into programmed and stochastic ones** (such as the free radical theory) **is outdated and obsolete.**" (Rattan, 2006)

47) - **Lifelong administration of nonenzymatic antioxidants have failed to provide consistent and reproducible life span extension.** (Selman et al, 2006) (Bayne, Sohal, 2002) (Bass et al, 2007) (Keaney, Gems, 2003)

48) - **Studies on heterozygous or homozygous mutant mice, in which the activities of antioxidant gene products were reduced or removed entirely, have results that were obtained have also been disappointing, and sometimes even surprising.** The *Sod2* [+/−] mutant mice, which to our point of view **is clearly incompatible with the MFRTA.** (Hekimi, 2006)

49) - **Hekimi's group provided further evidence for beneficial effects of mitochondrial oxidative stress. Mutational inactiva-tion of *clk-I* in *Caenorhabditis elegans*, and partial inactivation of *MclkI* in mice prolong average and maximum lifespan in these organisms.** (Liu et al, 2005)

50) - **A direct link between oxidative stress and aging has not as yet been established.** (Pedro de Magalha, Church, 2006)

51) - The **lifespan phenotype of these mitochondrial mutants, (heterozygous mice for thioredoxin 2, a small cysteine-rich protein with antioxidant properties localized to the mito-chondrial matrix, have been generated and are characterized by impaired mitochondrial function and high mitochondrial oxidative stress) have a preliminary report describes as sur-prisingly unaffected.** (Perez et al, 2008) (Jang, Remmen, 2009)

52) - **Non-targeted overexpression of catalase** (one of the big three antioxidant enzymes) **only or in combination with SOD2 has no effect on lifespan.** (Schriner et al, 2005) (Perez et a;. 2009)

53) - **In another study, P66(shc-/-) mice exhibited prolonged lifespan and increased resistance to oxidative stress, but un-expectedly, centenarians showed the highest basal levels of p66(shc) when compared with young people and the elderly.** (Pandolfi et al, 2005)

54) - **Not only have antioxidants failed to stop disease and ag-ing but also they may cause harm and mortality.** (Howes, 2006)

55) - **Directly targeting the mitochondria by feeding mice with coenzyme Q_{10}, a well-known mitochondrial antioxidant, has no effects on lifespan, even when mitochondrial coenzyme Q_{10} content was successfully increased.** (Sohal et al, 2006)

56) - <u>**Studies with the longest living rodents, the naked-mole rats (NMRs), have shown that rather than having low lev-els of oxidative stress, these animals exhibit higher levels of oxidative damage to lipids, DNA and proteins than mice at the same fraction of their maximum lifespan (physiologically matched) and equal to that of mice of the same chronological age**</u>. (Andziak et al, 2006)

57) - **Concentration of specific markers of lipid peroxida-tion are higher in young NMRs than in short-lived mice**

and, unexpectedly, did not accumulate with aging. (Andziak, Buffenstein, 2006)

58) - These data suggest that higher levels of oxidative stress markers are species specific and **the pronounced longevity of naked mole-rats is independent of oxidative stress parameters.** (Andziak, Buffenstein, 2006)

59) - **The oxidative hypothesis of senescence does not explain "premature" aging.** (van de ven et al, 2006)

60) - Lack of predictability. Some critics of the oxidative theory claim that the failure of antioxidant interventions to stop or reverse the aging process and to quell the current pandemic of age-related diseases (e.g. cardiovascular disease) **brings the oxidative hypothesis into question**. (Howes, 2006)

61) - **The over-expression of the mitochondrial superoxide dismutase (SOD2), which clearly represents the principal defense against mitochondrial superoxide, does not result in a lifespan extension in single transgenic mice or when over-expressed in combination with SOD1**. (Muller et al, 2007)

62) - **Glutathione peroxidase 1 (GPx1 knockout mice) are grossly phenotypically normal and have a normal lifespan** (Muller, 2007).

63) - **The main question is still without answer**: which of the mechanisms (oxidative damages, garbage catastrophe, mutation accumulation, antagonistic pleiotropy, etc.) proposed by scientists to cause senescence do cause aging in the natural population? (Gilca et al, 2007)

64) - **Further evidence against the MTA was provided by Vermulst et al., using a novel random mutation capture assay to quantify mutation burden in Polg$^{exo+/+}$ and Polg$^{exo+/-}$ mice. This strongly argues against a causal role for mtDNA mutations in natural aging.** (Vermulst et al, 2007)

65) - **The increased lifespan recently demonstrated for mice with partial inactivation of GPx4 represents an even greater challenge** (to the MFRTA). Indeed, **mice heterozygous for GPx4, the gene encoding the only mitochondrial enzymatic antioxidant that directly reduces membrane-bound lipid hydroperoxides, have an increased median lifespan despite higher levels of biomarkers of oxidative damage**. (Ran et al, 2007)

66) - In March 2007, Fox News.com presented a report for lay people entitled, "The Mega-vitamin Mega-myth," in which they stated, "**The conclusion that antioxidant supplements don't appear to help you live longer is likely on a sound footing. Even without statistically combining the studies through meta-analysis, it's fairly clear that antioxidant supplements are ineffective for increasing longevity.**"

67) - **Bjelakovic's analysis found that beta carotene, vitamin A and vitamin E, taken singly or combined with other antioxidant supplements, were associated with increased all-cause mortality. Conservatively, the supplements increase the likelihood of dying by about 5 percent.** Vitamin C and selenium appeared to have no impact on longevity. (Bjelakovic, February 28, 2007)

68) - **Treatment of nematodes with different antioxidants and vitamins prevents extension of life span**; whereas, increased EMOD formation and resulting in hormetic extension of life span, **questions current treatments of type 2 diabetes as well as the widespread use of antioxidant supplements. Ristow's group further demonstrated in their report that antioxidants and vitamins given to the worms erased the life-extending benefits of sugar deprivation, raising questions about the widespread use of antioxidant supplements.** (Schulz et al, 2007)

69) - **Impaired glucose metabolism extends life expectancy by inducing mitochondrial respiration** (EMOD formation). **The histone deacetylase Sir2.1 is found here to be dispensable for this phenotype, whereas disruption of aak-2, a homolog of AMP-dependent kinase (AMPK), abolishes extension of life span due to impaired glycolysis. Glucose restriction promotes mitochondrial metabolism, causing increased EMOD formation.** (Schulz et al, 2007)

70) - **A direct cause-and-effect relationship between the accumulation of oxidatively mediated damage and aging has not been clearly established.** (Kregel, Zhang, 2007)

71) - The longest-living rodent -Heterocephalus glaber- produces high levels of free radicals and has significant oxidative damage levels in proteins, lipids and DNA. **However, in contrast to MFRTA predictions, <u>high levels of oxidative damage in mtDNA do not decrease longevity in mice.</u> Available data concerning the role of free radicals in longevity control are contradictory,** and do not prove MFRTA. (Sanz and Stefanatose, 2008)

72) - **Resveratrol** (an antioxidant) **treatment in mice has failed to slow the rate of aging** in spite of some beneficial effects on health. (Pearson et al, 2008) (Wood et al, 2004)

73) - <u>**Significantly elevated mitochondrial ROS (EMOD) production was recently observed in the cardiovascular system of the long-lived Ames dwarf mice**</u> **when compared to wild-type littermates.** (Csiszar et al, 2008)

74) - **The longest living rodent, the naked mole-rat, lives in captivity for more than 28.3 years, approximately 9 times longer than similar-sized mice and has a very high level of oxidative stress. These animals have never been observed to develop any spontaneous neoplasm.** (Buffenstein, 2008)

75) - According to Lapointe and Hekimi, "The core statement of the theory (MFRTA) is wrong. **Yet, the theory is now being openly challenged by many.**" (de Magalhaes, Church, 2006) (Howes, 2006) (Blagosklonny, 2008) (Bonawitz, Shadel, 2007) (Buffenstien et al, 2008) (Gems, Doonan, 2009) (Fukui, Moraes, 2008)

76) - **Interventional trials have been controversial, with some positive findings, many null findings, and some suggestion of harm in certain high-risk populations.** Because of the mismatch between the epidemiologic studies and the interventional trials, **some researchers have advocated ending antioxidant work. Others have questioned the validity of the LDL oxidative hypothesis itself.** (Willcox et al, 2008)

77) - **"A balanced diet of moderate proportions and exercise remain today the only proven fountain of youth."** (Dominguez et al, 2009)

78) - **Recent years have seen an abundance of experimental evidence that contradicts the MTA in its present form.** (Alexeyev, 2009)

79) - **However, reports on age-related changes in the activity of these enzymes are often contradictory. For example, both an increase and a decrease in the activity of 8-oxoguanine DNA glycosylase, which is responsible for the removal of 8-oxodG from mtDNA, were associated with aging in the mitochondria. Opposing trends in the activity of Sod2 and GPx have also been reported with aging.** (Alexeyev, 2009)

80) - "**There is no single biological marker of aging.**" (Le Gall, Ardaillou, 2009)

81) - **The majority of the initial pioneering studies in mice to test the mitochondrial theory of aging have yielded results that either do not support the theory or remain inconclusive.** (Jang, Remmen, 2009)

82) - "**Genetic studies in invertebrates have provided a signifi- cant body of evidence that is inconsistent with predictions of the MTA.**" (Alexeyev, 2009)

83) - "**In summary, most experimental evidence to date does not support the MTA.**" (Alexeyev, 2009)

84) - **To date (2009), despite numerous experiments and clini- cal trials with promising compounds, there is no report of a successful study in mammals, and the results are strangely in- consistent in *Drosophila*.** (Howes, 2006) (Magwere et al, 2006)

85) - **It was recently shown that inactivation of the crucial mi- tochondrial antioxidant SOD-2 increases oxidative damage to proteins and general sensitivity to oxidative stress in *C. el- egans*, yet simultaneously prolongs lifespan of these animals.** (Van Raamsdonk, Hekimi, 2009). It has previously been shown that elim- ination of either cytoplasmic or mitochondrial SOD in yeast, flies, and mice results in decreased lifespan.

86) - **Hekimi et al. recently presented a new aging study with a large sample size in a mixed background that showed again that *Mclk1* +/- mutants live significantly longer than controls.** (Lapointe et al, 2009)

87) - **To date (2009), virtually all our findings resulting from the analysis of the phenotype of the long-lived *Mclk1* +/- mice appear irreconcilable with the MFRTA.** (Lapointe, Hekimi, 2008) (Lapointe et al, 2009)

88) - **Among participants with a dietary vitamin C intake above the median of 90 mg/day, vitamin E increased mortality among those aged 50-62 years by 19%.** (Hemila and Kaprio, 2009 Apr)

89) - **Esophageal cancer deaths increased 14% among those aged 55 years or older. Vitamin A and zinc supplementation**

was associated with increased total and stroke mortality. (Qiao et al, 2009)

90) - Thus, we believe that **it is reasonable to now consider the MFRTA as refuted.** (Lapointe, Hekimi, 2010)

91) - **Nutritional and genetic interventions to boost anti-oxidants have generally failed to increase life-span.** Furthermore, the free radical theory fails to explain why exercise causes higher levels of oxyradical damage, but generally promotes healthy aging." (Brewer, 2010)

92) - **The gold standard for determining whether aging is altered is life span, i.e., does altering oxidative stress/damage change life span? Mice with genetic manipulations in their antioxidant defense system designed to directly address this prediction have, with few exceptions, shown no change in life span. In environments with minimal stress, as expected under optimal husbandry, oxidative damage plays little role in aging.** However, under chronic stress, including pathological phenotypes that diminish optimal health, oxidative stress/damage plays a major role in aging. Under these conditions, enhanced antioxidant defenses exert an "antiaging" action, leading to changes in life span, age-related pathology, and physiological function as predicted by the oxidative stress theory of aging. (Salmon, et al, 2010)

93) - In **conflict with Harman's FRTA**, recent evidence suggests that calorie restriction and specifically reduced glucose metabolism induces mitochondrial metabolism to extend life span in various model organisms, including Saccharomyces cerevisiae, Drosophila melanogaster, Caenorhabditis elegans and possibly mice. **These effects may be due to increased formation of reactive oxygen species (ROS) (EMODs) within the mitochondria.** (Ristow, Zarse, 2010)

94) - **Consistently, abrogation of this mitochondrial ROS (EMOD) signal by antioxidants impairs the lifespan-extending and health-promoting capabilities of glucose restriction and physical exercise, respectively. ROS (EMODs) are essential signaling molecules which are required to promote health and longevity.** (Ristow, Zarse, 2010)

95) - **The generation of superoxide is elevated in the nuo-6 and isp-1 mitochondrial mutants. This elevation is necessary and sufficient to increase longevity, as it is abolished by the antioxidants NAC and vitamin C, and phenocopied by mild**

treatment with the prooxidant paraquat. These findings are not consistent with the mitochondrial oxidative stress theory of aging. Increased superoxide generation acts as a signal in young mutant animals to trigger changes of gene expression that prevent or attenuate the effects of subsequent aging. (Yang, Hekimi, 2010)

96) - *C. elegans isp-1* and *nuo-6* mutants, which carry point mutations in subunits of the mitochondrial electron transport chain (ETC) display an elevated generation of mitochondrial superoxide which appears to be causal to their increased lifespan. Indeed, antioxidants suppress the mutants' longevity and pro-oxidant treatment of the wild type phenocopies it. (Yang, Hekimi, 2010)

97) - The low plasma level of LPO in Okinawan centenarians, compared to younger controls, argues for protection against oxidative stress in the centenarian population and is consistent with the predictions of the Free Radical Theory of Aging. However, the present work does not strongly support a role for vitamin E in this phenomenon. (Suzuki et al. 2010)

98- Surprisingly, even double mutants, lacking both mitochondrial forms of SOD, show no reduction in lifespan. While we show a clear age-dependent, linear increase in oxidative damage in WT nematodes, we find no evidence for autocatalytic damage amplification as proposed by the "vicious cycle" theory. Comparing the SOD mutants with wild-type animals, we further show that oxidative damage levels in the mtDNA of SOD mutants are not significantly different from those in wild-type animals, i.e. even the total loss of mitochondrial SOD did not significantly increase oxidative damage to mtDNA." (Gruber et al, 2011)

99) Unfortunately, the use of antioxidant vitamins, as health promoting, disease-preventing and anti-aging agents, is based on a flawed theory. (Howes, *Antioxidant Failures and Dangers*, 2011)

100) - Several longevity-promoting interventions may converge by causing an activation of mitochondrial oxygen consumption to promote increased formation of reactive oxygen species (ROS) (EMODs). Antioxidant supplements that prevent these ROS (EMOD) signals interfere with the health-promoting and life-span-extending capabilities of calorie restriction and physical exercise. Taken together and consistent with ample published

evidence, **the findings summarized here question Harman's Free Radical Theory of Aging and rather suggest that ROS (EMODs) act as essential signaling molecules to promote metabolic health and longevity**. (Ristow, Schmeisser)

I could present many more but 100 should be enough for the open minded reader. For the sycophantic zealots blindly following the FRT, there will never be enough.

Also, please refer to the following book for references:

- Cancer and Longevity Answers: Naked mole rats, Exercise & EMODs (ROS). CreateSpace and Free Radical Publishing, © **2015.** (Howes, 2015, Cancer)

SUMMARY OF 150 ADDITIONAL FACTS
FOR BLIND ZEALOTS
INVALIDATING THE FRT
(FREE RADICAL THEORY)

150 Facts further nullifying the free radical theory

1- **Based on currently reported lifespan studies using mice with altered antioxidant defense, there is little evidence that oxidative stress plays a role in determining lifespan**. (Hamilton et al, 2012)

2- **Several experimental rodent models of antioxidant manipulation have failed to affect lifespan.** (Dai et al, 2014)

3- **In addition to effects on lifespan and aging, mitochondrial ROS (EMODs) have been shown to play a central role in health span of many vital organ systems.** (Dai et al, 2014)

4- **Skeletal muscle, like heart, relies on mitochondria to meet the majority of the ATP demands for sustained muscle contraction. Periods of increased mitochondrial ROS (EMOD) production are a normal part of the physiology of skeletal muscle**. (Anderson et al, 2009)

5- **These transient increases in oxidative stress modify muscle function and may play an important role in the beneficial adaptations to exercise training**. (Ristow et al, 2009)

6- **Increased ROS (EMODs) occurs in skeletal muscle and heart during exercise from a variety of sources, but the broad outcome of this oxidative stress is beneficial, resulting in the induction of mitochondrial biogenesis and aerobic capacity, augmented antioxidant capacity, improved vascularization, and insulin sensitivity**. (Alleman et al, 2014)

7- **There was evidence of oxidative stress after both exhaustive aerobic (AE) and isometric (IE) exercise. Lipid hydroperoxides, protein carbonyls, and total antioxidants increased after both IE and AE**.

8- **Most of the interventions based on antioxidant supplementation do not increase longevity, as would be predicted by the mitochondrial free radical theory of aging (MFRTA).** (Scialo et al, 2013)

9- **The antioxidant defenses never completely compensate for the increased formation of EMODs during exhaustive exercise**.

10- **Vitamin C supplementation seems at best to have limited clinically relevant effects on "the common man" and on athletes who are otherwise healthy and have a normal diet**. (Hemila, Chalker, 2013)

11- **Vitamin C and E do not seem to have appreciable/consistent ergogenic effects or effects on recovery from exercise**. (Clarkson, Thompson, 2000) (Braakhuis, 2012) (Bloomer, 2007) (Evans, 2000)

12- **Both animal and human studies have indicated negative effects on physiological adaptations to strength training when vitamin C and/or E are administered in high dosages.** (Paulsen et al, 2014)

13- **Vitamin C and E supplementation interfered with the acute cellular response to heavy-load resistance exercise and demonstrated tentative long-term negative effects on adaptation to strength training.** (Paulsen, Hammarsland, et al, 2014)

14- **There is now very compelling evidence that antioxidants exert negative effects under certain physiological contexts, and in some cases may actually do more harm than good**. (Ristow, 2014)

15- **New research at The University of Copenhagen surprisingly suggests that eating a diet rich in antioxidants may actually counteract many of the health benefits of exercise, including reduced blood pressure and cholesterol.**

16- **In older men, a natural antioxidant compound found in red grapes and other plants -- called resveratrol -- blocks many of the cardiovascular benefits of exercise, according to research published July, 22 2013 in** *The Journal of Physiology*.

17- **There is currently a lack of conclusive evidence that exercise performance or recovery would benefit in any significant way from dietary vitamin E supplementation. Most evidence suggests that there is no discernible effect of vitamin E supplementation on performance, training effect or rate of postexercise recovery in either recreational or elite athletes. There appears to be little reason for vitamin E supplementation among athletes.** (Tiidus, Houston, 1995)

18- **Vitamin E and C supplementation was found to be ineffective in preventing muscle damage following an ultra marathon (50 km) run in healthy participants**, although the supplements did decrease markers of lipid peroxidation and DNA damage. (Mastaloudis et al, 2004)

19- **The dogs ran, on average, 0.2 s slower when supplemented with 1 g of vitamin C**, equivalent to a lead of 3 m at the finish of a 500-m race. **Supplementation with vitamin C, therefore, appeared to slow racing greyhounds**. (Marshall et al, 2002)

20- **Supplementation with high (1000 IU) but not moderate (100 IU) daily doses of vitamin E appears to slow racing greyhounds.** (Hill et al, 2001)

21- Seven trained male cyclists **participated in 4 separate supplementation phases. They ingested 2 capsules per day containing vitamin C and Vitamin E treatments. However neither of these vitamins, either alone or in combination, will enhance exercise performance.** (Bryant et al, 2003)

22- Vitamin E supplementation had no effect on exercise performance or capacity in athletic students. (Gaeini et al, 2006)

23- Horses supplemented with vitamin E, at nearly 10-times the 1989 NRC recommended level, did not experience lower oxidative stress compared to control horses. (Williams, Carlucci, 2006)

24- Athletes (ultra-endurance runners) **with a regular intake of vitamin and mineral supplements in the four weeks before the race finished the competition no faster than athletes without an intake of vitamins and minerals.** (Knechtle et al, 2008)

25- Exercise-induced oxidative stress ameliorates insulin resistance and causes an adaptive response promoting endogenous antioxidant defense capacity. Supplementation with antioxidants may preclude these health-promoting effects of exercise in humans. (Ristow et al, 2009)

26- AOX (AOX; 272 mg of alpha-tocopherol, 400 mg of vitamin C, 30 mg of beta-carotene, 2 mg of lutein, 400 mug of selenium, 30 mg of zinc, and 600 mg of magnesium) **supplementation does not offer protection against exercise-induced lipid peroxidation and inflammation** and **may hinder the recovery of muscle damage**. (Teixeira et al, 2009)

27- In the Journal of the American Medical Association (JAMA), they published a review of 68 studies, containing 232,606 subjects, investigators found 66 studies reported no statistically significant association between supplement use and longevity. **The remaining two studies actually reported statistical increases in premature death with supplement use.**

28- Viewed as a whole, the data accumulated from a vast pool of data have too often failed to support the free radical theory. (Stuart et al, 2014)

29- Excellent, well controlled studies from the past decade in particular have isolated ROS (EMODs) as an experimental variable and have shown no relationship between its production or neutralization and aging or longevity. (Stuart et al, 2014)

30- Instead, a role for mitochondrial ROS (EMODs) as intracellular messengers involved in the regulation of some basic

cellular processes, such as proliferation, differentiation and death, has emerged. (Stuart et al, 2014)

31- The theory (MFRTA) has inevitably shown signs of fallibility, if not evidence of an outright midlife crisis. (Stuart et al, 2014)

32- We suggest that data gleaned from inter-species comparisons, dietary manipulations and genetic manipulations have collectively failed to offer sufficient support for the MFRTA, and have thus cast significant doubt on the validity of the theory. (Stuart et al, 2014)

33- The field has not succeeded in validating the original MFRTA. (Stuart et al, 2014)

34- Honda et al. investigated the relationship between environmental O_2 levels and lifespan, and found no effect when environmental O_2 was maintained at set values between 2% and 40% over the entire lifespan. (Honda et al, 1993)

35- Yanase and Ishii similarly found that daily exposure to 90% O_2 did not affect lifespan in wildtype C. elegans and actually extended it in some strains. (Yanase, Ishii, 2008)

36- In the strains of C. elegans in which high O_2 extended longevity, there was no evidence of an up-regulation of any of the superoxide dismutases in response to hyperoxia exposure. (Yanase, Ishii, 2008)

37- Similarly, genetic overexpression of these enzymes (SODs) is not associated with increased lifespan. (Doonan et al, 2008)

38- Higher levels of environmental O_2, which should translate directly into higher O_2 levels within the organism and therefore higher rates of O_2^- production in cells (if indeed antioxidant enzymes are not broadly induced), did not affect longevity in C. elegans. (Van Voorhies, Ward, 2000)

39- Some of the highest levels of O_2 exposure in mammals occur in the lungs (approximately 10 to 14%), and one might therefore predict that lung epithelium should be particularly vulnerable to the degenerative effects of aging, especially compared to tissues like cartilage, in which chondrocytes exist in a relatively hypoxic environment (<3% O_2). However, there is no evidence that this is so. (Stuart et al, 2014)

40- **If ROS, EMODs originating from mitochondria are responsible for aging then one would also predict that, since there should be more ROS (EMODs) produced within cardiomyocytes than in chondrocytes, the heart would age more rapidly** (superoxide dismutase levels are similar in heart and cartilage. (Frederiks, Bosch, 1997)

A recent epigenetic method for doing just this suggests that **heart tissue is actually typified by a particularly slow aging rate**. (Horvath, 2013)

41- **Some of the longest-lived endothermic vertebrate species for their respective body masses are birds and bats, even though both groups are generally characterized by relatively high mass-specific metabolic rates, and high mitochondrial abundance in heart and skeletal muscle tissues**. (Robb et al, 2014)

42- **In summary, the predicted relationships between either O_2 and aging rate or mitochondrial abundance within cells and aging rate have not been reliably identified**. (Stuart et al, 2014)

43- **The predicted simple relationships among O_2 exposure, mitochondrial abundance and aging/longevity do not exist**. (Stuart et al, 2014)

44- **Measurements of mitochondrial H_2O_2 production by isolated vascular tissues of the extremely long-lived naked mole rats and Damara mole rats also failed to uncover differences compared to shorter-lived guinea pigs and mice**. (Labinskyy et al, 2006)

45- *A similar absence of association between H_2O_2 generation was noted in comparisons of isolated heart mitochondria respiring on succinate (+/- the respiratory complex I inhibitor rotenone) between naked mole rats and mice.* (Brown, McClelland, et al, 2009) (Lambert et al, 2007)

46- **Rates of mitochondrial H2O2 production in Japanese quail were significantly higher than those in rats, despite the fact that these two species have similar maximum lifespans** (MLSPs). (Stuart et al, 2014)

47- **In a similar comparison between the long-lived house sparrow *Passer domesticus* and laboratory mice, the rates of**

isolated liver mitochondrial H_2O_2 production were significantly greater in the longer-lived species. (Brown et al, 2009)

48- **Brunet-Rossinni found no consistent association between MLSP and the rates of H_2O_2 production in mitochondria isolated from brain, heart and kidney of the little brown bat *Myotis lucifugus* (MLSP = 34 y), the white-footed mouse *Peromyscus leucopus* (MLSP = 8 y) and the short-tailed shrew *Blarina brevicauda* (MLSP = 2 y).** (Brunet-Rossinni et al, 2004)

49- **Under most experimental conditions, these investigators found few differences in H_2O_2 production rates between species and no association with MLSP.** (Lambert et al, 2007)

50- **Taken together, however, the collection of experimental results discussed above provides little support for the hypothesis that longer-lived organisms have adapted to produce less mitochondrial ROS (EMODs)**. (Brown et al, 2009) (Brunet-Rossinni et al, 2004) (Lambert et al, 2007)

51- **The caloric restriction studies, as a whole, do not offer strong support for the prediction of the MFRTA that mitochondrial ROS (EMOD) production will be reduced**. (Walsh et al, 2014)

52- **RMH Note: I have been aggressively pointing out the harmful consequences of the demonization of oxygen and its electronically modified derivatives (EMODs) for the past decade and a half. The FRT has delayed meaningful design and execution of laboratory studies for years and it has made authors try to fit their data into the framework of an invalidated theory. The FRT has even made investigators doubt their own laboratory results because their results were at odds with the flawed FRT.**

53- The manipulation of Reactive Oxygen Species (ROS, EMODs) can have a beneficial effect on various lung pathologies. However **indiscriminate uses of anti-oxidant strategies have not demonstrated any consistent benefit and may be harmful**. (Mannam et al, 2014)

54- **Antioxidant supplements that prevent these EMOD signals interfere with the health-promoting and life-span-extending capabilities of calorie restriction and physical exercise**. (Ristow, Schmeisser, 2011)

55- **Taken together and consistent with ample published evidence, the findings summarized here question Harman's Free Radical Theory of Aging** and rather suggest that **ROS (EMODs) act as essential signaling molecules to promote metabolic health and longevity**. (Ristow, Schmeisser, 2011)

56- **The second erroneous prediction arising from the MFRTA is that greater longevity should be associated with a greater capacity to neutralize mitochondrial ROS (EMODs)**. (Stuart et al, 2014)

57- **This analysis also failed to show a relationship between with MLSP, and therefore failed to support the second hypothesis relating to the MFRTA, that is, that the cellular capacity to neutralize ROS (EMODs) should be greater in longer-lived organisms**. (Robb et al, 2014)

58- **Overwhelmingly, the conclusions from these studies (mammalian lifespan studies have been conducted utilizing transgenic or knockout laboratory mouse models to increase or decrease gene expression of mitochondrial and other key intracellular antioxidant enzymes) has been that, although the expected increases and decreases in tissue oxidative damage biomarkers are usually observed in antioxidant enzyme gene under-expressing and overexpressing individuals, respectively, there are seldom corresponding effects on longevity. Thus, the results of experiments using this approach have most often yielded results that are inconsistent with the MFRTA**. (Stuart et al, 2014)

59- **Vitamin E has variously been shown to have no effect, a positive effect and even a negative effect on aging/lifespan. Certainly, no clear picture of an anti-aging activity emerges in the hundreds of studies that have been conducted**. (Stuart et al, 2014)

60- **Some human antioxidant supplement studies have been terminated prematurely due to adverse outcomes. A similar lack of consensus has emerged with respect to the anti-aging effects of a number of other vitamin antioxidant supplements, after many hundreds of experimental studies and clinical trials (for example, see the review by Dolora et al. 2012)**. (Bjelakovic et al, 2012)

61- **The dozens of experiments instigated by these findings failed to confirm any general positive longevity effects for resveratrol and a variety of plant-based molecules, including polyphenolic stilbenes**. (Stuart et al, 2014)

62- **While there is some evidence for increased lifespan with bioactive polyphenols in *C. elegans*, it is lacking in most other species**. (Stuart, Robb, 2013)

63- **The National Institutes of Health's Aging Intervention Testing Study (http://www.nia.nih.gov/research/dab/interventions-testing-program-itp/compounds-testing) has investigated the pro-longevity properties of a number of small molecule antioxidants, including vitamin E and resveratrol, in mice and reported no beneficial effects on lifespan**.

64- **Based on the results discussed above by Stuart et al, the evidence for an association between small molecule antioxidant supplementation and slowed aging and/or increased longevity is insufficient to support the MFRTA**. (Stuart et al, 2014)

65- **The anti-aging properties of MitoQ (an antioxidant conjugated to positively charged, membrane-permeant moieties) have been tested in *D. melanogaster*, where it failed to extend lifespan**. (Magwere et al, 2006)

66- **At this time there is no compelling evidence that reducing the rate of mitochondrial ROS (EMOD) production will slow aging or increase lifespan. Therefore, this line of investigation has failed to offer clear support for the MFRTA**. (Rodriguez-Cuenca et al, 2010)

67- **Taken together, the results discussed above suggest that if ROS (EMODs) participate in the biology of aging, it is not via the straightforward processes envisioned by the MFRTA**. (Stuart et al, 2014)

68- **It is important to note that overexpression of antioxidant enzymes that reduce intracellular ROS (EMOD) levels are not generally associated with increased longevity.** (Stuart et al, 2014)

69- **Within the context of the MFRTA, the ability of EMODs to regulate tissue-specific regenerative capacity could have important implications in maintaining organ function and thus animal health throughout the lifespan**. (Stuart et al, 2014)

70- **Virtually all attempts to control mitochondrial ROS, EMOD production or neutralization have yielded unexpected and even occasionally unwanted effects on aging and lifespan**. (Stuart et al, 2014)

71- **The MFRTA has as yet failed to offer a sufficient explanation of organismal aging as a phenomenon**. (Stuart et al, 2014)

72- **Whether considering the evolution of longevity by natural selection of specific traits, the extension of lifespan by caloric restriction, the ability of transgenes, gene knockouts or small molecule antioxidants to alter lifespan, the overall conclusion has been drifting toward 'no consistent relationship between mitochondrial ROS, EMODs and longevity'**. (Stuart et al, 2014)

73- **ROS, EMODs are recognized to impinge upon signaling pathways regulating all of the fundamental aspects of cell biology: the cell cycle, proliferation and differentiation, and life and death**. (Chiu, Dawes, 2012)

74- **The mitochondrial theory of aging, a mainstream theory of aging which once included accumulation of mitochondrial DNA (mtDNA) damage by reactive oxygen species (ROS) (EMODs) as its cornerstone, has been increasingly losing ground and is undergoing extensive revision due to its inability to explain a growing body of emerging data**. (Shokilenko, Wilson, Alexeyev, 2014)

75- **Meta-studies reveal no longevity benefit of increased antioxidant defenses**. (Shokilenko, Wilson, Alexeyev, 2014)

76- **Simultaneously, exciting new observations from both comparative biology and experimental systems indicate that increased ROS (EMODs) production and oxidative damage to cellular macromolecules, including mtDNA, can be associated with extended longevity**. (Shokilenko, Wilson, Alexeyev, 2014)

77- **Recent advances provide evidence against the existence of the "vicious" cycle of mtDNA damage and ROS, EMOD production and the MFRTA**. (Shokilenko, Wilson, Alexeyev, 2014)

78- **Regulation of EMODs has a vital role in maintaining "stemness" and differentiation of the stem cells.** (Chaudhari, Ye, Jang, 2014)

79- **The perspective of free radical theory of aging has become increasingly critical as the predicted beneficial effects of many antioxidant treatments and genetic manipulations have failed to materialize**. (Sanz, Pamplona, Barja, 2006) (Muller et al, 2007)

(Gruber, Schaffer, Halliwell, 2008) (Perez, et al, 2009 (Bratic, Larsson, 2013) (Barja, 2013) (Pulliam et al, 2913)

80- **Many of the manipulations that should decrease aging and increase longevity according to the classical versions of the mitochondrial free radical theory of aging have failed to do so, implying that the theory is wrong, or at best deeply flawed**. (Huang et al, 2000) (Bjelakovic et al, 2007) (Jang et al, 2009) (Perez et al, 2009)

81- **The mitochondrial free radical theory of aging is in crisis because recent studies have shown no relationship between free radicals and longevity**, and instead emphasize a role for mitochondrial reactive oxygen species as intracellular messengers. (Stuart et al, 2014)

82- **Our results are not consistent with a causal role for intracellular antioxidant enzymes in longevity**, similar to recent reports from studies utilizing genetic modifications of mice. (Perez et al, 2009)

83- **We found no evidence, in either the interspecific or the intraspecific comparisons, of a broad multi-tissue upregulation of antioxidant enzyme activities associated with the evolution of longevity**. (Page et al, 2010)

84- **Similar to CuZnSOD, we found no correlation between the activity of liver or heart MnSOD and animal MLSP**. (Page et al, 2010)

85- **There is little evidence that an upregulation of GPx/GR is associated with extended longevity in the Snell dwarf mice. Taken together with the results of published studies, our results suggest no link between GPx or GR activities and longevity**. (Page et al, 2010)

86- **Whilst it seems intuitive that this oxidative stress resistance might be achieved by increased expression of antioxidant enzymes in long-lived species, experimental evidence generally indicates that this does not occur.** (Andziak et al, 2005) (Page et al 2009b)

87- **This idea questions the FRTA and rather suggests that ROS (EMODs) act as essential signaling molecules to promote metabolic health and longevity**. (Sadowska-Bartosz, Bartosz, 2014)

88- **Up till now no prospective clinical intervention studies have been able to show a positive association between anti-oxidant supplementation and increased survival**. (Sadowska-Bartosz, Bartosz, 2014)

89- **Domination of the free radical theory has been little affected by an increasing number of studies that seem to contradict it.** (Blagosklonny, 2008) (Cabreiro et al, 2011) (Doonan et al, 2008) (Gems, Doonan, 2009) (Koc et al, 2004) (Lapointe, Hekimi, 2009) (Mockett, Sohal, Sohal, 2010) (Pani, 2010) (Perez et al, 2009) (Speakman, Selman, 2011) (Van Raamsdonk, Hekimi, 2012) (Van Raamsdonk, Hekimi, 2009)

90- **The free radical theory of aging is consistent with numerous studies, but many other reports clearly contradict this idea. Collectively, these studies argue against the universal role of oxidative damage in aging.** (Gladysjev. 2014)

91- **It is time to conclude that the oxidative (free radical) theory of aging limits further understanding of the aging process**. (Gladysjev. 2014)

92- **Recent work on a small European cave salamander (Proteus anguinus) has revealed that it has exceptional longevity, yet it appears to have unexceptional defenses against oxidative damage**. (Speakman, Selman, 2011)

93- **High dietary doses of vitamin C are ineffective at prolonging lifespan in mice because any positive benefits derived as an antioxidant are offset by compensatory reductions in endogenous protection mechanisms, leading to no net reduction in accumulated oxidative damage**. (Selman et al, 2006)

94- **At present, the free radical theory of aging is no longer considered to be true**. (Piotrowska, Bartnik, 2014)

95- **Studies that have attempted to modulate ROS-induced damage, either upwards or downwards, using antioxidant or genetic approaches, generally do not show a predictable effect on lifespan**. (Selman et al, 2013)

96- **Surprisingly, antioxidant supplementation significantly shortened lifespan in voles maintained under both cold (7 ± 2°C) and warm (22 ± 2°C) conditions**. (Selman et al, 2013)

97- **Several recent studies have raised reservations over the role of ROS (EMODs) in causing aging**. (Speakman, Selman, 2011) (Perez et al, 2009) (Gems, Doonan, 2009)

98- **The idea that supplementation with antioxidants such as vitamins E and C can decrease EMODs and oxidative damage, and hence increase lifespan is pervasive, despite a lack of convincing supportive data**. (Banks, Speakman, Selman, 2010)

99- **The effects of antioxidant supplementation on disease and mortality in humans are equally ambiguous, with some meta-analysis approaches even suggesting that mortality is increased following supplementation of certain antioxidants**. (Myung et al, 2013) (Bjelakovic et al, 2012) (Miller et al, 2005)

100- **Our data clearly demonstrates that dietary supplementation with either vitamin E or vitamin C dramatically shortened lifespan in voles**. (Selman et al, 2006)

101- **Both the negative impact of antioxidant supplementation and positive effect of cold exposure on lifespan cast further doubt on simplistic models of the free radical theory relating metabolism, ROS (EMOD) production and aging**. (Selman et al, 2012)

102- **Antioxidant efficacy in quenching ROS (EMODs) *in vitro* appears not to be predictive of lifespan in *Caenorhabditis elegans***. (Punn et al, 2010)

103- **In *Caenorhabditis elegans*, single or double SOD mutants have a normal lifespan, while mitochondrial SOD2 mutants (single or double with cytoplasmic SOD1) increased lifespan**. (Van Raamskonk, Hekimi, 2009)

104- **Later analyses suggested that over-expression of catalase, SOD1, or SOD2 using the genes' native promoters does not increase life span**. (Mockett et al, 1999) (Orr, Sohal, 2003)

105- **Elevated SOD2 did result in substantial life span increases**. (Landis, Tower, 2005)

106- **In transgenic mice, the overexpression of endogenous antioxidants, including CuZnSOD (SOD1, cytoplasmic), MnSOD (SOD2, mitochondrial), catalase, or combination of CuZnSOD/**

catalase and CuZnSOD/MnSOD failed to extend mouse lifespan. (Huang et al, 2000) (Jang et al, 2009) (Perez et al, 2009)

107- There was **no effect of antioxidant supplements on overall mortality, or even a significant increase in mortality in subjects receiving beta carotene, vitamin A, and vitamin E**. (Bjelakovic et al, 2007)

108- **Meta-analysis including 50 randomized controlled trials with 294,478 participants showed no evidence to support the use of vitamin and antioxidant supplements for prevention of cardiovascular diseases**. (Myung et al, 2013)

109- **The lack of anti-aging effect with antioxidant supplements led Harman to modify his original theory to specify mitochondria as both the primary sources of ROS (EMODs) and the primary targets of ROS damage**. (Harman, 1972)

110- **Glucose restriction in C. elegans extends lifespan by inducing mitochondrial respiration and increasing oxidative stress**, and **this AMPK-dependent lifespan extension is abolished by pre-treatment of antioxidant N-acetyl cysteine**, suggesting that **oxidative stress is required for lifespan extension of dietary restriction**. (Schulz et al, 2007)

111- Despite the evidence supporting the role of mitochondrial oxidative stress in experimental models of diabetes, **there are mixed results on the protective role of antioxidant treatments in diabetes or its complications from clinical trials**. (Johansen et al, 2005)

112- The HOPE trial showed **vitamin E treatment for 4.5 years fails to confer benefit in cardiovascular outcomes and nephropathy**. (Lonn et al, 2002)

113- **Results of SECURE trial and PPP trial also failed to demonstrate any protective effects with vitamin E treatment**. (Johansen et al, 2005)

114- **Meta-analyses of several clinical trials using antioxidant supplement have shown largely disappointing results**. (Bjilakovic et al, 2007)

115- **Surprisingly, Sod2(+/-)Gpx1(-/-) mice showed no reduction in life span, despite increased levels of oxidative damage**.

Thus, **these data do not support a significant role for increased oxidative stress as a result of compromised mitochondrial antioxidant defenses in modulating life span in mice and do not support the oxidative stress theory of aging**. (Zhang et al, 2009)

116- **Based on currently reported lifespan studies using mice with altered antioxidant defense, there is little evidence that oxidative stress plays a role in determining lifespan**. (Hamilton et al, 2012)

117- "**It may turn out that we have been systematically "poisoning" ourselves, increasing our disease risk and shortening our lifespan through antioxidant supplements.**" (Stefan Andrei Anghel, Harvard Science Review, 2010)

118- **Many long-living species such as birds, bats and mole-rats exhibit high-levels of oxidative damage, evident already at young ages**. (Rodriguez et al, 2011)

119- **The naked mole rat has proved Harman wrong on both counts, i.e., aging and cancer.** (RMH, 2015)

120- **If an organism has increased oxidative damage but exhibits no change in lifespan, the result falsifies the hypothesis of the FRT and the MFRTA. RMH Note: That is exactly what happens in the naked mole rat, i.e., it has increased oxidative damage, yet, it lives 8 times as long as other similar rodents.** (Buffenstein, 2008)

121- **A large cohort study showed that overexpression of CuZnSOD did not increase lifespan**. (Huang et al, 2000)

122- **Mice overexpressing CAT (2- to 4-fold) in the peroxisome did not show a significant extension of maximal lifespan**, although median lifespan showed a modest 10% increase. (Chen et al, 2004)

123- **No increases in lifespan was evident with overexpression of MnSOD**. (Perez et al, 2008)

124- **While lifespan studies have not been conducted on every antioxidant gene that is overexpressed, despite the many signs of enhanced protection, the available data show that the impact on lifespan is modest.** (Ishii, 2007)

125- **The cumulative indices of oxidative markers and oxidative stress in healthy humans related to aging and gender have been measured in multiple biological fluids and in many instances confounding results have been reported**. (Aejumelaeus et al, 1997) (Kim et al, 2001) (Meccocci et al, 2000) (Jones et al, 2002) (Erden-Inal et al, 2002) (Ozbay, Dulger, 2002) (Junqueira et al, 2004) (Gil et al, 2006) (Frisard et al, 2007) (Mendoza et al, 2007)

126- **Age-related changes in antioxidants (SOD, GPx and CAT, carotenoids and tocopherols) in humans do not show a consistent pattern**; generally erythrocytic activity of SOD and GPx increased while plasma values were unchanged. (Meccocci et al, 2000) (Erden-Inal et al, 2002) (Ozbay, Dulger, 2002) (Junqueira et al, 2004) (Frisard et al, 2007) (Mendoza et al, 2007)

127- **Direct measures of antioxidants, the results of their manipulations or correlations with disease and oxidant polymorphisms have not shown unequivocal support for the theory (MFTRA)**. (Ishii, 2007)

128- **Birds exhibit a 1.5-fold higher mass specific basal metabolic rate (BMR) than do similar-sized mammals and in contrast to the predicted detrimental effects on longevity caused by the inevitable ROS-induced damage due to oxygen consumption, some live approximately twice as long as do similar-sized mammals**. (Buttemer et al, 2008)

129- **Longevity in birds and mammals increased similarly with increasing body size, although birds generally live twice as long as similar-sized mammals**. (Lindstedt, Calder, 1976)

130- **When these effects of size and phylogeny on BMR are statistically corrected, the relationship between BMR and MLSP no longer holds in either birds or mammals**. (deMagalhães et al, 2007)

131- **Both these outcomes refute the explanatory power of the rate of living theory for MLSP.** (Lindstedt, Calder, 1976) (deMagalhães et al, 2007)

132- **There are also multiple exceptions to the presumed constant relationship between metabolic rate and lifespan posited by the rate of living theory. For example voluntary exercise and its associated increase in metabolic rate does not shorten**

lifespan of rats or humans and is generally thought to extend healthy lifespan. (Holloszy et al, 1985) (Lee, Hsieh, 1995)

133- **There is no inverse relationship between lifespan and mass-specific metabolic rates of individual mice, dogs or flies**. (Hulbert et al, 2004) (Speakman et al, 2003) (Speakman et al, 2004)

134- **There is no consistent stoichiometric relation between pro-oxidation or antioxidant measures, making inferences between species from limited measures of only a few antioxidants essentially meaningless.** (Perez-Campo et al, 1998)

135- **No consistent differences in known processes that remove radicals and repair the damage have been found to correlate with MLSP**. (Lambert et al, 2007) (Andziak, O'Connor, Buffenstein, 2005) (Brunet-Rossinni, 2004) (Andziak et al, 2006)

136- **These findings concur with studies showing that the effects of anti-oxidants on human health are equivocal as are the efficacy of pharmacological mimetics of antioxidants**. (Meydani et al, 1998) (Melov et al, 2000)

137- **Genetic overexpression of various antioxidants and their effects on lifespan in various animal models similarly yield conflicting results and knocking down antioxidant protection, while leading to more oxidative damage, does not impact upon longevity**. (Perez et al, 2009) (McCord, Fridovich, 1969)

138- **This observation correlates with the negative data from various dietary treatments with exogenous antioxidants that sometimes lead to extended median ages, but almost never extends MLSP**. (Perez-Campo et al, 1998) (Sanz, Pamplona, Barja, 2006) (Pamplona, Barja, 2007)

139- **The lack of a consistent pattern in these measures of oxidative damage and lifespan challenge the validity of this free radical theory**.

140- **The plethora of contradictory results together with the lack of a general consensus among multiple species across the animal kingdom as well as among genetically manipulated mice in which oxidative stress is altered strongly suggest that species MLSP is unrelated to any of the oxidative stress parameters currently being measured**. (Rodriguez et al, 2011)

141- **Similarly, high levels of oxidative damage to lipids, proteins and DNA in the naturally long-lived naked mole-rat coupled with low levels of Gpx that are not compensated for by other enzymatic antioxidants, do not negatively impact on their exceptional longevity.** (Rodriguez et al, 2011) **This may limit the role of oxidative stress in leading to diseases including cancer, myopathy, vascular disease and neurodegeneration known to result from unchecked ROS (EMODs).**

142- **Investigators explored how different species, including the longest lived rodent, the naked mole-rat, have defied the most predominant free radical theory of aging.** (Lewis et al, 2013)

143- **Lewis et al have previously reported that catalase activity did not correlate with maximum lifespan in bats and rodents with the highest levels evident in both short-lived rats (MLSP 4 years) and long-lived vampire bats (MLSP 34 years).** (Buffenstein, Edrey, Yang, Mele, 2008)

144- **Concurring with these findings of no correlation between catalase levels and longevity is a recent study using five species of birds with a seven-fold range in longevity and no indications that catalase correlates either positively or negatively with longevity.** (Montgomery et al, 2012)

145- **Mice heterozygous for Gpx4 are more sensitive to oxidative stress, but surprisingly defy predictions based upon the oxidative stress theory of aging and show an increase in median lifespan and delay in cancer incidence.** (Lewis et al, 2013)

146- **Antioxidant status concur with studies in multiple tissues in species representative of the major phylogenetic groups (yeasts, worms, insects, amphibians, birds, reptiles, and mammals); little to no correlation occurs between antioxidant status (i.e., catalase, Sod, and Gpx) and lifespan.** (Lewis et al, 2013)

147- **Studies involving genetic manipulation of antioxidant expression of antioxidants Sod1, Sod2, and catalase reveal no lifespan extension. Conversely, when these genes are knocked-out of mice, lifespan is unaffected, although these animals often show an increase in oxidative damage in multiple tissues.** (Perez et al, 2009)

148- **These data, together with similar observations in birds and other mammals, support the counterintuitive notion of** pro-oxidative cellular environments being associated with long lifespan. (Lewis et al, 2013)

149- **long-lived vampire bats and many longer lived birds have higher levels of oxidative damage to DNA than do shorter lived mammals measured under identical conditions**. (Buffenstein, Edrey, Yang, Mele, 2008)

150- ***At best, naked mole-rats provide only equivocal support for the oxidative stress theory of aging***. (Lewis et al, 2010)

RMH Note: the findings in the naked mole rat repeatedly undermine the teachings and foundations of the free radical theory, the mitochondrial free radical theory of aging and the mitochondrial theory of aging. (Howes, 2015, cancer)

Oxidative damage or oxidative bliss

The simplest free radical is an atom of the element hydrogen, with one proton and a single electron. Free radicals may also be nitrogen- or carbon-centered but O_2-centered radicals are the most important ones in aerobic organisms.

Reactive oxygen species (EMODs), produced under normal aerobic metabolism, are essential for cell signaling, for bacterial defense and a host of other critical metabolic pathways.

In respiring cells, there appears to be a so-called "leakage of electrons" from the mitochondrial electron transport chain, to eventually yield a variety of such free radicals and active oxygen derivatives that are collectively and inaccurately called reactive oxygen species, ROS.

RMH Note: A more accurate term is electronically modified oxygen derivatives, EMODs.

Under normal conditions about 1% - 5% of reactive oxygen species daily escapes the control of the endogenous anti-oxidant defenses and performs its protective roles or homeostatic functions in surrounding tissues.

Please keep the following dogma in mind: it is claimed that, "If the body or cell capacity to neutralize reactive oxygen species is altered, then they will produce acute damage to vital proteins, lipids and DNA. In humans, unbalance between reactive oxygen species production and endogenous antioxidants has been involved in the generation or worsening of more than a hundred pathologic conditions." (Gutteridge, 1993)

Measuring the free radical activity *in vivo* (i.e., increased reactive oxygen (EMOD) production) is confronted with practical and analytical problems: we are left with the surrogate determinations of the end products of oxidation.

In fact, the oxidative damage is commonly determined by the quantity of nucleic acid that is damaged with the Comet assay, the amount of end products of lipid peroxidation or of protein oxidation. (Cesari et al, 2005) (Hartmann et al, 2003) (Sakamoto et al 2002)

RMH Note: There has been little concordance amongst the various 30+ test to measure in vivo oxidative damage and the results have been confusing and conflicted.

There is a substantial lack of data regarding the effects of acute or chronic exercise in aging animals or humans. Inconsistent results (partly also due to methodological limitations in the reactive oxygen species measurements) do not allow a clear interpretation of studies regarding exercise-related DNA and protein oxidation, and lipid peroxidation.

RMH Note: Actually, there is a lot data on the effects of exercise in humans but it presents a so-called "paradox" because the high levels of EMODs generated by exercise decrease the risks of most common diseases and extend the lifespan.

This, alone, should negate the free radical theory.

Current literature seems to show an increased resistance to oxidative damage with chronic exercise and increased lipid, DNA or protein oxidation after an acute bout of maximal exercise. (Polidori et al, 2000)

RMH Note: Counter to the advise of the FRT, regular physical activity and exercise are recommended for the maintenance of an optimal health status and the prevention or management of chronic diseases. (DHHS, 1995)

Regular physical activity has shown to reverse age-related body composition modifications in older subjects (ie, by increasing lean mass and reducing adipose tissue) (Fiatarone Singh

1998) (Fiatarone et al, 1994) (Polidori et al 2000), **and to confer significant protection against several age-related diseases (eg, non-insulin-dependent diabetes (Hughes et al, 1995)** (Hughes et al, 1995); **cancer** (Ji et al, 1991); **hypertension** (Dengel et al, 1998); **and osteoporosis.** (Evans, 1999)

Yet, animal as well as human models have demonstrated that acute bouts of eccentric exercise produce higher oxidative damage to muscles in aged mice and men compared to young animals or human subjects. (Zerba et al, 1990) (Quindry et al, 2003) (Tozzi-Ciancarelli, Penco and Di Massimo, 2002) (Watson et al, 2005)

In fact, and even more impressively against the FRT, **even if exercise is associated with an abnormal production of free radicals, physically active older persons benefit from exercise-induced adaptations in the cellular antioxidant defense systems.** (Fulle et al 2004)

RMH Note: Investigators can not bring themselves to admit or suggest that EMODs can be beneficial to overall health. They struggle to misinterpret the data.

Physical exercise may lead to an increase in antioxidant defenses of the organism in younger as well as in older subjects. (Lawler and Powers 1998) (Leeuwenburgh and Heinecke 2001)

This is probably due to the higher rate of oxidative stress occurring in older persons, partly explained by increased number of concurrent clinical conditions and the sedentary lifestyle. (Ames, 1989) (Facchini et al, 2000) (Greco et al, 2000) (Olinski et al, 2003)

RMH Note: Data in centenarians do not agree with Ames and show that EMOD production is low in the elderly.

No significant difference in the antioxidant enzyme response between old and young animals has been suggested. (Fiebig et al, 1994) (Ji, 1996) (Lawler and Powers, 1998)

Moreover, endurance training has shown to increase antioxidant enzyme activities even in the senescent muscle. (Ji et al, 1991)

Antioxidants are substances, which inhibit or delay oxidation of a substrate while present in minute amounts. Endogenous antioxidant defenses are both non-enzymatic (e.g., uric acid, glutathione, bilirubin, thiols, albumin, and nutritional factors, including vitamins and phenols) and enzymatic (e.g., the superoxide dismutases, the glutathione peroxidases [GSHPx], and catalase).

In the normal subject the endogenous antioxidant defenses balance the reactive oxygen species production, but for the above-mentioned 1% daily leak. **The most important source of antioxidants is provided by nutrition, many belonging to the phenol family**.

RMH Note: Please remember that polyphenols are poorly absorbed and minimally bioavailable.

Nutritional antioxidants act through different mechanisms and in different compartments, but are mainly free radical scavengers: 1) they directly neutralize free radicals, 2) they reduce the peroxide concentrations and repair oxidized membranes, 3) they quench iron to decrease reactive oxygen species production, 4) via lipid metabolism, short-chain free fatty acids and cholesteryl esters neutralize reactive oxygen species. (Berger, 2005)

RMH Note: Technically, not much of the above is true because they are flip sides of the same redox coin. Most antioxidants can or will become prooxidants once they donate their electrons to oxygen. Please check out my other books on the subject.

- Antioxidant Overkill, CreateSpace and Free Radical Publishing, © **2011.** (Howes, 2011, Overkill)

The tissue levels of the various antioxidants remains limited to research protocols as tissue biopsies are required. Ascertaining these levels is fraught with errors.

Compared with α-tocopherol, γ-tocopherol is a slightly less potent antioxidant with regard to electron-donating propensity, but is superior in detoxifying electrophiles, such as reactive nitrogen oxide species. (Jiang et al, 2001)

The most known and studied carotenoid is the β-carotene, a potent antioxidant able to quench singlet oxygen rapidly. (Di Mascio et al, 1991)

ß-carotene, α-carotene, ß-cryptoxanthin, lycopene, and lutein/ zeaxanthin have all been found associated with inflammation. (Hu et al, 2004)

Melatonin is a mammalian hormone synthesized from serotonin, mainly in the pineal gland. Besides of its widely documented action regulating the circadian rhythm, **it has been reported that melatonin**

contributes to the reduction of oxidative damage in both the lipid and the aqueous environments of the cell. (Aydogan et al, 2006)

The powerful antioxidant capacity of melatonin is exerted by stimulating the expression and activity of glutathione peroxidase, superoxide dismutase, NO synthetase. (Nishida, 2005) (Pieri et al, 1995)

Interestingly, **melatonin concentrations are particularly high in mitochondria and the cell nucleus**, where major oxidation reactions occur.

RMH Note: Please read and remember the following: The balance between oxidant and reducing forces is subtle. Trace elements with antioxidant properties such as copper and selenium, may become strongly pro-oxidant both *in vivo* and *in vitro*, as a consequence of their physical properties. (Terada et al, 1999)

This is also the case with vitamins A, C, E, which may become pro-oxidant under defined conditions. (Berger, 2005)

Vitamin E can also become a pro-oxidant in isolated lipoprotein suspensions (e.g., parenteral nutrition solutions in clinical conditions. (Neuzil et al 1995)

The pro-oxidant effects of selenium have been investigated on cultured vascular cells exposed to parenteral nutrition containing various forms and quantities of selenium. (Terada et al 1999)

In a recent study, Nakamura and colleagues (Nakamura et al 2006) **suggested that Vitamin C may play an important role to prevent the prooxidant effect of Vitamin E in LDL oxidation.**

Antioxidant supplementation

At the beginning of the Nineties, Renaud and de Lorgeril created the so-called "French Paradox", describing how, despite the high intake of saturated fat, the French population presents a low incidence of coronary heart disease events. (Renaud and de Lorgeril, 1992)

Even if their study raised a huge controversy, it has been suggested that beneficial effects from red wine consumption might be related to its high content of antioxidants. (Heller et al, 1998)

Resveratrol, a phytoalexin found in several plants (in particular, red grapes), has shown to be able to up-regulate the nuclear Liver X receptor α and its target genes in macrophages, and to reduce the expression of lipoprotein lipase and scavenger receptor All. (Sevov et al, 2006)

Through these mechanisms, resveratrol seems to limit cholesterol accumulation in human macrophages.

A recent study conducted in cultured human coronary artery endothelial cells has also demonstrated a beneficial effect of polyphenols (i.e., catechin and quercetin) on the expression of the plasminogen activator inhibitor-1 gene, potentially providing a further biological explanation to the cardiovascular protective role of these molecules (Pasten et al 2007). However, **no definite conclusion can still be drawn given the complex mechanisms in which polyphenols (e.g., resveratrol) are involved and which may influence the net results of their supplementation.** (Iannelli et al, 2006)

In 1999, an American Heart Association Science Advisory recommended that the general population consume a balanced diet with emphasis on antioxidant-rich fruits, vegetables, and whole grains. (Krauss et al, 2000)

Given the absence of data from randomized, controlled clinical trials at the time, **no recommendations were made regarding the use of antioxidant supplementation**.

In a more recent American Heart Association Science Advisory, **current evidence about the beneficial effects of antioxidant vitamins (such as vitamin E, vitamin C, and ß-carotene) on cardiovascular risk has been revised and discussed.** (Kris-Etherton et al, 2004)

Consistently with previous recommendations from the American Heart Association, scientific data do not yet justify the use of antioxidant vitamin supplements for cardiovascular risk reduction. (Mosca et al, 2004) and the American College of Cardiology. (Gibbons et al, 2003)

Recently, Pham and Plakogiannis have reviewed evidence on the effects of vitamin E supplementation and cardiovascular and cancer prevention. Their meta-analysis showed that **contradicting results regarding the benefits of vitamin E in the prevention of cardiovascular disease and cancer from the considered studies. Authors assured the presence of adequate evidence from large, well-designed**

studies to discourage the use of vitamin E in the primary pre-vention of cardiovascular disease. (Pham and Plakogiannis 2005)

It is important to underline how positive findings are mostly from observational studies, so that the relationship between vitamin E supplementation (the most promising antioxidant in the prevention of atherosclerotic disease) and lower rates of cardiovascular disease may just reflect an overall healthy lifestyle and dietary intake of supplement users rather than a real protective effect.

Oxidative stress has been implicated in mechanisms leading to neuronal cell injury in various pathological states of the brain. (Calabrese et al, 2003)

Increasing evidence has recently indicated oxidative dam-age as a potential cause of Alzheimer's disease pathogenesis. (Onyango and Khan 2006)

In a recent review, Vina and colleagues demonstrate that the **cognitive function in Alzheimer's disease patients is inversely correlated with systemic oxidative stress.** They also confirm the idea that vi-tamin E may be considered as an effective treatment of Alzheimer's disease. (Vina et al, 2004)

However, the effect of vitamin E on Alzheimer's disease pa-tients shows considerable variations both in its antioxidant function and in its capacity to improve cognitive functions. Therefore, consistently with previous recommendations (Kris-Etherton, and for the Nutrition Committee of the American Heart Association Council on Nutrition Physical Activity and Metabolism 2004), Authors suggest that the determination of the oxidant-antioxidant status of the patient is particularly important to test the effect of antioxidants on given functions.

RMH Note: Here are the excuses as to why the antioxi-dant supplements have not been proven to prevent or cure Alzheimer's disease.

A major limitation present in most of the intervention studies ex-ploring the effects of antioxidants supplementation (eg, vitamin E) on Alzheimer's disease outcomes is that they have been conducted on subjects who already have been diagnosed with this clinical condition. Therefore, it is difficult to assess the full potential of the specific sub-stances in the prevention of Alzheimer's disease.

Moreover, antioxidants are often tested as single agents, while it is becoming clearer that combinations of antioxidants are more effective. As for evidence related to cardiovascular disease, a large part of studies on the topic (mostly from epidemiologic reports) has shown that individuals, who consume higher amounts of fruits and vegetables, as well as vitamin supplement users, have lower rates of Alzheimer's disease.

Some reports have suggested that combinations of vitamins with antioxidant properties (in particular, vitamin C and vitamin E) have shown the greatest benefits. (Frank and Gupta, 2005)

Cancer

Recently, the supplementation en vitamines et mineraux antioxydants (SU.VI.MAX) study, a randomised, double-blind, placebo-controlled primary prevention trial, tested the efficacy of supplementation with a combination of antioxidant vitamins and minerals, at nutritional doses, in reducing the incidence of cancer in a general population not selected for risk factors. (Hercberg et al, 2004)

After a 7.5-year follow-up, antioxidant supplementation was associated with a reduction in cancer incidence in men only.

Authors also warned that high dosage antioxidant supplementation 1) may be deleterious in subjects in whom an initial phase of carcinogenesis has already started, and 2) could be ineffective in well-nourished subjects with adequate antioxidant status. (Hercberg et al, 2006)

Consistent with these findings, a trial aimed at evaluating the lung cancer incidence showed that selenium supplementation was beneficial only among individuals with low baseline selenium concentrations. (Reid et al, 2002)

In the cancer prevention study II nutrition cohort, the authors examined the association between multivitamin supplementation and incidence of colorectal cancer. **Results were consistent with the hypothesis that past, but not recent, multivitamin use may be associated with a modest lower risk of colorectal cancer**. (Jacobs et al, 2003)

A recent review of randomized trials comparing antioxidant supplements to placebo/no intervention for the incidence

of gastrointestinal cancers has found no evidence that anti-oxidant supplements prevent gastrointestinal cancers. On the other hand, antioxidant supplements seem to increase overall mortality. (Bjelakovic et al, 2004)

Similarly to what obtained for the cardiovascular disease out-come, Pham and Plakogiannis found no sufficient evidence that vitamin E is able to reduce the risk of cancer, concluding that vitamin E supplementation for cancer prevention is not recommended. (Pham and Plakogiannis, 2005)

Physical performance and muscle strength

Whether higher antioxidant intake is beneficial in promot-ing better physical performance and muscular strength is still controversial. Findings of some studies have shown improvements. (Gao et al, 2004) (Hauer et al, 2003) (Takanami et al, 2000) (Upritchard et al 2003) (Wijnen et al, 2001)

However, **other studies do not support beneficial effects of increased antioxidant intakes on physical performance.** (Avery et al, 2003) (Balakrishnan and Anuradha, 1998) (Barnett and Conlee, 2003) (Clarkson, 1995) (Konig et al, 2001) (Oostenbrug et al, 1997) (Van der Beek, 1991)

Physical activity

Regarding antioxidants supplementation (eg, vitamin C, vi-tamin E or glutathione) and their potential protective role against exercise-related oxidative damage, results are again highly inconsistent and/or not adequate, especially in human models. (Tiidus and Houston, 1995)

Therefore, the paradox of physical activity (which is certainly beneficial at all ages, but simultaneously potentially harmful if not adequately performed due to the free radical excessive production) can not be clarified at the present time.

Several current guidelines recommend regular physical activity in the older persons (Department of Health and Human Services, Centers for Disease Control and Prevention, and National Center for Chronic Disease Prevention and Health Promotion 1996; Pate et al 1995)

Please refer to my book, **- Sports, Athletes, Exercise Facts and Antioxidant Myths,** CreateSpace and Free Radical Publishing, © **2011.** (Howes, 2011, Sports)

Longevity

Nutritional supplementation, especially with antioxidants, has been frequently indicated as a potential mean to improve health status and increase longevity. (Harman, 1962)

However, **only limited evidence about the protective effects of specific micronutrients is available. Moreover, it is still unclear whether the health benefits from diets at high consumption of fruit and vegetables can be replicated by antioxidant supplementations.** (van Poppel and van den Berg, 1997) (Potter, 1997)

The theoretical basis supporting a possible relationship between antioxidant supplementation and longevity are mainly from the evidence showing a relationship of the latter with the rate of mitochondrial oxygen radical generation and the degree of unsaturation of membrane fatty acids. (Barja 2002)

In fact, these two molecular traits are significantly lower in all the relatively long-lived homeothermic vertebrates, and may be main causes of the low rate of aging of long-lived animals.

In an animal model, Lipman and colleagues showed no effect on age-associated lesions patterns, lesion burden or longevity in ad libitum mice fed with a the diet supplemented with antioxidants (vitamin E and glutathione) and initiated during middle age. (Lipman et al, 1998)

Results from the SU.VI.MAX study, consistently with findings obtained on incidence of cancer, showed a possible protection for overall mortality in men enrolled in the intervention group. However, **no definite conclusion was provided by authors regarding this possible association.** (Hercberg et al, 2004)

A great interest has been attracted by the potential capacity of melatonin to extend life span. (Anisimov, 2003)

Melatonin is a potent free radical scavenger, especially towards highly toxic hydroxyl radicals. Moreover, melatonin additionally stimulates a number of antioxidative enzymes. **Unfortunately, current data do not still allow to conclude that melatonin may have a role in extending normal longevity. Moreover, as for many other antioxidants, melatonin can act as a prooxidant under certain conditions.** (Anisimov, 2003) (Clapp-Lilly et al, 2001) (Osseni et al, 2000)

Antioxidant supplementation issues

Moreover, several other potential explanations should be considered when analyzing the lack of agreement between the predicted positive benefits and the results of the clinical trials conducted to date.

An important part of the evidence supporting the beneficial effects of antioxidant supplementation is based on animal data. Results from these studies need to be considered cautiously.

The belief that if enough of an essential nutrient is good, then more is better is wide spread. Nevertheless, this may not be true. For example, zinc supplements using doses >50 mg/day have been associated with depressed immune response (Chandra and McBean, 1994), and chronic exposure to selenium compounds is associated with several adverse health effects. (Chandra and McBean, 1994) (Vinceti et al, 2001)

Even if some epidemiological studies shown that antioxidant supplementation may decrease the risk of several clinical conditions, such observations are usually not universal. (Butler et al 2002)

The only capability of reducing oxidative damage is through antioxidant supplementation and it is limited.

For example, **McCall and Frei stated that "except for supplemental vitamin E, and possibly vitamin C, being able to significantly lower lipid oxidative damage in both smokers and non-smokers, the current evidence is insufficient to conclude that antioxidant vitamin supplementation materially reduces oxidative damage in humans".** (McCall and Frei, 1999)

The further step of assessing whether the modification of a biological mechanism (eg, decrease of lipid oxidative damage levels) is able to provide a clinical benefit (eg, reduction of cardiovascular events) is still far to be ascertained.

In conclusion, <u>current evidence does not allow to recommend antioxidant supplementation as a useful mean to prevent age-related pathophysiological modifications and clinical conditions</u>. Several concerns are present not only about their efficacy, but also on their safety. (Fusco et al, 2007)

SECTION TWO

POMEGRANATE

[14th century. From Old French *pome grenate*, literally "seedy apple."]

Currently, there is a push to aggressively market pomegranate products, especially because it is claimed to be an "antioxidant superpower."

Pomegranate Juice for Prostate Cancer Prevention?

August 28, 2015   Gerald Chodak, MD

Dr Gerald Chodak, for Medscape, talked about the possible role of pomegranate juice or extract in men with rising prostate-specific antigen (PSA) levels after local therapy for prostate cancer.

A randomized study has finally been done and now we have some data on the PSA doubling time in men who took a placebo, a liquid extract of pomegranate juice, or pomegranate juice itself. (Pantuck et al, 2015) (Pantuck AJ, Pettaway CA, Dreicer R, et al, A randomized, double-blind placebo-controlled study of pomegranate extract on rising PSA levels in men following primary therapy for prostate cancer. Prostatic Dis.l 2015. July 14 [Epub ahead of print])

In approximately 180 men who were enrolled in this trial, the authors found that the PSA doubling time increased in the placebo and treatment groups, but **the differences between the three groups were not statistically significant**. They did find a slightly better effect of pomegranate juice compared with pomegranate extract. However, there were only 17 men in the extract subgroup, and it is unclear why they received it in the first place.

So, although it certainly tastes good and some preliminary studies have suggested a role for pomegranate juice on the progression of prostate cancer, **this study suggests that there isn't much of a benefit**.

PSA doubling time tells us nothing about survival. It is a much longer-term event, but it is unlikely that this study is going to be continued long enough to know whether there is a true impact on overall survival.

However, the investigators did find something interesting. They measured manganese superoxide dismutase and found that **the PSA doubling time in men who were positive for that marker (mg-SOD) actually was much greater than the overall effect in all men, with and without that marker**.

RMH Note: Please remember that SOD produces hydrogen peroxide.

So, further analysis and more time will be necessary to identify whether this dismutase plays a role in determining whether men may benefit from the ingredients that are present in pomegranate juice or extract.

There was certainly a lot of excitement early on about pomegranate juice and its potential role. However, **in May 2012, the Federal Trade Commission found that the makers of pomegranate juice were making unfounded claims about the potential role of pomegranate juice in prostate cancer**.

They were claiming things that were just not proven to be true.

Now, **with a randomized trial in place looking at an endpoint of PSA doubling time, we are not seeing a significant impact from pomegranate juice**.

Will longer follow-up make a difference? Perhaps, but for the moment, the impact of pomegranate juice extract on men with rising PSA levels after prostate cancer therapy is not significant, and **for now it is hard to make an argument that it should be used**.

POM Wonderful loses bid to block deceptive ad claims

POM boasts that its juice is **"crazy healthy"** and it is **"the antioxidant superpower"**.

Bloomberg News - January 31, 2015

WASHINGTON — **POM Wonderful's claims that its pomegranate products combat heart disease, prostate cancer and erectile dysfunction aren't adequately backed by research, a federal appeals panel ruled, upholding a Federal Trade Commission ban on deceptive advertising by the company**.

"We see no basis for setting aside the commission's conclusion that many of POM's ads made misleading or false claims," U.S. Circuit Judge Sri Srinivasan wrote for a three- judge panel in Washington. "The FTC proscribes - and the First Amendment does not protect - deceptive and misleading advertisements."

The ruling, made Friday, is a setback in POM's aggressive marketing of pomegranates, which includes a successful challenge in the Supreme Court to Coca-Cola, the world's largest beverage company, over its labeling of products containing the juice of the heavily seeded fruit. POM had sued Coca-Cola claiming a label on one of its drinks promoting pomegranate was misleading and the Supreme Court ruled in June the lawsuit could proceed.

"Consumers know that pomegranate juice is inherently healthy, and POM Wonderful has always communicated with consumers in a transparent, honest manner, delivering valuable information about the potential health benefits of our products," Rob Six, a spokesman for POM, said in an emailed statement on Friday's appeals court ruling.

POM's owners, Stewart and Lynda Resnick, introduced the garnet-red juice in the curvy little bottle in 2002, touching off a marketing craze of flavored fruit teas, martinis and salad dressings. The Resnicks are the biggest U.S. growers of pomegranates and pistachios.

The POM boom was fueled by advertising claims, challenged by the FTC, that described pomegranates as "the antioxidant superpower" offering protection against heart and prostate maladies as well as some of the enhancement attributes of Viagra.

The FTC in January 2013 upheld the findings of an administrative law judge that POM's advertising was deceptive and ordered the company to stop claiming that its products are effective in treating, curing or preventing any disease "unless the claim is supported by two randomized, well-controlled, human clinical trials."

Friday's ruling pared back the FTC's study requirement for POM to one clinical trial. Mandating more than one such study "exacts considerable costs" and could deny consumers accurate information about a product's disease-prevention attributes documentable in a single, large, well-designed clinical trial, according to Srinivasan's ruling.

"We are grateful that the court substantially reduced the requirement that the FTC tried to enforce on us," Six said in his statement.

POM reported spending at least $34 million researching the health benefits of pomegranates by the time the FTC filed its complaint against the Los Angeles-based company in 2010.

POM "routinely distorted the scientific record and omitted the negative results" of its studies, according to an FTC filing in the court case. **"POM had not substantiated any of its disease claims with positive results from even one well-controlled clinical trial,"** FTC lawyers said in the filing.

POM countered that at most its claims are only "potentially misleading" and the FTC was obliged to apply constitutional free-speech protections to advertising "based upon accurate and verifiable information that did not actually mislead any consumer," company lawyers wrote.

Peter Kaplan, a spokesman for the FTC, didn't respond to an e-mail seeking comment on the decision.

In the Supreme Court case, POM, in an 8-0 vote, was allowed to revive a six-year-old false-advertising lawsuit against Coca- Cola for its labeling of Pomegranate Blueberry Flavored Blend of Five Juices, a concoction that is 99.4 percent grape juice.

The label is deceptive because the larger lettering of 'pomegranate' belies the tiny amount of pomegranate juice in the product, POM contended.

Coca-Cola, based in Atlanta, argued that POM's suit was out of bounds because the name and label of its product meet Food and Drug Administration regulations.

The Supreme Court ruling gives companies more room to police competing products for misleading claims and allows them to pursue false advertising suits even when the FDA regulates a product.

© 2015 The Daily Herald Co., Everett, WA

Here is another report on the same litigation.

Court upholds deceptive ad claims against POM

1-30-15

WASHINGTON (AP) — **A federal appeals court said that many advertising claims for POM Wonderful juice were deceptive in asserting that it curbs the risk of heart disease, prostate cancer and erectile dysfunction and is clinically proven to work.**

In a 3-0 decision, the U.S. Court of Appeals for the District of Columbia Circuit upheld a conclusion reached earlier by the Federal Trade Commission that many of POM's ads made misleading or false claims.

The ads appeared in national publications, on Internet sites, bus stops, billboards, newsletters and on tags attached to the products.

POM Wonderful LLC produces a number of pomegranate-based products.

"We see no basis for setting aside the commission's conclusion that many of POM's ads made misleading or false claims about POM products," wrote appeals judge Sri Srinivasan, an appointee of President Barack Obama.

The Federal Trade Commission Act does not allow, "and the First Amendment does not protect — deceptive and misleading advertisements," Srinivsan wrote.

The other two judges in the case were chief appeals judge Merrick Garland and appeals judge Douglas Ginsburg. Garland was nominated by President Bill Clinton, Ginsburg by President Ronald Reagan.

The court upheld the commission's requirement that POM gain the support of at least one randomized, controlled, human clinical trial before claiming a causal relationship between consumption of POM products and the treatment or prevention of any disease.

Ruling against the FTC on one point, the appeals court said it found inadequate justification for the commission's blanket requirement of at least two such studies as a precondition to any disease-related claim.

The appeals court examined studies the company used — an early one that was favorable to POM and two later, larger ones that were not.

The court said that a POM newsletter omitted any mention of the unfavorable studies and trumpeted the findings of the favorable study.

"A consumer reading POM's promotional materials after 2006 would not have known of those studies or that they cast doubt" on the prior findings, the appeals court stated.

POM had won its own false advertising case against a competitor last June, when the Supreme Court ruled in its favor. The justices ruled 8-0 that POM could proceed with a lawsuit alleging that **the label on a "Pomegranate Blueberry" beverage offered by Coca-Cola Co.'s Minute Maid unit is misleading because 99 percent of the drink was apple and grape juice.** The Supreme Court found that the juice label may technically comply with Food and Drug Administration rules but still may be misleading to consumers.

At that time, I had written several letters to the editor concerning the false claims regarding pomegranate products.

Letter to the editor: The Pundit Speaks

Pomegranate Claims Violate The Law

Recently, I read an advertisement in *Discover* magazine for pills made from pomegranate juice, which called their "pompills or POMx" the "Antioxidant Superpill." It went on to say that they have spent $34 million in medical research, documented POMx's unique and superior antioxidant power and "revealed promising results for prostate and cardiovascular health." WOW!

However, in very small print at the bottom of the page, they state, **"These statements have not been evaluated by the FDA. This product is not intended to diagnose, treat, cure or prevent any disease."**

Yet, their logo replaces the "O" in POM with a symbol of the human heart and their article is written as though pomegranate juice or POM pills can prevent prostate cancer and protect against heart disease.

Neither of these insinuations are true.

In fact, the FDA says, "Pomegranates may be full of antioxidants, but there is no evidence that POM Wonderful's pomegranate products prevent heart disease, prostate cancer or erectile dysfunction."

In February of 2010, the FDA issued a warning about the health claims the POM company made online about its products, which stated that its 100% pomegranate juice was shown to reduce blood pressure and reduce the risk of prostate cancer in scientific studies, using language that is only permissible for FDA-approved drugs and therefore in violation of the Federal Food, Drug and Cosmetic Act.

In September of 2010, the Federal Trade Commission (FTC) filed a complaint against POM Wonderful for its printed health ads claiming its product produces a "30% decrease in arterial plaque and promotes healthy blood vessels."

The FTC says these overstated claims are both false and unsubstantiated.

According to the Chicago *Tribune*: "The labor-intensive and messy pomegranate was stuck on the sidelines of the American fruit market until 2002 when Beverly Hills billionaires **Stewart and Lynda Resnick** planted enough of the fruit to quadruple the market, simultaneously introducing POM Wonderful juice to consumers." In short, **they jumped on the "antioxidant band wagon."**

The Director of the FTC's Bureau of Consumer Protection said, "**Any consumer who sees POM Wonderful products as a silver bullet against disease has been misled**." As expected, the POM company disagrees with these charges.

If you want to know the truth about antioxidants, read my book, *Death In Small Doses? Antioxidant Vitamins A, C & E in the 21st Century: A Health Impact Statement.* Randolph M. Howes, M.D., Ph.D. (Howes, Book 1, 2010)

It is available at Amazon.com, Barnes and Nobles and Borders bookstores and online. Let the truth protect you and do not be a chump for clever marketing and false claims. Many will lie to you for profit but I will tell you the scientific truth and let you decide for yourself.

I always present both sides of the story.

Prof Randolph M. Howes MD, PhD

Food Supplement Linked to Lower PSA in Prostate Cancer

Kate Johnson - June 10, 2013

A commercially available **food supplement that contains pome-granate, broccoli, green tea, and turmeric significantly lowers prostate-specific antigen (PSA) levels**, compared with placebo, in patients with prostate cancer, **a double-blind placebo-controlled randomized trial** has shown.

The study results, presented here at the 2013 Annual Meeting of the American Society of Clinical Oncology (ASCO®), made headlines around the world and caused the **polyphenol-rich supplement, known as *Pomi-T*** (nature Medical Products), to sell out within hours.

This is a "promising new therapy," said Tomasz Beer, MD, professor of medicine and director of the prostate cancer research program at the Oregon Health and Science University in Portland, during a "highlights of the day" session.

"We have been staggered by the level of interest...from medical professionals and the public," Marcus Williams, owner and director of nature Medical Products, told *Medscape Medical News*. As soon as the results of this study were released, the company, based in Porthcawl, South Wales, United Kingdom, **received a rush of orders from customers** in Australia, Canada, the United Kingdom, and the United States.

"It's awesome," the study's lead investigator, Robert Thomas, MD, a consultant oncologist at Bedford Hospital and Addenbrooke's Hospital, in the United Kingdom, told *Medscape Medical News*.

"We didn't expect such a big response. People are seeing that this can change practice...because men and their doctors do look at their PSA as a deciding factor in whether to stop active management," he explained.

Significantly Different Than Placebo

The study involved **203 men** (average age, 74 years) with a PSA relapse after radiotherapy or surgery for localized prostate cancer. The men,

94

who were being managed with active surveillance, were **randomized** to receive the supplement 3 times a day for 6 months or placebo.

At 6-month follow-up, the median increase in PSA was 63.8% lower in the supplement groups than in the placebo group. In addition, PSA levels were stable or lower than baseline more often in the supplement group (46% vs 14%; P = .00001).

Fewer men in the supplement group than in the placebo group went on to receive brachytherapy, radiotherapy, surgery, or androgen-deprivation therapy.

At the end of the study, more men in the supplement group than in the placebo group continued on active surveillance (92.6% vs 74.0%). "This is an end point we feel is important: more men were choosing to stay on treatments with less toxicity," Dr. Thomas noted.

There were no differences between the supplement and placebo groups for baseline and serial measurements of cholesterol, blood pressure, serum glucose, C-reactive protein, or adverse events.

"Pomi-T was well tolerated," he said. "More men experienced nonsignificant bloating or diarrhea, but 15% of men reported beneficial effects, including better digestion and improvement of urinary symptoms."

Previous research has shown that the polyphenols and antioxidants in pomegranate, broccoli, green tea, and turmeric have individual anticancer properties, but "we believe there's a synergistic effect in the supplement," said Dr. Thomas.

Please refer to my book, - **Chocolate & Red Wine Antioxidants (Polyphenols, Flavonoids & Resveratrol): Facts vs. Falsehoods.** CreateSpace and Free Radical Publishing, © **2015.** (Howes, 2015, Chocolate)

In addition, the fact that each ingredient originates from a separate food category (fruit, vegetable, herb, and spice) might prevent potential adverse effects from the over consumption of one particular type of polyphenol, he noted.

In the lab, polyphenols have been shown to have antiproliferative, antiangiogenic, proadhesion, antimetastatic, and proapoptotic properties, and notably, they have no phytoestrogenic or

hormonal effects. "We specifically chose to steer away from anything that might have a hormonal effect."

Because of the supplement's effect is likely not hormonal, future trials will involve men with different stages of prostate cancer and those receiving androgen-deprivation therapy, he said. In addition, the researchers hope to look at the impact of the supplement on other slow-growing cancers and even on cancer prevention.

The study received no funding from the manufacturer of the supplement; however, **the company worked very closely with the research team to develop the product,** said Williams. "Unlike other nutritional supplement products, the manufacture of this supplement was significantly more time-consuming because Dr. Thomas and colleagues, for whom this was initially made, insisted on a great deal of quality assurance, over and above that normally required by the US Food and Drug Administration or European Commission, particularly in terms of purity and authenticity."

He said the study signals "**a new era for the nutritional supplement industry,** which has previously relied on advertising and marketing rather than evidence of benefit. Clearly, it's the latter that the public wants."

Dr. Beer noted that the product's significant effect on adherence to active surveillance is "potentially clinically meaningful... If this can be confirmed, this is really interesting," he said, although he added that "these patients were more severe than the sort of patients that we would follow [with active surveillance] here in the United States."

Prostate Cancer UK reacted more cautiously to the news, releasing a statement saying that "there is not yet enough evidence that Pomi-T food supplements have a significant impact."

Kate Holmes, MD, head of research at Prostate Cancer UK, said in a statement that "there is increasing evidence showing that men who have a healthy lifestyle, including a balanced diet and regular exercise, have better prostate cancer outcomes than those who do not. At this stage, however, **we simply do not have enough evidence to suggest that any particular foods or supplements have a significant impact and these should certainly not be substituted for conventional treatments."**

"We **would not encourage** any man with prostate cancer to start taking Pomi-T food supplements on the basis of this research. Anyone with any concerns about prostate cancer should discuss them with their doctor or call Prostate Cancer UK's helpline," she added.

2013 Annual Meeting of the American Society of Clinical Oncology. Abstract 5008. Presented June 3, 2013.

The following was adapted from the thesis of Valeriya Karasovskaya. (Karasovskaya, 2012)

Antioxidant Properties of Berries

Antioxidant Properties of Berries: Review of Human Studies and their Relevance in the Context of the European Food Safety Authority

Valeriya Krasovskaya
2012228, June 2012
Hogeschool van Amsterdam
Bacheloropleiding Voeding en Diëtetiek

Student number: 500630231
Number thesis: 2012228
Thesis supervisor: Willem Gerritsen

My summary of the Krasovskaya thesis: **More than 10,000 phytochemicals have been identified to date. Several thousand polyphenols have been identified. There have been identified approximately 8,000 individual flavonoids.**

Research teams worldwide have no consensus as how to assess metabolism of (berry) flavonoids and their impact on health. The research team concluded that "The potential systemic biological effects of pomegranate juice ingestion should be attributed to the colonic microflora metabolites rather than to the polyphenols present in the juice." For now, the consumers should be aware that sound claims of marketers on

Prof Randolph M. Howes MD, PhD

antioxidative properties of berries are not (sufficiently) sub-stantiated from the scientific perspective.

Abstract

Berries have been traditionally consumed worldwide to prevent and treat diverse ailments. In the last decennium some of the berry products, traditionally used in certain parts of the world, have appeared on market shelves of the other parts under the label "superfoods". The efficient marketing policies, making use of selected scientific research, have resulted in rapidly increasing sales numbers. A great number of health claims is ascribed to berries and their constituents. The marketers largely stress antioxidant properties of berries. There is an outstanding number of research available on antioxidant activity of different berries. However, most of the research is represented by in vitro experiments, followed by animal studies. Human research is still scarce and often operate with the markers which are not considered reliable enough to substantiate health claims.

The European Food Safety Authority (EFSA) is the body responsible for authorization of health claims within the European Union. **The authorization of 222 out of 2758 health claims and their adoption by the European Commission on May 16 2012 has raised sound discussions within food industry**. Discussed are both the EFSA methodology and the consequences of the regulation for food producers. **None of the submitted berry claims have been authorized.** This paper provides an overview of the research available on five popular berries: açaí, blueberry, cherry, goji and pomegranate and links it to the EFSA evaluation criteria.

So far, for none of the studied berries there is a satisfactory (from the EFSA perspective) body of research available for substantiation of health claims related to antioxidant activities. Research on pomegranate and its products (juice, polyphenolic extracts) is the most pertinent, compared to the other four berries, but still more human long-term well-designed studies should take place before any antioxidant-related claim can get the green light in the European Union.

A great amount of in-vitro research and considerably smaller amount of human trials are obtainable through academic databases. Nevertheless, both consumers and trained nutritionists lack the accessible overview of the data available on the health benefits of the berries/their constituents. The European Food Safety Authority (EFSA) is the body responsible for authorization of all health claims made on foods within the European Union. Recent authorization of 222 out of 2758 (8%) health claims by EFSA and their adoption by the European Commission on May 16 2012 has raised sound discussions within food industry. Discussed are both the methodology hunted by the EFSA and the consequences of the regulation for food producers. Approximately forty of those 2758 claims are related to different berries, half of which are related particularly to antioxidative effects. **None of them have been authorized by EFSA**.

Since the beginning of the 21st century some of the berry products, traditionally used in certain parts of the world, migrated to other parts under the brand **"superfoods"**. Examples include goji berries, pomegranate juice, freeze-dried açaí berry. The efficient marketing strategies led to that they have reached broad audiences thanks to the appraisal in media and advertisements for their outstanding qualities. These products are sold as health food articles, and the marketers are willingly making use of the selected research, mostly in vitro (in laboratory conditions) experiments, that stress the antioxidative, anti-inflammatory and other beneficial effects of the berries.

The available experimental data have led to a vast number of health claims ascribed to berries by the marketers, presenting them as "cure all" products.

Definitions and Essential Concepts

The human body uses oxygen for routine metabolic reactions. Free radicals are usually created in the body during normal metabolic processes, and they can be introduced from the outside, such as by exposure to radiation (Sun rays, X-Ray), toxins, pollution, smoke, alcohol and unsaturated fats consumption and other factors.

A free radical is readily formed when a covalent bond between entities is broken: basically, it is, by definition, an atom or a group of atoms with at least one unpaired electron in the outermost shell. An electron without a pair can be unstable and highly reactive, but some are not.

A free radical involving oxygen can be referred to as reactive oxygen species (ROS) or more accurately, as **an electronically modified oxygen derivative, EMOD**.

A free radical accepts an electron from a neighboring molecule, and thus a new free radical is formed in its place. The newly formed radical again accepts an electron from another molecule, and a chain reaction can occur, which, if not intercepted by the antioxidative network, may lead to oxidative damage.

ROS have the potential to damage vital biological systems and are incriminated to contribute to the aging process and to over a hundred of disease conditions.

An oxidant is a compound that oxidizes other compounds.

Oxidation is a chemical reaction involving transportation of electrons from a substance to an oxidizing agent. The peroxyl radical (ROO') is a product of lipid peroxidation.

A hydroxyl radical removes a hydrogen atom from one of the carbon atoms in the fatty acid chain forming a molecule of water and leaving the carbon atom with an unpaired electron; thus, now a radical. One of the most probable things to happen next is it reacts with a molecule of oxygen forming a peroxyl radical. This may then steal a hydrogen atom from a nearby side chain making it now a radical also.

Oxidative stress is a condition when the production of oxidants and free radicals exceeds the ability of the body to cope with them in order to prevent damage. Halliwell & Gutteridge **defined an antioxidant as 'any substance that, when present at low concentrations compared with that of an oxidizable substrate, significantly delays or inhibits oxidation of that substrate'.**

Antioxidant is a generic name for all elements of so-called antioxidant defense system. These elements elsewhere can also be called free radical scavengers, chain terminators, or reductants. The antioxidant defense system is (allegedly) responsible for cellular protection against oxidative stress.

The major biological process leading to oxygen-derived O_2 generation is electron transport associated with the mitochondrial membranes. The attack of free radicals can damage the polyunsaturated fatty acids in lipoproteins and in cell membranes, thus disrupting the transportation of substances into and out of cells.

Free radicals can also damage DNA, RNA and proteins, contributing to cell distraction and disease development. By donating one of their own electrons, antioxidants may neutralize free radicals and end the chain reaction.

Under normal conditions the antioxidant defense system within the human body easily copes with the free radicals produced. The body produces several antioxidant enzymes, including superoxide dismutase, catalase, and glutathione peroxidase, that neutralize free radicals. The proper action of these enzymes depends on the minerals selenium, copper, manganese and zinc.

In addition the body uses vitamins that can act as antioxidants in their own right: vitamin C, vitamin E and vitamin B2. All these elements are part of a so-called primary antioxidant defense system. Secondary defense mechanisms involve lipolytic enzymes, phospholipases, proteolyticenzymes, proteases, peptidases, DNA repair enzymes, endonuclease, exonuclease, and ligase.

Polyphenols exhibit evident antioxidant properties as well.

Antioxidant scavenging enzymes

Superoxide dismutase (SOD), Catalase (CT), Glutathione peroxidise (GSH-PX)

Superoxide dismutase (SOD)

Dismutation of the superoxide anion to H_2O_2 by SOD occurs. SODs are categorized into three groups depending on the metal ion content: Cu/ZnSOD, Mn SOD, and Fe SOD. Although some of the SOD activity appears to be extracellular, most of the activities are localized intracellularly, divided between the mitochondrial (Mn SOD) and cytostolic compartments (Cu/Zn SOD).

Catalase (CT) is another major antioxidant defense component whose primarily function is to catalyse the decomposition of H_2O_2. CT performs this activity together with another enzyme, **Glutathione peroxidise (GSH-PX)**. Both enzymes detoxify oxygen reactive radicals by catalysing the formation of H_2O, derived from oxidant superoxide. Most species exhibit GSH-PX intracellularly located in the cytosol and mitochondrial matrix. Next to canalization of the reduction of H_2O, GSH-PX also catalyses the reduction of organic hydroperoxides.

Gallic acid (3,4,5-Trihydroxybenzoic acid) is a type of phenolic acid found in many plants. It is used as a standard for determining the phenolic content of plant constituents by the FolinCiocalteau assay; results are reported in gallic acid equivalents (GAE).

Phytochemicals are bioactive non-nutrient plant compounds. **More than 10,000 phytochemicals have been identified to date**, but a large percentage still remains unknown. Phytochemicals are responsible for food's color, flavor, aroma, taste and other characteristics. In human body phytochemicals can mimic hormones, act as antioxidants and probably suppress development of diseases.

Polyphenols (previously called collectively Vitamin P) are plant secondary metabolites. They are physiologically essential for processes as plants' growth, pigmentation, lignification, pollination, allelopathy to name a few. **Several thousand polyphenols have been identified to date**, and several hundred of them have been found in edible plants. The antioxidant characteristics of the polyphenols are due to the hydrogen of thephenoxyl groups that is prone to be donated to a radical, and by the ensuing structure that is chemically stabilized by resonance.

Flavonoids are a chemically defined class of polyphenols and several subclasses of flavonoids are characterized by a substitution pattern in the B- and C-rings. **There have been identified approximately 8,000 individual flavonoids**. Most of the flavonoids are present in plants with sugars attached (glycosides), although occasionally they are found as aglycones. Most of the research is concentrated on flavonoids with a common C6-C3-C6 structure consisting of 2 aromatic rings linked through an oxygenated heterocycle. The main subclasses include flavan-3-ols (catechin, epicatechin), flavanones (hesperetin), flavones (luteolin, apigenin), isoflavones (genistein), flavonols (quercetin, kaempferol, myricetin), and anthocyanidins.

European Food Safety Authority and Health Claims Authorization

European Food Safety Authority (EFSA) is the body responsible for the verifying the scientific substantiation of health claims submitted for authorization in the EU. One of the key objectives of the EFSA activity is to ensure that any claim made on a food label in the EU is clear and substantiated by scientific evidence.

Antioxidant activity assays

ORAC, TEAC, TRAP, FRAP, and FOX

With regard to claims on antioxidant status and antioxidant defense, as far as EFSA concerns, assays which measure the overall antioxidant capacity of plasma, are not a reliable indication of any health benefits for humans.

ORAC, TEAC, TRAP, FRAP, and FOX assays which assess changes in the antioxidant capacity of plasma are often used for research purposes; these assays are explicitly mentioned in the Guidance with the remark that **"It is not established that changes in the overall antioxidant capacity of plasma exert a beneficial physiological effect in humans as required by Regulation (EC) No 1924/2006."**

Further, those changes "do not predict a role of the food/constituent in the protection of body cells and molecules such as DNA, proteins and lipids from oxidative damage in vivo, and therefore are not suitable outcome measures for the scientific substantiation of the claimed effect."

Therefore, **claims supported by the data referring to any of the above mentioned assays are (going to be) assessed by the EFSA with unfavorable outcome**. The mechanism of action of these assays, as well as often used CAP-e and Folin–Ciocalteu assays is briefly outlined beneath.

ORAC refers to Oxygen Radical Absorbance Capacity. The concept of ORAC assay is based on the measurement of how effectively a compound eradicates the peroxyl radical as compared to the ability of Trolox (a vitamin E analogue) to act as antioxidant. The ORAC assay depends on the free radical damage to a fluorescent probe, such as fluorescein, to result in a downward change of fluorescent intensity. The assumption is that the degree of change is correlated to the degree of radical damage. The outcomes of the ORAC assay are expressed in micromoles of Trolox equivalents (TE) per gram. Indicator above one TE unit suggests that the compound has a stronger radicals scavenging activity. Food industry agents operate with so-called ORAC scores (elsewhere ORAC units or ORAC values), which are basically the outcomes of the measurements of antioxidant capacity of foods/food constituents expressed in mmol TE/g or converted into TE/ 100 g. The higher ORAC values, the higher the potential antioxidative effect of the compound. ORAC is used not only for measuring the antioxidant capacity of human plasma, but also for measurement of antioxidant capacity of food/ food constituents.

Recently the USDA's Nutrient Data Laboratory (NDL) removed the USDA ORAC Database for Selected Foods from its website "due to increasing evidence that the scores indicating antioxidant capacity have no direct link to the effects of specific bioactive compounds, including polyphenols, on human health."

TEAC refers to Trolox Equivalent Antioxidant Capacity. The TEAC assay is based on the measurement of an antioxidant ability to scavenge the relatively stable ABTS radical. The ABTS is intensely colored, and when it reacts with an antioxidant the decolorization takes place. The reference compound is, as in the case of ORAC, Trolox, which has a TEAC score of 1.

FRAP refers to the ferric reducing ability of plasma assay of Benzie and Strain. This assay also uses Trolox as the standard. The assay measures the ability of a sample to reduce $Fe3+$-TPTZ complex to the ferrous form at low pH. No oxidants are applied in the assay.

TRAP refers to total radical trapping antioxidant parameter. This assay is based on the ability of azo-initiators to decompose, producing a peroxyl radical flow at a constant temperature dependent rate. This flow has enough energy to abstract hydrogen from a substrate, thus initiating a (lipid) peroxidation chain. In TRAP the consumption of dissolved oxygen is the marker of the rate of lipid peroxidation and thus an indirect measure of plasma's ability to inhibit the oxidation. Trolox is used as the standard.

FOX refers to ferrous oxidation of xylenol orange (an organic reagent). This assay uses dye xylenol orange to form a blue-purple complex with a maximum absorption at 560 nm. The method is based on the principle of the rapid peroxide-mediated oxidation of $Fe2+$ to $Fe3+$ under acidic conditions. The latter, in the presence of xylenol orange, forms a $Fe3+$-xylenol orange complex which can be measured spectrophotometrically.

CAP-e refers to cell-based antioxidant protection in erythrocytes. During the measurement procedure, the red blood cells are first incubated with a test sample at a range of concentrations. The erythrocytes are then combined with fluorescein, which is subjected to oxidation, and the antioxidant activity of the tested substance is measured based on the degree of fluorescein inhibition, which is an indirect and nonspecific measure of reactive oxygen species production.

Interestingly enough, The CAP-e assay was developed by Alexander Schauss and Gitte Jensen, both of whom are devoted to the study of the properties of açaí berry.

The Total Phenolic Assay by Folin–Ciocalteu, also called the Gallic Acid Equivalence method, is a colorimetric assay of measurement of phenolic content in plants. It works by measuring the amount of the tested substance needed to inhibit the oxidation of the Folin-Ciocalteu reagent.

Summary: Nine steps to have your antioxidant claims authorized

These summarized guidelines, with the exception of Step seven, which is of particular interest for antioxidant activity related claims, are relevant for all health claims applicants under article 13.1. General health claims of the EU Regulation No 1924/2006.

Step one. The product should be sufficiently characterized. Information on the characteristics of the food/constituent for which a health claim is made should be provided. Where applicable, this information should contain aspects considered pertinent to the claim, such as the composition, physical and chemical characteristics, manufacturing process, stability, and bioavailability.

Step two. The wording of the health claim should be proposed. Where appropriate, this includes specification of conditions of use, such as the target population and population who should avoid using the product; the quantity of the food/constituent and pattern of consumption required to obtain the claimed effect, and whether this quantity could reasonably be consumed as part of a balanced diet; restrictions and directions of use.

Step three. The beneficial effect of the product consumption should be specified. Reference to general, non-specific benefits of the food/food constituent for overall good health or health-related well-being may only be made if accompanied by a specific health claim. Examples of general and non-specific claim are "premature aging" and "healthy aging".

Step four. The specified health effect should be beneficial for the human health. The claimed effect should be considered beneficial in the context of the specific claim and taking into account the population group for whom the claim is intended.

Step five. The claim should be accompanied by (all available) pertinent scientific data. The application must contain all relevant scientific data (published and unpublished) in favor as well as not in favor of the claim. The data provided forms the basis for substantiation of the health claim.

Step six. Human studies addressing the relationship between the consumption of the food/constituent and the claimed effect should be provided. Because of the scientific uncertainties in extrapolating non-human data to humans, data from studies in animals or in vitro experiments may be included only as supporting evidence. Human studies are central for the substantiation of health claims. Randomized controlled studies are prioritized.

Step seven. The provided human studies should operate with reliable biomarkers. Studies measuring (changes in) antioxidant capacity of plasma will not be regarded as pertinent. EFSA suggests the following biomarkers for measurements of oxidative damage to proteins, lipids and DNA: oxidative damage to proteins: direct measurements in vivo (e.g. measurement of oxidative changes of amino acids in proteins) by means of HPLC-MS and other methods, as long as identification and separation of such molecules in plasma from other substances is successfully achieved (e.g. from protein tyrosine nitration products); oxidative damage to lipids: measurements of changes in F2-isoprostanes in 24-h urine samples, using gas-chromatography techniques, of which mass spectrometry is preferred. Other acceptable markers are PCOOH; oxidative damage to DNA: direct measurements of oxidative damage to DNA in vivo using modifications of the comet assay, which allow the detection of oxidized DNA bases (e.g. use of endonuclease III to detect oxidized pyrimidines).

Step eight. Design and quality of the provided studies should allow conclusions to be drawn for the scientific substantiation of the claim. This presupposes that the provided data should be consistent in establishing a cause and effect relationship between the consumption of the food/constituent and the claimed effect. Further, the specific study group(s) in which the evidence was obtained should be representative of the target population for which the claim is intended.

Step nine. The quantity of the product and pattern of consumption required to obtain the claimed effect should reasonably be achieved as part of a balanced diet. This boils down to that the consumer should be able to introduce the proposed food/food constituent in their daily diet with ease. For instance, the claim "Walnuts contribute to the improvement of the elasticity of blood vessels" may be used only for a product which provides a daily intake of 30 g of walnuts. In order to bear the claim, information shall be given to the consumer that the beneficial effect is obtained with a daily intake of 30 g of walnuts.

Authorized antioxidant claims

ESFA has authorized claims on copper, manganese, riboflavin (Vitamin B2), selenium, vitamin C, vitamin E, and zinc with the wording contributes to the protection of cells from oxidative stress *. All of these claims were authorized, because the EFSA concluded that the role of the reference vitamins and minerals as (indirect) components of the antioxidant defence system had been well established. The EFSA, therefore, was engaged in a profound examination of available research confirming the antioxidant activity of these micronutrients. The only authorized of all the proposed claims on antioxidant activity of food/food constituents so far is the claim on polyphenols in olive oil, with the wording Contribute to the protection of blood lipids from oxidative stress.

EFSA issued a number of opinions where it summarized the outcomes of the scientific assessment of the proposed antitoxin activity related claims in batches. Claim on the antioxidant activity of pomegranate gained a separate opinion. *The claim may be used only for food which is at least a source of the constituent as referred to in the claim SOURCE OF [NAME OF VITAMIN/S] AND/OR [NAME OF MINERAL/S] as listed in the Annex to Regulation (EC) No 1924/2006.

The case of pomegranate

The pomegranate (Latin name Punica granatum) is a fruit of a deciduous shrub belonging to Punicaceae family that grows up to 7 meters height. Inside the fruit, which on average is of an apple size, there are arils with 300-400 of edible seeds. The taste of the seeds varies depending on the sort and ripeness from sour to sweet with a hint of astringent taste deriving from the tannins.

Pomegranate juice is consumed world-wide, and is gaining more and more popularity. **The highest antioxidant activity among pomegranate polyphenols was observed for punicalagin (the pomegranate ellagitannin**). Synonyms Anardana, Dadim, **Fruit of the Dead**, Granada, Grenade, Roma, Shi Liu Gen Pi.

Interesting facts

The fruit is present in Persian and Greek mythologies, as well as in Hinduism and Chinese folklore, symbolizing life, marriage, fertility, prosperity and regeneration; in Christianity its seeds are a symbol of individual worshipers gathered in one community of faith, while **In Islam, the Quran indicates that pomegranates grow in the gardens of paradise**.

Many scholars believe that the forbidden fruit that Eve seduced Adam with in the Garden of Eden was actually not an apple but a pomegranate.

The sales of pomegranate juice increased from $84,507 in 2001 to $66 million in 2005 in the United States.

Health claims most often attributed to pomegranate by suppliers

Weight reduction, cholesterol, control free radicals scavenging, skin nourishment, antiwrinkle effects, protection against Alzheimer's disease, protection against rheumatoid arthritis, and increased libido.

Antioxidant profile

Antioxidant properties of pomegranate are attributed to its polyphenolic complex including fatty acids, punicalagins (pomegranate ellagitannins), hydrolyzed tannins, ellagic acid and anthocyanins, delph-inidin, cyanidin, and pelargonidin being predominant in the last group.

Ellagitannins are the major polyphenols in the pomegranate fruit and juice (juice pressed whole fruit, arils, and seeds) and account for >90% of the antioxidant activity of the juice. **The research demonstrates low bioavailability of the pomegranate polyphenols. It is there-fore speculated that the health benefits of pomegranate are due to its metabolites (e.g., urolithins) rather than the com-pounds of the intact fruit.**

Alpha-punicalagin Commercial pomegranate juices have shown an antioxidant activity three times higher (18- 20 TEAC) than those of red wine and green tea (6-8 TEAC). **The activity was remarkably higher in juices extracted from whole pomegranates than in experimental juices obtained from the arils only**.

Pomegranate in PubMed The term 'pomegranate' yielded 28 re-sults, 'pomegranate' + 'antioxidant' − 11 results, 5 of which are defined as randomized controlled trials. All these trials are outlined in the ap-pendix Pomegranate Research Review, although some of them are of obviously less relevance than the others. Five more clinical human stud-ies found through Google Scholar are described there as well.

Research on pomegranate Studies of Michael Aviram

The protective qualities of pomegranate juice against atherogenesis have been extensively studied in the last decade by Aviram's and co-workers in Haifa, Israel. He took active part in the four following in vivo trials and in one ex-vivo trial, outlined below in the correspond-ing paragraph. In a three-year long study of Aviram et al. the effects of pomegranate juice (PJ) consumption by atherosclerotic patients with carotid artery stenosis (CAS) on the progression of carotid lesions and changes in oxidative stress and blood pressure was investigated. Ten patients were supplemented with PJ for 1 year and five of them contin-ued for two more years. After 1 year the PJ group participants' serum paraoxonase 1 (PON 1) activity was increased and LDL-oxidation was decreased significantly, and serum total antioxidant status (TAS) was increased by 130%.

An increase in the (carotid) lesion glutathione(GSH) content, by 2.5-fold, was observed after PJ consumption for 3 or 12 months. In support to these results, LDL oxidation by lesions was significantly decreased (43% after 3 months, 32% after 12 months) in comparison to the control group. The author states that increase of PON 1 activity and decrease in LDL-oxidation were correlated. **Serum paraoxonase 1 (PON 1) is a HDL-associated paraoxonase, which, according to the EFSA Guidelines*, is not a reliable in vivo marker of lipid peroxidation**.

EFSA states that "decrease in glutathione is considered a beneficial physiological effect only if such changes provide (additional) protection of cells and molecules from oxidative damage, which should be demonstrated in vivo in humans. "The amount of LDL-associated lipid peroxides in the study was measured by the method of El-Saadani et al., which is a spectrophotometric assay for lipid peroxides in serum lipoproteins **and is not mentioned in the Guidelines as a reliable assay for measurement of lipid peroxidation**. Further, it should be taken into account that the use of a small number of patients in this study could cause a statistical error.

Conclusions from the summarized above could be that **the biomarkers observed during the study and the method of measurement of (lipid) peroxidation cannot be considered a convincing evidence for antioxidant activity of PJ**.

But this study can probably be used as a supporting evidence next to research focusing on other biomarkers.

In a study of Rosenblat, Hayek and Aviram 20 subjects whereof 10 healthy (controls) and 10 non-insulin dependent diabetes mellitus (NIDDM) patients participated. Both groups consumed 50 ml PJ per day for 3 months. In the patients versus controls serum levels of lipid peroxides and thiobarbituric acid reactive substances (TBARS) were both increased, whereas serum SH groups content and paraoxonase 1 (PON1) activity, were both decreased (measured before the intervention, which indicated oxidative stress in diabetic patients). In the patients versus controls (HMDM), increased level of cellular peroxides and decreased glutathione content was observed (before the intervention).

After PJ consumption the lipid peroxides and TBARS levels were decreased by 56% and 28%, respectively, as compared to the levels observed in the patients' serum prior to consumption, whereas serum total sulfhydryl groups content and PON1 activity, significantly increased by 12% and 24%, respectively. PJ consumption also significantly reduced cellular peroxides (by 71%), and 51 increased glutathione levels (by 141%) in the patients' HMDM. The patients' versus control HMDM took up oxidized LDL (Ox-LDL) at enhanced rate, and PJ consumption significantly decreased the extent of Ox-LDL cellular uptake in vitro. **It was thus concluded that PJ consumption by diabetic patients resulted in anti-oxidative effects on serum and macrophages**.

In a recent study (2011) of Aviram and Dornfeld the effect of pomegranate juice consumption (50 ml daily, 1.5mmol of total polyphenols) for 2 weeks by hypertensive patients (n=10) on their blood pressure and on serum angiotensin converting enzyme (ACE) activity was tested. A 36% decrement in serum ACE activity and a 5% reduction in systolic blood pressure were noted. **The results of the study cannot receive direct interpretation in the antioxidant activity context**.

In a recent (2011) pilot study of Balbir-Gurman et al. 6 subjects with rheumatoid arthritis consumed POMx preparation (10 ml daily) for 12 weeks. The daily dose of preparation (10 ml) contained 1300 mg GAE and consisted of 95% polymolecular mixture ellagitannins, mainly punicalagin, and 5% ellagic acid. The intervention significantly reduced the composite Disease Activity Index (DAS28) by 17%, and the tender joint count (by 62%). These results were associated with a significant reduction in serum oxidative status and a moderate but significant increase in serum high density lipoprotein-associated PON1 activity. The addition of POMx to serum from the participants reduced free radical induced lipid peroxidation by up to 25%.

Other human studies

A randomized controlled clinical trial of Hashemi et al. was conducted among 30 adolescents (12–15 y) with metabolic syndrome. The participants had to drink either pomegranate or grape juice daily during 30 days. The biomarkers of endothelial function (basal brachial artery dimension and flow-mediated dilation) and endothelial-dependent dilation were measured. After receiving nitroglycerin spray, these markers were evaluated by high resolution mode (ultrasonography) after 4 hours post-consumption and after 1 month. Flow-mediated dilation improved significantly within 4 hours of drinking juice in both groups. **There was also significant improvement after 1 month of regular consumption of the aforementioned juices in both groups**, but basal brachial dimension only improved significantly after 1 month of regular consumption of grape juice.

The authors suggested therefore that consumption of antioxidant-rich drinks may improve endothelial function in children with metabolic syndrome.

In the study of Summer et al. the effects of daily consumption of pomegranate juice for 3 months were studied in a **randomized, placebo-controlled, double-blind study**. 45 patients with ischemic coronary heart disease (CHD) were involved, and the affect on myocardial perfusion was investigated. After 3 months, the extent of stress-induced ischemia decreased in the pomegranate group but increased in the control group.

In the study of Abidov et al, the effects of **Radical Fruits TM (RF)** supplement were studied on plasma cholesterol and urinary 8-epi PGF2a and 11-dehydro-TXB2 concentrations in 52 hypercholesteremic men (n=44). The RF supplement was composed of the following concentrated ingredients: prune, pomegranate, apple, grape, raspberry, blueberry, white cherry and strawberry. The RF group took 900 mg of the supplement 3 times daily before meals during 4 weeks. **The results of the intervention indicate a significant inverse correlation between consumption of RF supplement and total plasma cholesterol concentration, as well as reduction of plasma LDL and increase in plasma HDL concentrations.**

A pilot study of Heber et al. involving 22 overweight subjects was designed for antioxidant activity assessment by administration of a pomegranate ellagitannin-enriched polyphenol extract (POMx). Two POMx capsules were provided per day, containing 1000 mg of extracts (610 mg of gallic acid equivalents (GAEs). Measurement of antioxidant activity in plasma were done before and after POMx supplementation. **There was evidence of antioxidant activity through a significant reduction in TBARS, a biomarker of oxidative stress, measuring products of lipid oxidation in the blood.**

In a 5-week **randomized, double-blind, placebo-controlled trial** of Cerda et al. the effect of pomegranate juice (PJ) supplementation on patients with stable chronic obstructive pulmonary disease (COPD) (n=30) was investigated. The daily dose of PJ was 400 ml and contained 2.66 g polyphenols and provided 4 mmol/l TEAC. None of the polyphenols present in PJ were detected in plasma or in urine of the subjects. **The most abundant PJ polyphenols, ellagitannins**, were metabolized by the colonic microflora of the patients to yield two major metabolites in both plasma and urine (dibenzopyranone derivatives) with no TEAC. **There was no difference with the control group for any of the evaluated parameters.**

The results suggest that PJ supplementation adds no benefit to the standard therapy in patients with stable COPD, and that "the high TEAC of PJ cannot be extrapolated in vivo probably due to the metabolism of its polyphenols by the colonic microflora."

Di Silvestro et al. researched effects of pomegranate rinsing in relevance with gingivitis risk (**randomized, single-blinded controlled intervention**; n=32). Among other findings, it was concluded that thrice daily pomegranate mouth rinsing during 4 weeks resulted in increase of activities of the antioxidant enzyme ceruloplasmin (which is believed to give protection to oral oxidant stress) and increased radical scavenging capacity (though this increase was significant only by nonparametric statistical analysis).

Supporting ex-vivo and animal studies

In a comparative 4 weeks study of Guo et al. on the effects of apple and pomegranate juice on antioxidant status of plasma, involving 26 elderly subjects, increased plasma antioxidant capacity and decreased plasma carbonyl content were demonstrated after daily consumption of pomegranate juice (250 ml).

In a study of Aviram et al. potent antioxidative effects of pomegranate juice against lipid peroxidation in whole plasma and in isolated lipoproteins (HDL and LDL) were assessed in humans and in E0 mice after pomegranate juice consumption. The human study consisted of two parts, first one involving 13 healthy subjects (consuming daily 50 mg PJ during 2 weeks) and the second involving 3 subjects (consuming daily 20-80 ml/d of PJ during 10 weeks). The human studies were conducted ex-vivo.

Human plasma obtained after 2 wk of PJ consumption showed 6 % decreased susceptibility to AAPH induced lipid peroxidation. Additionally, a 9% increase in plasma total antioxidant status was observed after 2 weeks of PJ consumption. Following supplementation with 20 ml PJ/d for 1 week (n=3) resulted in a 11% decrease in plasma lipid peroxide content. Supplementation with 50 ml PJ/d for 1 more week resulted in a further 21% decrease in plasma lipid peroxidation, while yet an additional increase in PJ supplementation to 80 ml PJ/d for an additional week did not inhibit plasma susceptibility to lipid peroxidation further.

The inhibitory effect of PJ consumption on plasma lipid per-oxidation was maintained for 2 weeks after PJ supplementation ended.

In E0 mice, LDL oxidation by peritoneal macrophages was reduced by up to 90% after PJ administration, and this effect was associated with reduced cellular lipid peroxidation and superoxide release. The uptake of oxidized LDL and native LDL by peritoneal macrophages obtained after pomegranate juice administration was reduced by 20%. Finally, **pomegranate juices supplementation reduced the size of the mice' athero-sclerotic lesions by 44% and also the number of foam cells.**

It is therefore speculated by the research team that **pomegranate juice "had potent antiatherogenic effects in healthy humans and in atherosclerotic mice that may be attributable to its antioxidative properties".**

Bioavailability of pomegranate polyphenols

Pomegranate ellagitannins (ETs) comprise on average 70% of the poly-phenols in commercial PJ (3), but are assumed to be non-absorbable due to the large size of the ET molecules.

The study of Mertens-Talcott et al. investigated the absorption and an-tioxidant effects of a standardized extract from pomegranate in healthy volunteers **(n=11)** after the acute consumption of 800 mg of extract. **(RMH Note: this is an extremely small study)**

Results showed that ellagic acid (EA) from the extract was bioavailable. The antioxidant capacity of plasma using ORAC Assay was measured and it was maximally increased after 0.5 h (31.8%). The second peak in antioxidant capacity was measured after 6 h (31.7%). No change in the reactive oxygen species generation was observed.

In a study of Seeram et al. one person consumed 180 ml of PJ contain-ing 25 mg ellagic acid (EA) and 318 mg hydrolyzable ellagitannins (ETs), and the bioavailability of EA and ETs was accessed. (20) ETs were not detected in plasma, while EA was.

Following study of Seeram et al., this time involving **18 subjects**, fur-ther investigated the bioavailability of ETs. After an acute single oral dose of PJ concentrate (180 ml containing 318 mg punicalagins and 12 mg of free EA), EA increased rapidly and was cleared from plasma samples of all volunteers by 5 hours.

These findings correspond with the outcomes of the research of Cerda et al. who studied the bioavailability of the pomegranate ellagitannines in vitro and in humans. The volunteers (n=6) consumed 1 liter of pomegranate juice (5.6 g of **polyphenols including ellagitannins, ellagic acid derivatives and anthocyanins**). Neither punicalagin nor ellagic acid present in the PJ were detected in both plasma and urine, but at least 3 microbial ellagitannin-derived metabolites were detected. The metabolites did not show significant antioxidant activity compared to punicalagin from PJ.

The research team concluded that "The potential systemic biological effects of pomegranate juice ingestion should be attributed to the colonic microflora metabolites rather than to the polyphenols present in the juice."

Pomegranate and EFSA

There have been 12 applications made on pomegranate related health claims. The overview of the entries can be found in appendix Overview non-authorized antioxidant activity related claims on berries/berry products. Four of these entries were related to antioxidative properties of pomegranate/pomegranate juice. The EFSA Panel on Dietetic Products, Nutrition and Allergies (NDA) was asked to provide a scientific opinion on the pomegranate related health claims. The NDA issued its opinion in 2010.

The active food constituents were defined as punicalagin/ellagic acid, and claimed effects were "antioxidative function", "antioxidant properties", and "antioxidants and immunity". The NDA assumed that the claimed effects related to the protection of lipids from oxidative damage caused by free radicals, which is a beneficial physiological effect.

In its opinion the NDA Panel summarized the provided human data for the proposed claims as follows: A single arm, uncontrolled intervention study in 13 healthy male volunteers which assessed the effects of pomegranate juice consumption (50 mL per day containing 1.5 mmol total polyphenols) for two weeks on changes in the ex vivo activity of serum paraoxonase (an HDL associated esterase), in plasma lipid peroxides (AAPH induced spectrophotometric method), and in the oxidation lag time of low-density lipoproteins (LDL) ex vivo was provided (Aviram et al., 2000).

A second single arm (Rosenblat et al., 2006), uncontrolled intervention study in 10 healthy subjects and 10 non-insulin dependent diabetes mellitus (NIDDM) patients under pharmacological treatment was provided with the consolidated list. All subjects consumed 50 ml per day of pomegranate juice containing 1979 mg/l of tannins (1561 mg/L of punicalagin and 417 mg/l of hydrolysable tannins), 384 mg/l of anthocyanins (delphinidin 3,5-diglucoside, cyanidin 3,5-diglucoside, delphinidin-3-glucoside, cyanidin 3-glucoside and pelargonidine 3-glucoside) and 121 mg/l of ellagic acid derivatives for three months. Serum concentrations of lipid peroxides, thiobarbituric acid reactive substances (TBARS), serum SH groups, serum paraoxonase 1 (PON1) activity, cellular peroxides and glutathione content in monocytes-derived macrophages (HMDM), and oxidized LDL uptake by HMDM were measured at the beginning and end of the intervention.

The NDA Panel considered that no conclusions could be drawn from these small and uncontrolled studies for the scientific substantiation of the claimed effect, and concluded that a cause and effect relationship was not established between the consumption of punicalagin/ellagic acid in pomegranate/ pomegranate juice and the protection of lipids from oxidative damage.

The NDA Panel did not take into consideration a 3 year-long study of Aviram et al., 2004, which investigated the effects of regular PJ supplementation on the thickness of carotid intima-media, blood pressure and LDL oxidation, and which yielded positive results. Small number of participants and the choice of markers (which, if used alone, cannot be used for substantiation of health effects) will not allow the study to be qualified as a reliable scientific substantiation by the EFSA. But this study can probably be used as supporting evidence next to research focusing on other biomarkers.

At the moment the research on pomegranate is actively going on (for instance in Rappaport Institute Haifa, Israel). It is not excluded that in the years to come enough evidence is piled to substantiate a claim related to antioxidative properties of pomegranate.

Concluding Remarks

Berries have been traditionally consumed everywhere in the world to prevent and cure diverse diseases. **Centuries-long observations make the establishment of the connection between ingestion of certain berries and (improvement of) certain conditions possible: pomegranate as part of the Mediterranean diet and lower incidence of cardiovascular diseases in the region; improvement of gout condition with abundant cherry consumption. These observations often become the point of departure for scientific research**.

In the last two decennia there is a an obvious exploding interest for health benefits of berries from scientific perspective. Berry polyphenols are generally considered to be nontoxic and beneficial for health, although **the precise mechanisms of their metabolism and action remains largely unclear**.

Absorption peculiarities and routs of biological activity probably depend on the individual structure of polyphenols, as well as on humans inter-individual variation in their metabolism. Most studies report low flavonoid excretions, being particularly poor for anthocyanins, which are considered to play the major role in antioxidative mechanisms of berries (for instance in blueberries they are supposedly responsible for >50% of antioxidant activity).

Therefore, it could be suggested that not all of the flavonoids' metabolites might have been identified yet, and that their bioavailability might be underestimated. **Most of the berries studies available to date are in vitro experiments**. Laboratory trials are on the lowest scale of the EFSA hierarchy of scientific data which can be used as substantiation for health claims on foods/foods constituents.

An outstanding amount (for some berry types, for instance blueberries) of animal studies is not of much relevance for EFSA either, as it also can play only a supportive role in substantiation of health claims. **That what needs to be supported – human data – is scarce**.

Moreover, in most cases the researchers operate with the markers which, to EFSA point of view, can only be supportive to primary markers of direct measurements (of oxidative damage), while those primary markers are missing in the research.

What needs to be noted is that **research teams worldwide have no consensus as how to assess metabolism of (berry) flavonoids and their impact on health**.

Further (human) research is needed in order to design a reliable model for assessment of utilization of berries active compounds by the humans and their alleged benefits.

Of the five berries examined in this paper, pomegranate shows to be the most promising in the sense, that the number of the human research available is the greatest for this fruit (although still not really impressive: 10 controlled clinical trials) and that some of the studies are long-term and/or operate with reliable markers (of oxidation).

It is not excluded that in the near future enough evidence is piled together to substantiate a claim related to **36 antioxidative properties of pomegranate**.

For now, the consumers should be aware that sound claims of marketers on antioxidative properties of berries are not (sufficiently) substantiated from the scientific perspective.

As berries are a safe, tasty and nutrient-dense, their consumption should be encouraged, and the years to come probably will shed more light on their benefits for human health.

PJ does not affect fasting glucose or insulin

Pomegranate juice does not affect fasting plasma glucose or the insulin resistance index.

Abstract

BACKGROUND:

Diabetes causes the increased concentration of circulatory cytokines as a result of inflammation. Considering that pomegranate juice (PJ) is known to have antioxidant and anti-inflammatory properties, the purpose of this study was to determine the effects of PJ consumption on markers of inflammation in patients with type 2 diabetes (T2D).

MATERIALS AND METHODS:

In a randomized, double-blind clinical trial study, 50 patients with T2D (40-65 years old) were randomly assigned to one of two groups. Participants in each group received either 250 mL/day PJ or a control beverage for 12 weeks. Biochemical markers including fasting plasma glucose (FPG), insulin and inflammatory markers were assayed on the baseline and follow-up blood samples.

RESULTS:

In all, 44 patients in two groups were included in the analysis: PJ (n = 22) and placebo (n = 22). After 12 weeks of intervention, in the PJ group, there were 32% and 30% significant decreases in plasma C-reactive protein (hs-CRP) and Interlukin-6, respectively ($P < 0.05$). The mean ± SD plasma interlukin-6 (7.1 ± 5.6 vs. 11.9 ± 14.4 mg/L) and hs-CRP (1791 ± 1657 and 1953 ± 1561 ng/mL) concentrations in the PJ group were significantly lower than the placebo group after intervention ($P < 0.05$).

CONCLUSION

PJ consumption by patients with T2D does not affect FPG or the insulin resistance index (HOMA-IR), whereas **it does reduce Interlukin-6 and hs-CRP concentrations in plasma.** Therefore, PJ consumption may have an anti-inflammatory effect in patients with T2D. (Sohrab et al, 2014)

PJ does not affect pulse wave velocity and plasma FRAP

Pomegranate juice does not affect pulse wave velocity and plasma FRAP.

Abstract

Pomegranate juice may improve cardiovascular risk because of its content of antioxidant polyphenols. We conducted a **randomized**

placebo-controlled parallel study to examine the effect of pomegranate juice on pulse wave velocity (PWV), blood pressure (BP) and plasma antioxidant status (ferric reducing power; FRAP) in 51 healthy adults (30-50 years). Participants consumed 330 ml/day of pomegranate juice or control drink for four weeks. Measurements were made at baseline and at four weeks.

There was no effect of the intervention on PWV and plasma FRAP. However,**there was a significant fall in systolic blood pressure (-3.14mmHg, P<0.001), diastolic blood pressure (-2.33mmHg P<0.001) and mean arterial pressure. Change in weight was similar in the two groups over the intervention period.**The fall in BP was not paralleled by changes in concentration of serum angiotensin converting enzyme.We conclude that **pomegranate juice supplementation has benefits for BP in the short term, but has no effect on PWV.**The mechanism for the effect is uncertain. (Lynn et al, 2012)

PJ does not decrease postprandial plasma TAG concentrations

Pomegranate juice does not decrease postprandial plasma TAG concentrations.

Abstract

We investigated whether a test drink enriched in pomegranate polyphenols, consumed with a high-fat meal, can reduce postprandial lipaemia and improve vascular function and blood pressure compared to placebo. Nineteen young, healthy men completed a randomized, controlled crossover trial.The active drink (containing a pomegranate extract) was consumed during a high-fat meal (ET-DUR) or 15 min before (ET-PRE), and the placebo drink (no pomegranate extract) was consumed during the high-fat meal (CONTROL). Postprandial lipaemia was assessed by venous plasma TAG 0-2 h, and capillary plasma TAG 0-4 h. Blood pressure and digital volume pulse, to measure reflection index (DVP-RI) and stiffness index (DVP-SI), were monitored at baseline, 2 and 4 h. There was no inhibition of postprandial lipaemia by the active drink compared to CONTROL. ET-PRE caused a greater increase in the venous plasma TAG at 2 h compared to CONTROL and ET-DUR (treatment effect P = 0.001). The incremental area under the curve 0-4 h for capillary plasma TAG was not significantly different between treatments. Systolic blood pressure (SBP) increased in the ET-PRE and ET-DUR groups to a lesser extent than the CONTROL group (treatment effect P = 0.041). There were no treatment effects for DVP-RI, DVP-SI or diastolic blood pressure. In conclusion, **the consumption of a single drink containing ET-rich pomegranate extract did not decrease postprandial plasma TAG concentrations, but suppressed the postprandial increase in SBP following the high-fat meal**. (Mathew et al, 2012)

PJ polyphenols lower lipid peroxidations

Pomegranate polyphenols lower lipid peroxidation in adults with type 2 diabetes but have no effects in healthy volunteers.

Abstract

Aims: To examine the antioxidant and anti-inflammatory effects of pomegranate polyphenols in obese patients with type 2 diabetes (T2DM) (n = 8) and in healthy nondiabetic controls (n = 9). Methods. Participants received 2 capsules of pomegranate polyphenols (POMx, 1 capsule = 753 mg polyphenols) daily for 4 weeks. Blood draws and anthropometrics were performed at baseline and at 4 weeks of the study. Results. Pomegranate polyphenols in healthy controls and in T2DM patients did not significantly affect body weight and blood pressure, glucose and lipids. Among clinical safety profiles, serum electrolytes, renal function tests, and hematological profiles were not significantly affected by POMx supplementation. However, aspartate aminotransferase (AST) showed a significant increase in healthy controls, while alanine aminotransferase (ALT) was significantly decreased in T2DM patients at 4 weeks (P < 0.05), though values remained within the normal ranges. Among the biomarkers of lipid oxidation and inflammation, oxidized LDL and serum C-reactive protein (CRP) did not differ at 4 weeks in either group, while pomegranate polyphenols significantly decreased malondialdehyde (MDA) and hydroxynonenal (HNE) only in the diabetic group versus baseline (P < 0.05).

CONCLUSION

POMx reduces lipid peroxidation in patients with T2DM, but with no effects in healthy controls, and specifically modulates

liver enzymes in diabetic and nondiabetic subjects. Larger clinical trials are merited. (Basu et al, 2013)

Efficacy and safety of PJ medicinal products for cancer

Abstract

Preclinical in vitro and in vivo studies demonstrate potent effects of pomegranate preparations in cancer cell lines and animal models with chemically induced cancers. We have carried out one systematic review of the effectiveness of pomegranate products in the treatment of cancer and another on their safety. The PubMed search provided 162 references for pomegranate and cancer and 122 references for pomegranate and safety/toxicity. We identified 4 clinical studies investigating 3 pomegranate products, of which one was inappropriate because of the low polyphenol content. **The evidence of clinical effectiveness was poor because the quality of the studies was poor.** Although there is no concern over safety with the doses used in the clinical studies, pomegranate preparations may be harmful by inducing synthetic drug metabolism through activation of liver enzymes.** We have analyzed various pomegranate products for their content of anthocyanins, punicalagin, and ellagic acid in order to compare them with the benchmark doses from published data. **If the amount of coactive constituents is not declared, patients risk not benefiting from the putative pomegranate effects.** Moreover, pomegranate end products are affected by many determinants. Their declaration should be incorporated into the regulatory guidance and controlled before pomegranate products enter the market. (Vlachojannis et al, 2015)

PJ and prostate cancer

Abstract

Two exploratory clinical studies investigating proprietary pomegranate products showed a trend of effectiveness in increasing prostate-specific antigen doubling time in patients with prostate cancer. A recent clinical study did not support these results. We therefore analyzed a lot of the marketed pomegranate blend for co-active pomegranate compounds. The high-performance liquid chromatography method was used to detect punicalagin, ellagic acid and anthocyanins. Total polyphenoles were determined by the Folin-Ciocalteu method using gallic acid as reference. **The results show that the co-active compounds in the daily dose of the pomegranate blend were far below those previously tested and that the photometric assessment is not reliable for the standardization of study medications.**

Not pomegranate but the low amount of co-active compounds in the proprietary pomegranate blend was responsible for its clinical ineffectiveness. (Chrubasik et al, 2014)

PJ and type 2 diabetes

Abstract

Over the last decade, various studies have linked pomegranate (Punica granatum Linn), a fruit native to the Middle East, with type 2 diabetes prevention and treatment. This review focuses on current laboratory and clinical research related to the effects of pomegranate fractions (peels, flowers, and seeds) and some of their active components on biochemical and metabolic variables associated with the pathologic markers of type 2 diabetes. This review systematically presents findings from cell culture and animal studies as well as clinical human research. **One key mechanism by which pomegranate fractions affect the type 2 diabetic condition is by reducing oxidative stress and lipid peroxidation.**

This reduction may occur by directly neutralizing the generated reactive oxygen species, increasing certain antioxidant enzyme activities, inducing metal chelation activity, reducing resistin formation, and inhibiting or activating certain transcriptional factors, such as nuclear factor κB and peroxisome proliferator-activated receptor γ.

Fasting blood glucose levels were decreased significantly by punicic acid, methanolic seed extract, and pomegranate peel extract.

Known compounds in pomegranate, such as punicalagin and ellagic, gallic, oleanolic, ursolic, and uallic acids, have been identified as having anti-diabetic actions.

Furthermore, **the juice sugar fraction was found to have unique antioxidant polyphenols (tannins and anthocyanins), which could be beneficial to control conditions in type 2 diabetes**. These findings provide evidence for the anti-diabetic activity of pomegranate fruit; however, before pomegranate or any of its extracts can be medically recommended for the management of type 2 diabetes, controlled, clinical studies, are needed. (Banihani et al, 2013)

Mixed pro- and anti-oxidative effects of PJ polyphenols in cultured cells

Abstract

In recent years, the number of scientific papers concerning pomegranate (Punica granatum L.) and its health properties has increased greatly, and there is great potential for the use of bioactive-rich pomegranate extracts as ingredients in functional foods and nutraceuticals. To translate this potential into effective strategies it is essential to further elucidate the mechanisms of the reported bioactivity.

In this study HepG2 cells were supplemented with a pomegranate fruit extract or with the corresponding amount of pure punicalagin, and then subjected to an exogenous oxidative stress. **Overall, upon the oxidative stress the gene expression and activity of the main <u>antioxidant enzymes appeared reduced</u> in supplemented cells, which were more prone to the detrimental effects than unsupplemented ones**.

No differences were detected between cells supplemented with the pomegranate juice or the pure punicalagin. Although further studies are needed due to the gaps existing between in vitro and in vivo studies, **our results suggest caution in the administration of high concentrations of nutraceutical molecules, particularly when they are administered in concentrated form**. (Danesi et al, 2014)

The following article was adapted from: Potent health effects of pomegranate.

Potent health effects of pomegranate

Abstract (Zarfeshany et al, 2014)

INTRODUCTION

Punica granatum L. (Pomegranate) is a long-lived and drought-tolerant plant. Arid and semiarid zones are popular for growing pomegranate trees. They are widely cultivated in Iran, India, and the Mediterranean countries such as Turkey, Egypt, Tunisia, Spain, and Morocco. (Ercisli et al, 2011)

However, **pomegranate is categorized as a berry** but it belongs to its own botanical family, *Punicaceae*. The only genus is *Punica*, with one predominant species called *P. granatum*. (Newman, 2011)

The trees can grow up to 30 feet in height. The leaves are opposite, narrow, oblong with 3-7 cm long and 2 cm broad. It has bright red, orange, or pink flowers, which are 3 cm in diameter with four to five petals. Edible fruit has a rounded hexagonal shape, with 5-12 cm in diameter and weighing 200 g. The thick skin surrounds around 600 arils, which encapsulates the seeds. (Newman, 2007)

CHEMICAL COMPOSITION

Seed

About 18% of dried and cleaned white seeds are oil. The oil is rich in punicic acid (65%), which is a triple conjugated 18-carbon fatty acid. **There are some phytoestrogen compounds in pomegranate seeds that have sex steroid hormones similar to those in**

humankind. The 17-alpha-estradiol is a mirror-image version of estrogen. (Newman, 2007)

Juice and peel

Pomegranate juice is a good source of fructose, sucrose, and glucose. It also has some of the simple organic acids such as ascorbic acid, citric acid, fumaric acid, and malic acid. In addition, it contains small amounts of all amino acids, specifically proline, methionine, and valine.

Both the juice and peel are rich in polyphenols. The largest classes include tannins and **flavonoids** that indicate pharmacological potential of pomegranate due to their **strange antioxidative and preservative activities.** (Newman, 2007)

Ellagitannin is a type of tannin; it can be broken down into hydroxybenzoic acid such as ellagic acid. **It is widely used in plastic surgeries, which prevents skin flap's death due to its antioxidant activity.**

Two other ellagitannins that are found in both pomegranate juice and peel are punicalagin and punicalin. Several classes of pomegranate flavonoids include anthocyanins, flavan 3-ols, and flavonols. **Pomegranate juice and peel have catechins with a high antioxidant activity.**

They are essential compounds of anthocyanin's production with antioxidant and inflammatory role. Anthocyanins cause the red color of juice, which is not found in the peel.

All pomegranate flavonoids show antioxidant activity with indirect inhibition of inflammatory markers such as tumor necrosis factor-alpha (TNF-α). (Newman, 2007)

Bark and roots

The pomegranate tree's bark and roots are rich sources of chemicals called alkaloids. They are carbon-based substances; they were used to treat worms in the human gastrointestinal tract in traditional medicine. (Newman, 2007) (Jurenka, 2010)

Health effects

Prostate cancer

After lung cancer, the second leading cause of male cancer death is prostate cancer worldwide. Its progress before onset of symptoms is slow; therefore, pharmacological and nutritional interventions **could** affect the quality of patient's life by delaying its development. (Malik et al, 2005)

It was shown that pomegranate fruit **could** be used in the treatment of human prostate cancer because it **could** inhibit cell growth and induce apoptosis. (Rettig et al, 2008)

It leads to induction of pro-apoptotic proteins (Bax and Bak) and downregulation of anti-apoptotic proteins (Bcl-xL and Bcl-2). (Rettig et al, 2008)

Moreover, **the presence of NFκB and cell viability of prostate cancer cell lines has been inhibited when using pomegranate fruit extract, because it blocks NFκB**. (Albrecht et al, 2004)

Polyphenols of fermented juice and pomegranate oil can inhibit the proliferation of LNCaP (epithelial cell line derived from a human prostate carcinoma), PC-3, and DU145 human prostate cancer cell lines. These effects were the result of changes in cell cycle distribution and apoptosis induction. (Rettig et al, 2008)

In addition, it is reported that pomegranate fruit extract oral administration in nude mice implanted with androgen-sensitive CWR22RV1 cells caused significant decrease in serum prostate-specific antigen (PSA) level and inhibited tumor growth. (Albrecht et al, 2004)

Besides, the observed increase in NFκB activity during androgen dependence to androgen independence transition in the LAPC4 xenograft model was terminated. (Kim et al, 2002)

RMH Note: Still, there is no confirmation of these results in humans using randomized controlled trials in patients with prostate cancer. These are speculative in vitro studies.

Breast cancer

Fermented pomegranate juice has double the antiproliferative effect compared to fresh pomegranate juice in human breast cancer cell lines MCF-7 (breast cancer cell line isolated in 1970 from a 69-year-old Caucasian woman) and MB-MDA-231. In addition, pomegranate seed oil caused 90% prevention of proliferation of MCF-7 cells. (Mehta, Lansky, 2004) (Khan et al, 2007)

RMH Note: Again, there is no confirmation of these results in humans using randomized controlled trials in patients with breast cancer. These are also speculative in vitro studies.

Lung cancer

Pomegranate fruit extract can inhibit several signaling pathways, which can be used in the treatment of human lung cancer. Pathways include Mitogen-activated protein kinases (MAPK) PI3K/Akt and NFκB. In addition, there was a 4 day delay in the appearance of tumors (from 15 to 19 days) in mice implanted with A549 cells. (Khan et al, 2007)

These studies indicate the **speculative** chemopreventive effects of pomegranate fruit extract.

RMH Note: Again, there is no confirmation of these results in humans using randomized controlled trials in patients with breast cancer. These are also speculative in vitro studies.

Colon cancer

Adams et al. have reported the anti-inflammatory effects of pomegranate juice on the signaling proteins in HT-29 human colon cancer cell line. Reduction in phosphorylation of the p65 subunit of NFκB, its binding to the NFκB response, and 79% inhibition in TNF-α protein expression have been observed with 50 mg/L concentration of pomegranate extract. (Adams et al, 2006)

RMH Note: Again, there is no confirmation of these results in humans using randomized controlled trials in patients with breast cancer. These are also speculative in vitro studies.

Skin cancer

It has been demonstrated that pomegranate oil has chemopreventive efficacy **in mice**. Reduced tumor incidence (7%), decrease in tumor numbers, reduction in ornithine decarboxylase (ODC) activity (17%), significant inhibition in elevated Tissue plasminogen activator (TPA)-mediated skin edema and hyperplasia, protein expression of ODC and COX-2, and epidermal ODC activity have been reported with pomegranate oil treatments. (Hora et al, 2003) (Syed et al, 2006)

Pomegranate extract in various concentrations (5-60 mg/L) was effective against UVA- and UVB-induced damage in SKU-1064 **fibroblast cells** of human, which was relevant in reducing NFκB transcription, down regulating proapoptotic caspase-3, and elevating the G0/G1 phase associated with deoxyribonucleic acid (DNA) repair. (Pacheco-Palencia et al, 2008)

RMH Note: Again, there is no confirmation of these results in humans using randomized controlled trials in patients with breast cancer. These are also speculative in vitro studies.

Cardiovascular diseases

Pomegranate juice is an affluent source of polyphenols with high antioxidative potential. Moreover, **its antiatherogenic, antihypertensive, and anti-inflammatory effects have been shown in limited studies in human and murine models**. (Gil et al, 2000)

Hypertension is the most common disease in primary care of patients. It is found in comorbidity with diabetes and cardiovascular disease, and the majority of patients do not tend to be medicated. **Pomegranate juice prevents the activity of serum angiotensin-converting enzyme and reduces systolic blood pressure**. (Stowe, 2011)

Angiotensin II acute subcutaneous administration causes increased blood pressure in **diabetic Wistar rats**. It has been shown that pomegranate juice administration (100 mg/kg) for 4 weeks **could reduce the mean arterial blood pressure**. (Mohan, Waghulde, Kasture, 2010)

Pomegranate juice consumption resulted in 30% decrease in carotid intima-media thickness after 1 year. The patient's serum paraoxonase 1 (PON 1) activity showed 83% increase, whereas both serum low density lipoprotein (LDL) basal oxidative state and LDL susceptibility to copper ion significantly decreased by 90% and 95%, respectively. (Aviram et al, 2004)

Punicic acid, which is the main constituent of pomegranate seed oil, has antiatherogenic effects. In a study on 51 hyperlipidemic patients, pomegranate seed oil was administered twice a day (800 mg/day) for 4 weeks. **There was a significant decrease in triglycerides (TG) and TG: High density lipoprotein (HDL) cholesterol ratio by 2.75 mmol/L and 5.7 mmol/L, respectively**, whereas serum cholesterol, LDL-C, and glucose concentration remained unchanged. (Mirmiran et al, 2010)

High plasma LDL concentration is the major risk factor for atherosclerosis. Therefore, LDL modifications, including oxidation, retention, and aggregation, play a key role in atherosclerosis as well. Studies have shown that consuming pomegranate juice for 2 weeks resulted in declined retention and aggregation of LDL susceptibility and increased activity of serum paraoxonase (a protective lipid peroxidation esterase related to HDL) by 20% in humans.

Pomegranate juice administration **in mice** for 14 weeks showed reduced LDL oxidation by peritoneal macrophages by more than 90%, which was because of reduced cellular lipid peroxidation and superoxide release. The uptake of oxidized LDL showed 20% reduction in mice. **The size of atherosclerotic lesions reduced by 44% after pomegranate juice supplementation**. (Aviram et al, 2000)

Moreover, pomegranate juice administration to **apolipoprotein E-deficient mice** with advanced atherosclerosis for 2 months reduced oxidized LDL (31%) and increased macrophage cholesterol efflux (39%). (Kaplan et al, 2001)

In **cultured human endothelial cells and hypercholesterolemic mice**, both pomegranate juice and fruit extract reduced the activation of ELK-1 and p-CREB (oxidation-sensitive responsive genes) and elevated the expression of endothelial nitric oxide synthase. It is **suggested** that polyphenolic antioxidant compounds in pomegranate juice are responsible for the reduction of oxidative stress and atherogenesis. (de Nigris et la, 2007)

In another study, concentrated pomegranate juice was shown to reduce heart disease risk factors. Administration of concentrated pomegranate juice to 22 **diabetic type 2 patients with hyperlipemia** could significantly reduce TC, LDL-C, LDL-C: HDL-C ratio, and TC: HDL-C ratio. **However, it was unable to decrease serum TG and HDL-C concentrations**. (Esmaillzadeh et al, 2006)

Oral administration of pomegranate flower aqueous extract in streptozotocin (STZ)-induced **albino Wistar rats** in both 250 mg/kg and 500 mg/kg doses for 21 days could significantly reduce fibrinogen (FBG), TC, TG, LDL-C, and tissue lipid peroxidation level and increased the level of HDL-C and glutathione content. (Bagri et al, 2009)

Heart fibrosis increases among diabetics, which results in impairing cardiac function. Endothelin (ET)-1 and NFκB are interactive fibroblast growth regulators. It is suggested that pomegranate flower extract (500 mg/kg/day) in **Zucker diabetic fatty rats** could reduce the ratios of van Gieson-stained interstitial collagen deposit area to a total left ventricular area and perivascular collagen deposit areas to coronary artery media area in the heart and diminishes cardiac fibrosis in these rats. In addition, overexpressed cardiac fibronectin and collagen I and II messenger RNAs (mRNAs) were inhibited. It also decreased the up-regulated cardiac mRNA expression of ET-1, ETA, inhibitor-κBβ, and c-jun. Pomegranate flower extract is a dual activator of peroxisome proliferator-activated receptor (PPAR)-α and γ and improves hyperlipemia, hyperglycemia, and fatty heart in diabetic fatty Zucker rats. (Huang et al, 2005) (Huang et al, 2005, BJP)

Punicic acid caused a dose-dependent increase in PPAR alpha and gamma reporter activity in 3T3-L1 cells. Dietary punicic acid reduced plasma glucose, suppressed NFκB activation and unregulated TNF-α expression and PPAR-α/γ responsive genes in adipose tissue and skeletal muscle. (Hontecillas et al, 2009)

Pomegranate leaf extract was administered (400 and 800 mg/kg/day) to **high-fat-diet-induced obese and hyperlipidemic mouse models** for 5 weeks. The results indicated significant reduction in body weight, energy intake (based on food intake), serum total cholesterol (TC), TG, FBG, and TC/HDL-C ratio. Intestinal fat absorption was inhibited as well. (Lei et al, 2007)

Prof Randolph M. Howes MD, PhD

The high fat diet (HFD) with 1% pomegranate seed oil (rich source of punicic acid) was administered for 12 weeks to induce obesity and **insulin resistance in mice**. The pomegranate seed oil-fed group exhibited lower body weight (4%) and body fat mass (3.1%) compared with only HFD-fed mice. A clear improvement was observed in peripheral insulin sensitivity (70%) **in pomegranate seed oil-administered rats**. (Vroegrijk et al, 2011)

Fatty liver is the most common abnormal liver function among diabetics. Pomegranate flower was examined for its antidiabetic effects on **diabetic type II and obese Zucker rats**. Rats fed with 500 mg/kg/day of pomegranate flower extract for 6 weeks showed decreased ratio of liver weight to tibia length, lipid droplets, and hepatic TG contents. In addition, it increased PPRA-α and Acyl-COA oxidase mRNA levels in HepG2 cells. (Xu et al, 2009)

In a study by de Nigris *et al.*,[31] they compared the influence of pomegranate fruit extract with pomegranate juice on nitric oxide and arterial function in **obese Zucker rats**. They have demonstrated that both pomegranate fruit extract and juice significantly reduced the vascular inflammatory markers expression, thrombospondin, and cytokine TGFP 1. Increased plasma nitrite and nitrate were observed with administration of either pomegranate fruit or juice. (de Nigris et al, 2007, NO)

Many studies have reported the anti-inflammatory potential of pomegranate extract. In a study on 30 **Sprague-Dawley rats with acute inflammation** due to myringotomy, it was observed that 100 µl/day of pomegranate extract could significantly reduce reactive-oxygen species (ROS) levels. The extract was administered 1 day before and 2 days after surgery. Reduced thickness of lamina propria and vessel density was reported as well. (Kahya et al, 2011)

Both ellagitannins and ellagic acid are the main components of pomegranate extract, which have anti-inflammatory properties. They are metabolized by gut microbiota to yield urolithins. It is suggested that urolithins are the main components responsible for the anti-inflammation properties of pomegranate. It is **suggested** that NFκB activation, MAPK downregulation of COX-2, and mPGES-1 expression were inhibited through a decrease in PGE2 production. (Gonzalez-Sarrias et al, 2010)

Neutrophils play key roles in inflammatory processes by releasing great amounts of ROS (EMODS) generated by NADPH-oxidase and myeloperoxidase. It is indicated that punicic acid exhibited a potent anti-inflammatory effect via prevention of TNF-α-induced priming of NADPH oxidase by targeting the p38MAPKinase/Ser 345-p 47 phox-axis and releasing MPO. (Boussetta et al, 2009)

Hyperglycemia results in oxidative stress in diabetes mellitus, which is a major factor in the pathogenesis of cardiovascular disease.

Results suggested that pomegranate extract, owing to its polyphenol-rich antioxidants (oleanolic, ursolic, and gallic acids), could prevent cardiovascular complications through decrease in LDL, increase in HDL, serum paraoxonase I stability and activity, and nitric oxide production. (Katz et al, 2007) (Rock et al, 2008) (Fenercioglu et al, 2010)

RMH Note: Again, there is no confirmation of these results in humans using randomized controlled trials in patients with cardiovascular disease. All of the above studies on cardiovascular disease are highly speculative.

Osteoarthritis

The most common forms of arthritis are osteoarthritis and its major progressive degenerative joint disease, which could affect joint functions and quality of life in patients. It is mediated by proinflammatory cytokines such as IL-1 and TNF-α. MAPKs are important due to their inflammatory and cartilage damage regulation. (Rasheed, Akhtar, Haqqi, 2010)

P38-MAPKs are responsible for regulating cytokine production, neutrophils activation, apoptosis, and nitric oxide synthesis. The MAPK family phosphorylates a number of transcription factors such as runt-related transcription factor-2 (RUNX-2). (Lee et al, 1994) (Kumar et al, 2001) (Loeser et al, 2008)

Pomegranate extract, with its rich source of polyphenols, can inhibit IL-1 β-induced activation of MKK3, DNA-binding activity of RUNX-2 transcription factor, and p38 α-MAPK isoform. (Rasheed, Akhtar, Haqqi, 2010)

Rheumatoid arthritis

Rheumatoid arthritis is an autoimmune disease that affects 0.5-1% of people worldwide. Women are afflicted more than men. This inflammatory disease is characterized by inflammation and bone erosion. (Rasheed, Akhtar, Haqqi, 2010) (Lee et al, 1994)

133

Critical mediators in the pathogenesis of rheumatoid arthritis are TNF-α, IL-1 β, MCP1, Inducible nitric oxide synthase (iNOS), and COX-2-agents, which are stimulated by p38-MAPK and NFκB activation.

It is shown that pomegranate extract could reduce the onset and incidence of collagen-induced arthritis in mice. Severity of arthritis, joint inflammation, and IL-6 level were significantly reduced in pomegranate extract-fed **mice**. (Shukla et al, 2008)

Antimicrobial/fungal effect

Since bacterial resistance to antimicrobial drugs is increasing, medicinal plants have been considered as alternative agents. Pomegranate has been widely approved for its antimicrobial properties. (Lansky, Shubert, Neeman, 2004) (Satish et al, 2007)

It has been shown that dried powder of **pomegranate peel has a high inhibition of Candida albicans.** (Mithun et al, 2010)

In addition, antimicrobial effects of both methanol and dichloromethane pomegranate extracts have been demonstrated on the *Candida* genus yeast as pathogen-causing disease in immunosuppressive host. (Hofling et al, 2010)

Methicillin-resistant *staphylococcus aureus* (MRSA) and methicillin-sensitive *staphylococcus aureus* (MSSA) (multiple antibiotics resistant) produce panta valentine leukocidin (PVL) toxin, which can lead to higher levels of morbidity and mortality. (Ferrara, 2007) (Wenzel, Bearman, Edmond, 2007)

It is indicated that a combination of pomegranate peel extract with Cu (II) ions exhibit enhanced antimicrobial effects against isolated MSSA, MRSA, and PVL. (Gould et al, 2009)

One of the leading etiological bacteria of urinary tract infections is *Escherichia Coli*. Strong antibacterial activity of ethanol extract against *E. coli* has been shown. (Sharma et al, 2010)

Skin

Solar ultraviolet radiations are the primary causes of many biological effects such as photoaging and skin cancer. These radiations resulted in DNA damage, protein oxidation, and matrix metalloproteinases induction. In one study, the effects of pomegranate juice, extract, and oil were examined against UVB-mediated damage. These products caused a decrease in UVB-induced protein expression of c-Fos and phosphorylation of c-Jun. (Afaq et al, 2009)

On the other hand, production of proinflammatory cytokines IL-1 β and IL-6 was decreased by topical application of 10 micromol/L of ellagic acid. The inflammatory macrophages infiltration was blocked in the integuments of SKH-1 hairless UVB-exposed mice for 8 weeks. (Bae et al, 2010)

Dental effects

The interbacterial coaggregations and these bacterial interactions with yeasts are related to the maintenance of oral microbiota. It is indicated that dried, powdered pomegranate peel shows a strong inhibition of *C. albicans* with a mean zone of 22 mm. (Pai et al, 2010)

In another study, the antiplaque effect of pomegranate mouth rinse has been reported. (Bhadbhade et al, 2011)

In addition, hydroalcoholic extract of pomegranate was very effective against dental plaque microorganisms (84% decrease (cfu/ml)). (Menezes et al, 2006)

Reproductive system

One of the main constituents (16%) of the methanolic pomegranate seed extract is beta-sitosterol. It is suggested that the extract is a potent phasic activity stimulator in rat uterus, which happens due to the non-estrogenic effects of beta-sitosterol on inhibiting sarco-endo-plasmic reticulum Ca^{2+} -ATPase (SERCA) and K channel, which resulted in contraction by calcium entry on L-type calcium channels and myosin light chain kinase (MLCK). (Promprom et al, 2010)

It is demonstrated that pomegranate fruit extract has an embryonic protective nature against adrianycin-induced oxidative stress (adri-anycin is a chemotherapeutic drug used in cancer treatment). (Kishore et al, 2009)

Moreover, pomegranate juice consumption could increase epididymal sperm concentration, motility, spermatogenic cell density, diameter of seminiferous tubules and germinal cell layer thickness. (Turk et al, 2008)

Alzheimer's disease

Hartman *et al.* showed that mice treated by pomegranate juice have 50% less soluble Abeta 42 accumulation and amyloid deposition in the hippocampus, which could be considered for Alzheimer's disease im-provement. (Hartman et al, 2006)

Malaria

In the presence of pomegranate fruit rind, the induced MMP-9 mRNA levels by haemozoin or TNF was decreased, which may be attributed to the antiparasitic activity and the inhibition of the proinflammatory mechanisms responsible in the onset of cerebral malaria. (Dell'Agli et al, 2009) (Dell'agli et al, 2010)

HIV

The anti-HIV-1 microbicide of pomegranate juice blocks virus binding to CD4 and CXCR4/CCR5, thereby preventing infection by primary virus clades A to G and group O. (Neurath et al, 2005)

Wound healing

Use of pomegranate extract and flower showed significant reduction in wound area and increased the well-organized bands of collagen, fibroblasts, and few inflammatory cells. (Piralouti et al, 2010) (Pirbalouti et al, 2010)

Properties of elevated wound contraction and the period of epithelialization, collagen, and protein synthesis were reported in hydroalcoholic pomegranate extract. (Hayouni et al, 2011)

Mechanisms of action

Pomegranate can induce its beneficial effects through its various metabolites. The antioxidant and anti-atherosclerotic potentials of pomegranate are mainly relevant to the high polyphenol concentrations in pomegranate fruit such as ellagitannins and hydrolysable tannins. (Gil et al, 2000)

COX-1 and COX-2 enzymes and IL-1 β activity can be inhibited by pomegranate fruit extract. (Tao et al, 1998)

It is suggested that pomegranate can antagonize the stimulation of mRNA of MMP-9 in THP-1/monocytes. The whole fruit and compounds inhibit TNF-induced MMP-9 promoter activity.

Urolithins are metabolites that are metabolized by the human intestinal microflora. These compounds decreased MMP-9 sretion and mRNA levels induced by HZ or TNF. It is suggested that ellagitannins are responsible for the control of excessive production of MMP-9, which could result in decreased production of noxious cytokine TNF. (Cerda et al, 2003)

TNF cytokines promote NFκB binding to target sequences while inducing transcription of several genes such as the MMP-9 gene. (Prescott, Fitzpatrick, 2000)

Ellagitannins prevent NFκB promoter activity by blocking NFκB-driven transcription and affecting the entire cytokine cascade. Ellagitannins inhibit the activation of inflammatory pathways such as MAPK.

In addition, pomegranate compounds could inhibit angiogenesis through the downregulation of vascular endothelial growth factor in cancers.

Drug interactions involving pomegranate

Therapeutic benefits of pomegranate in various diseases would lead to an increase in its consumption. (Mena et al, 2011)

It is important that pomegranate consumption does not affect the oral bioavailability of drugs. (Shravan et al, 2011)

A study on human liver microsomes has shown the inhibitory effect of pomegranate juice on CYP2CP (a gene that codes for an enzyme to break down warfarin in the body) and increased bioavailability of tolbutamide (substrate for CYP2CP) in rats. Moreover, it is suggested that pomegranate may inhibit cytochrome P450-3A (CYP3A)-mediated carbamazepine metabolism. (Nagata et al, 2007) (Misaka et al, 2011)

Pomegranate safety

Many studies have been carried out on the different components derived from pomegranate but no adverse effects have been reported in the examined dosage.

Histopathological studies on both sexes of OF-1 mice confirmed the non-toxic effects of the polyphenol antioxidant punicalagin. Besides, in a study on 86 overweight human subjects who received 1420 mg/day of pomegranate fruit extract in tablet form for 28 days, no side effects or adverse changes in urine or blood of individuals were reported. (Vidal et al, 2003)

Products and supplementation

Apart from fruit, pomegranate is available in various forms such as bottled juice (fresh or concentrated), powdered capsules, and tablets, which are derived from seed, fermented juice, peel, leaf and flower, gelatin capsules of seed oil extracts, dry or beverage tea from leaves or seeds, and other food productions such as jams, jellies, sauces, salad dressings, and vinegars. Anardana, which is the powdered form of pomegranate seed, is used as a form of spice.

CONCLUSION

Pomegranate is a potent antioxidant. This fruit is rich in flavonoids, anthocyanins, punicic acid, ellagitannins, alkaloids, fructose, sucrose, glucose, simple organic acids, and other components **and has anti-atherogenic, anti-hypertensive, and anti-inflammatory properties**.

Allegedly, pomegranate can be used in the prevention and treatment of several types of cancer, cardiovascular disease, osteoarthritis, rheumatoid arthritis, and other diseases.

In addition, it improves wound healing and is beneficial to the reproductive system.

Pomegranate can induce its beneficial effects through the influence of its various bioavailable constituents and metabolites on gene expression. Although many *in vitro*, animal and clinical trials have been carried out to examine and prove the therapeutic effects of these compounds, **further human trials and studies are necessary to understand the therapeutic potentials of pomegranate**. (Zarfeshany et al, 2014)

Pomegranate: a fruit that ameliorates metabolic syndrome

Abstract

Pomegranate is an ancient fruit that is still part of the diet in the Mediterranean area, the Middle East, and India. Health-promoting effects have long been attributed to this fruit. **Modern research corroborates the use of pomegranate as a folk remedy for diabetes and metabolic syndrome**, and is responsible for a new evaluation of nutritional and pharmaceutical aspects of pomegranate in the general public. In the last decade, industry and agricultural production have been adapted to meet higher market demands for pomegranate.

In vivo and in vitro studies have demonstrated that **pomegranate exerts hypoglycemic effects, including increased insulin sensitivity, inhibition of α-glucosidase, and impact on glucose transporter type 4 function, but is also responsible for a reduction of total cholesterol, and the improvement of blood lipid profiles, as well as anti-inflammatory effects through the modulation of peroxisome proliferator-activated receptor pathways.**

These effects may also explain how pomegranate-derived compounds function in the amelioration of adverse health effects caused by metabolic syndrome. Pomegranate contains polyphenols such as ellagitannins and anthocyanins, as well as phenolic acids, fatty acids and a variety of volatile compounds. Ellagitannins are some of the most prevalent compounds present in pomegranate, and may be responsible for certain benevolent characteristics associated with pomegranate. **Although the fruit is consumed in many countries, epidemiological and clinical studies are unavailable.** Additional research is necessary to corroborate the promise of current in vivo and in vitro findings. (Medjakovic, Jungbauer, 2013)

The following was adapted from Life Extension Magazine November 2014. Even though this article contains references, it seems to be more of an **"advertorial."**

Enhance Endothelial Health By James Harrison

Pomegranate extracts are proving to be an effective means of protecting our delicate endothelium. **Studies show that pomegranate works on a number of levels to ensure cardiac health by reducing cellular cholesterol accumulation, protecting LDL from oxidation, and in lab studies, shrinking atherosclerotic plaque.** (Kaplan et al, 2001) (Rosenblat, Volkova, Aviram, 2010) (Aviram, Rosenblat, 2013)

In addition, **pomegranate promotes supple arteries that maintain healthy blood flow and pressure to all of your tissues and organs**. (Aviram, Rosenblat, 2013) (Asgary et al, 2014)

Best of all, **research concludes that by improving** endothelial **health, pomegranate supplementation lowers risk factors for heart attacks, strokes, and other cardiovascular events.** (Asgary et al, 2014) (Aviram et al, 2004) (Davidson et al, 2009)

Your chances of having a heart attack or a stroke depend a great deal on the health of your **endothelium.**

The endothelial cells use the free radical, *nitric oxide,* to signal the need for relaxation to arterial muscle cells.

As we age and develop pathological conditions such as atherosclerosis, our ability to produce and respond to *nitric oxide* rapidly diminishes. (Edsmyr et al, 1981)

Research demonstrates that **pomegranate** extracts enhance the body's natural protective responses to prevent endothelial dysfunction, promote healthy mechanisms, and even remove oxidized LDL from arterial walls.

Pomegranate extracts directly aid your own body's defense mechanisms and prevent catastrophic outcomes. Pomegranate extracts:

- *Enhance* cholesterol outflow from inflammatory white blood cells, helping to reduce the risk of plaque formation. (Fuhrman et al, 2005)
- *Protect* vulnerable LDL molecules from the oxidation that leads to arterial wall inflammation and promotes plaque generation. (Rosenblat, Volkova, Aviram, 2010)
- *Boost* natural antioxidant systems, particularly *superoxide dismutase* (SOD), protecting vital nitric oxide and allowing the endothelium to recover from the effects of chronic oxidative and inflammatory stresses. (Dong et al, 2012) (Shaban et al, 2013)

RMH Note: By FDA regulations, they can use any words except the following four: diagnose, treat, prevent or cure. So, they use enhance, protect and boost.

Pomegranate's Endothelial Defense Mechanisms

Pomegranate contains a number of extremely potent antioxidant molecules including *tannins* and *anthocyanins*, which have been shown to exert important endothelial-protective, anti-atherosclerosis effects. (Aviram, Rosenblat, 2012)

Pomegranate contains particularly potent polyphenols that protect against LDL and HDL oxidation, which helps minimize **endothelial dysfunction** in its earliest stages.

A unique property of pomegranate is its ability to boost activity of a beneficial enzyme called *paraoxonase-1* (PON-1), which is found in beneficial HDL and accounts for many of its "good cholesterol" features by breaking down oxidized lipids, even those that have already been taken up into plaques. (Aviram, Rosenblat, 2013) (Kaplan et al, 2001)

In a **mouse** model of coronary heart disease, treatment with pomegranate extract had a number of benefits to reduce atherosclerotic plaque. (Al-Jarallah et al, 2013)

The previous two studies show pomegranate's great promise in preventing atherosclerosis and protecting heart muscle from oxidant damage, if you are a rat or a mouse.

A third study, however, illustrates that **pomegranate juice can, in fact, slow development of even advanced atherosclerosis.** Here, scientists used young **mice** genetically programmed to develop atherosclerosis, treating them with pomegranate juice or placebo for two months. (Houston, 2014)

Pomegranate juice intake led to increased *paraoxonase-1* **(PON-1)** activity, which protects the function of HDL in transporting cholesterol out of arteries and back to the liver for disposal. PON-1 also reduced the amount of oxidized LDL taken up by **31%** in certain inflammatory white blood cells compared with controls.

PON-1 allegedly blocks destructive lipid peroxidation reactions. (Sobieszczyk, Beckman, 2006) (Lorenz et al, 2007) (Mirmiran et al, 2010)

A late 2013 study reveals still more about the potential role of pomegranate juice and extracts in protecting endothelial health. An early stage in the development of atherosclerosis is the accumulation of oxidized LDL in inflammatory cells called *macrophages*. Israeli scientists found that **by adding pomegranate juice to such inflammatory cells in combination with a statin drug (*simvastatin*), they could significantly improve the statin's ability to block production of cholesterol in the cells**. (Rosenblat et al, 2013)

Moreover, **pomegranate increased the statin's ability to diminish oxidative stress, which would mean that it would also reduce the levels of nitric oxide**.

Pomegranate supplementation can boost superoxide dismutase (SOD) levels and this would also increase the levels of hydrogen peroxide which has been formed from the dismutation of superoxide anion.

Pomegranate extracts act via several different, but complementary mechanisms to restore the body's endothelial defenses, lowering risk factors for a cardiovascular event, and helping to keep arteries supple and youthful. Pomegranate extracts have been shown to promote cholesterol outflow from macrophages, to enhance natural antioxidant systems like superoxide dismutase (SOD), and to directly protect LDL from oxidant damage and resulting inflammation.

A robust form of the antioxidant enzyme SOD has been developed that enhances SOD activity beyond what is provided by pomegranate. Studies show that this oral supplement product, which is protected from stomach acid digestion, **GliSODin**®, survives passage through the stomach to boost SOD levels, which may reduce cardiovascular risk by improving endothelial health. (Vouldoukis et al, 2004)

Enhance Endothelial Health - How Pomegranate Protects Against Atherosclerosis

Human Studies Support Pomegranate

Pomegranate's ability to mobilize the body's own self-defense forces against endothelial dysfunction are validated by human studies. A dose of **150 mL** of fresh pomegranate juice once daily for two weeks in patients with hypertension demonstrated reductions in both systolic (top number) and diastolic (bottom number) blood pressures. These changes were accompanied by significant decreases in levels of *vascular cell adhesion molecule-1* (VCAM-1), an important endothelial-produced inflammatory protein.

These changes after such a short period indicate the potential for long-term benefit of pomegranate supplementation on blood pressure and the inflammation that raises risk for heart attack and stroke.

In a study of pomegranate juice supplementation in a group of people who already had increased *intima-media thickness* (IMT), the results showed those who did not consume the pomegranate had a **9%** increase in IMT over one year. Those who did drink pomegranate juice had an average reduction in IMT of up to **30%**. (Aviram et al, 2004)

This was accompanied by an **83%** increase in the patients' levels of the beneficial antioxidant enzyme PON-1. Additionally, levels of oxidized LDL dropped by **90%**, further reducing risk of heart attack or stroke, probably related to the fact that total antioxidant status was increased by **130%** after a year of pomegranate supplementation. These beneficial changes were accompanied by a **12%** reduction in systolic blood pressure over one year. (Aviram et al, 2004)

A subsequent study revealed that pomegranate supplementation also reduced progression of IMT thickening in those subjects with the worst oxidative stress and highest triglyceride/lowest HDL groups. These studies provide direct evidence of how pomegranate ramps up the body's protective responses to reduce the risk of cardiovascular disease.

In a remarkable **2014** study, researchers found that adding pomegranate extract to the cholesterol-lowering drug *simvastatin* lowered dangerous production of *reactive oxygen species* in white blood cells from patients with high cholesterol by **30%**, compared with only an **18%** decrease in those on the drug only.[37] Similarly, the pomegranate-plus-*simvastatin* group saw a significant **48%** reduction in triglyceride levels, which did not fall in the drug-only group.[37]

Pomegranate seed oil contains *punicic acid*, a beneficial fatty acid unique to pomegranate. Lab studies have shown it to have powerful anti-atherogenic effects. A human study demonstrated that after four weeks of pomegranate seed oil, **400 mg** twice daily in people with high cholesterol, their triglyceride levels fell from **306 mg/dL** to **244 mg/dL**, and their ratios of triglyceride to HDL cholesterol (an important measure of cardiovascular risk) fell from **7.5** to a safer **5.7**. Supplemented patients also had a beneficial increase of **5 mg/dL** in HDL-cholesterol, which fell by **0.77 mg/dL** in placebo recipients. (Mirmiran et al, 2010)

My conclusions on pomegranate are as follows:

Research teams worldwide have no consensus as how to assess metabolism of (berry) flavonoids and their impact on health. The research team concluded that "The potential systemic biological effects of pomegranate juice ingestion should be attributed to the colonic microflora metabolites rather than to the polyphenols present in the juice." For now, the consumers should be aware that sound claims of marketers on antioxidative properties of berries are not (sufficiently) substantiated from the scientific perspective.

ORAC, TEAC, TRAP, FRAP, and FOX assays which assess changes in the antioxidant capacity of plasma are often used **for research purposes**; these assays are explicitly mentioned in the Guidance with the remark that **"It is not established that changes in the overall antioxidant capacity of plasma exert a beneficial physiological effect in humans as required by Regulation (EC) No 1924/2006."**

Further, those changes **"do not predict a role of the food/constituent in the protection of body cells and molecules such as DNA, proteins and lipids from oxidative damage in vivo, and therefore are not suitable outcome measures for the scientific substantiation of the claimed effect."**

Recently the **USDA's Nutrient Data Laboratory (NDL)** removed the **USDA ORAC Database for Selected Foods** from its website "due to increasing evidence that the scores indicating antioxidant capacity have no direct link to the effects of specific bioactive compounds, including polyphenols, on human health."

The research demonstrates low bioavailability of the pomegranate polyphenols. It is therefore speculated that the health benefits of pomegranate are due to its metabolites (e.g., urolithins) rather than the compounds of the intact fruit.

Pomi-T - A commercially available **food supplement that contains pomegranate, broccoli, green tea, and turmeric significantly lowers prostate-specific antigen (PSA) levels**, compared with placebo, in patients with prostate cancer, **a double-blind placebo-controlled randomized trial** has shown.

Based on the above statements, pomegranate's medicinal benefits still await further investigation; however, some of the scientific studies in this section lend support to its possible clinical potential contributions. We wait for additional studies.

SECTION THREE

BROCCOLI

Sulforaphane (SF)

https://lahey.org/Departments_and_Locations/Departments/Nephrology/Ebsco_Content/Kidney_Failure.aspx?chunkiid=111823

Sulforaphane is a chemical found in broccoli sprouts, as well as other cabbage-family vegetables such as broccoli, Brussels sprouts, cabbage, cauliflower, and kale. Some evidence hints that sulforaphane might help prevent cancer.

Requirements/Sources

Sulforaphane is not an essential nutrient. It is found in especially high levels in broccoli sprouts.

Therapeutic Uses

Numerous observational studies have found that a high consumption of vegetables in the cabbage family is associated with a reduced risk of cancer, especially breast, prostate, lung, stomach, colon, and rectal cancer. (van Poppel et al, 1999)

On this basis, scientists have looked for anticancer substances in these foods.

Sulforaphane is one such candidate substance (indole-3-carbinol, I3C, is another).

In test-tube and animal studies, sulforaphane exhibits properties that suggest it could, indeed, help prevent many forms of cancer. (Singh et al, 2005) (Sulforaphane-induced cell death in human prostate cancer cells is initiated by reactive oxygen species.) (Joseph et al, 2004) (Johnston, 2004) (Pham et al, 2004) (Tseng et al, 2004) (Myzak et al, 2004) (Fahey et al, 2002) (Hecht, 1999) (Verhoeven et al, 1997) (Talalay, Zhang, 1996) (Nestle, 1998) (Nestle, 1997) (Fahey, Talalay, 1999) (Gamet-Payrestre et al, 2000) (Solowiej et al, 2003)

(Frydoonfar, McGrath, Spiegelman, 2003) (Chiao et al, 2002) (Levi et al, 2001) (Brooks, Paton, Vidanes, 2001) (Conaway et al, 2001) (Steinkellner et al, 2001) (Kelloff et al, 2000)

However, it is a long way from such studies to reliable evidence of benefit.

Observational studies are notoriously poor guides to treatment, sometimes leading to conclusions that are the reverse of what is ultimately found to be correct. (Kunz, Oxman, 1998) (Kramer, 2004)

The problem is that they can't show cause-and-effect—they only show association. It is possible, for example, that people who consume more cabbage-family vegetables share other traits that are responsible for reduced cancer rates. Consider the history of hormone replacement therapy.

In the 1990s, scientists had concluded that estrogen prevents heart disease, based largely on observational studies that showed menopausal women who use hormone replacement have lower heart disease rates.

When double-blind, placebo-controlled studies were performed, however, they showed that **hormone replacement therapy actually increases heart disease risk**. For all we know, we could be making a similar mistake with cabbage-family vegetables.

Certainly, it is too great a leap to jump to one constituent of such vegetables and advocate that substance for preventing cancer. **Thousands of substances show anticancer properties in the test tube and fail to pan out in real life**.

The beta-carotene story is another instructive example. Not only did observational studies show that people who consume foods high in beta-carotene have less lung cancer, test-tube studies found that **beta-carotene has anti-cancer properties. However, subsequent large double-blind studies found that beta-carotene supplements do not help prevent lung cancer, and might even increase risk**.

The bottom line: **At present, we cannot recommend sulforaphane for preventing cancer**.

Therapeutic Dosages

The proper daily intake (if there is any) of sulforaphane is not known. Typical recommendations range from 200 to 400 mcg daily.

Safety Issues

No major adverse effects have been reported with sulforaphane supplements, but comprehensive studies have not been performed. Maximum safe doses in young children, pregnant or nursing women, or people with severe liver or kidney disease are not known.

NOTE: **Sulforaphane has shown the potential for interacting with numerous medications**. (Kall, Vang, Clausen, 1997)

For this reason, we recommend that people taking any oral or injected medication that is critical to their health or well-being avoid using sulforaphane supplements until more is known.

Potential health benefits of sulforaphane: A review

Potential health benefits of sulforaphane: A review of the experimental, clinical and epidemiological evidences and underlying mechanisms

Prof Randolph M. Howes MD, PhD

(Elbarbry, Elrody, 2011)

Extensive epidemiological evidence and animal experimental studies suggest that cruciferous vegetables may prevent or delay various inflammatory disorders, including cancers. Much of this chemopreventive effect has been attributed to the physiological effect of the isothiocyanates, especially sulforaphane (SF).

Sulforaphane has been proven as a potent protector against oxidative damage and carcinogens.

A plethora of clinical effects are reported in various experimental diseases as well as human clinical studies.

This review summarizes the present knowledge about the health effects of sulforaphane with possible underlying mechanisms for these effects based on the reported in vitro and in vivo studies. These studies suggest that SF has the potential to reduce risk of various types of cancers, diabetes, atherosclerosis, respiratory diseases, neurodegenerative disorders, ocular disorders, and cardiovascular diseases.

Traditionally, Nrf2-mediated induction of phase 2 detoxification enzymes has been recognized as the major mechanism by which SF protects cells.

However, several recent studies have reported multiple other mechanisms involved in response to SF, including inhibition of cytochrome P450 enzymes, induction of apoptosis and cell cycle arrest, and antiinflammatory effect. **It is suggested that these mechanisms work synergistically to provide the observed health effects of sulforaphane.**

There is a growing interest in the use of herbal medicine as part of the complementary and alternative medicine (CAM). In the United States, approximately 40% of adults and approximately 12% of children are using some form of CAM. (Jung et al., 2002)

Several epidemiological studies have shown that consumption of large quantities of fruits and vegetables, especially cruciferous vegetables (e.g. Broccoli and Brussels sprouts), can protect against carcinogenesis, mutagenesis, drug toxicities, and other chronic diseases. (Conaway et al., 2002)

(Shapiro et al., 2001)

Induction of apoptosis is hypothesized to be through intracellular activation of a family of cysteine proteases, named caspases, responsible for initiation and execution of apoptosis. Such ability of SF to induce apoptosis in various cancerous cells makes it a potential candidate against secondary and possibly recurrent cancers. Several mechanisms, including both caspase-dependent and independent, have been proposed to explain the induction of apoptosis by SF and have been reviewed. (Juge et al., 2007) (Myzak and Dashwood, 2006)

Cruciferous vegetables are a rich source of glucosinolates, which, upon chewing, are enzymatically hydrolyzed by the plant-specific myrosinase (ß-thioglucoside N-hydroxysulfates; EC 3.2.3.1) and release isothiocyanates. (Fahey et al., 2001) (Fahey et al., 1997) (Shapiro et al., 2001)

The un-hydrolyzed glucosinolate can be degraded by thioglucosidase activity of the flora present in the human gut, but are not likely to get absorbed into systemic circulation. (Vermeulen et al., 2008)

The most abundant glucosinolate in broccoli is glucoraphanin, which upon hydrolysis by myrosinase or intestinal flora yields the isothiocyanates, sulforaphane (R-1-isothiocyanato-4-methylsulfinyl butane, SF).

Sulforaphane is the most extensively studied isothiocyanates, and **most studies attribute the health benefits of cruciferous vegetables to their high content of SF.** (Fahey et al., 1997) (Matusheski et al., 2001)

Several recent human studies have also reported the potential effect of SF for the eradication of H. pylori infection. (Galan et al., 2004) (Fahey et al. 2002)

Although, significant oxidative damage is observed in Alzheimer's disease and leads to extracellular deposition of β-amyloid as senile plaques, very little, if any, research has been conducted to investigate the beneficial effect of SF in this NDD. A recent review by Mukherjee et al. (2007) showed that **broccoli's glucosinolate content has an anti- acetylcholinesterase (AChE) activity and could have a potential to treat symptoms of Alzheimer's disease.** (Mukherjee et al., 2007)

In vitro experiments, *in vivo* animal studies and a smaller number of clinical trials with humans have suggested that the dietary SF is a safe, cheap and effective strategy to reduce the risk of atherosclerosis, cancer, diabetes, gastric, heart, neurodegenerative, ocular and respiratory diseases. These findings are consistent with epidemiological observations that high intake levels of SF and SF-rich diets are correlated with low rates of these diseases.

SF-drug interactions should be carefully addressed in the context that **SF is a potent inhibitor for CYP enzymes and inducer for phase 2 enzymes involved in drug metabolism**. Studies in our lab show that SF is a potent inhibitor for human CYP3A4, an enzyme involved in metabolism of almost 50% of drugs available on the market (data not published). Such decrease in metabolism of these drugs can result in toxicity problems when drug concentrations get too high.

While the major function of CYP enzymes is drug metabolism, some CYP enzymes are involved in maintenance of the homeostasis of endogenous molecules such as cholesterol and vaso-active agents and play a critical role in the regulation of vascular function. The potential inhibitory effect of SF on these CYP enzymes should be investigated as it may affect the normal cellular functions.

SF induces cell cycle arrest and apoptosis in leukemia cells

Sulforaphane Induces Cell Cycle Arrest and Apoptosis in Acute Lymphoblastic Leukemia Cells

Acute lymphoblastic leukemia (ALL) is the most common hematological cancer in children. Although risk-adaptive therapy, CNS-directed chemotherapy, and supportive care have improved the survival of ALL patients, disease relapse is still the leading cause of cancer-related death in children. Therefore, new drugs are needed as frontline treatments in high-risk disease and as salvage agents in relapsed ALL.

Many standard chemotherapeutic agents have been discovered from natural sources (e.g., daunorubicin and cytarabine). Sulforaphane (SF) is a dietary isothiocyanate found in cruciferous vegetables and is endowed with both preventive and therapeutic activities in solid tumors. **Epidemiological studies conducted in the US found that individuals who consumed a diet rich in cruciferous vegetables (i.e., broccoli and cabbage) had a lower incidence of breast, lung, prostate, and colon cancer**.

Furthermore, the consumption of raw cruciferous vegetables inversely correlates with the risk of bladder cancer. This cancer chemopreventive property has been largely attributed to the activity of isothiocyanates derived from the metabolism of glucosinolates that accumulate in cruciferous vegetables.

In this study, we report that **purified sulforaphane, a natural isothiocyanate found in cruciferous vegetables, has anti-leukemic properties in a broad range of ALL cell lines and primary lymphoblasts from pediatric T-ALL and pre-B ALL patients**. The treatment of ALL leukemic cells with sulforaphane resulted in dose-dependent apoptosis and G2/M cell cycle arrest, which was associated with the activation of caspases (3, 8, and 9), inactivation of PARP, p53-independent upregulation of p21[CIP1/WAF1], and inhibition of the Cdc2/Cyclin B1 complex.

Interestingly, sulforaphane also inhibited the AKT and mTOR survival pathways in most of the tested cell lines by lowering the levels of both total and phosphorylated proteins.

Finally, the administration of sulforaphane to the ALL xenograft models resulted in a reduction of tumor burden, particularly following oral administration, suggesting a potential role as an adjunctive agent to improve the therapeutic response in high-risk ALL patients with activated AKT signaling.

This is the first report on the anti-leukemic property of SF in hematological malignances, supporting its use as an adjunctive chemotherapy in ALL. (Suppipat et al, 2012)

SF antitumor activity and ROS

Cytotoxic and Antitumor Activity of Sulforaphane: The Role of Reactive Oxygen Species (ROS)

(Sestili, Fimognari, 2015)

According to recent estimates, cancer continues to remain the second leading cause of death and is becoming the leading one in old age. Failure and high systemic toxicity of conventional cancer therapies have accelerated the identification and development of innovative preventive as well as therapeutic strategies to contrast cancer-associated morbidity and mortality.

In recent years, increasing body of in vitro and in vivo studies has underscored the cancer preventive and therapeutic efficacy of the isothiocyanate sulforaphane.

In this review article, we highlight that sulforaphane cytotoxicity derives from complex, concurring, and multiple mechanisms, among which **the generation of reactive oxygen species has been identified as playing a central role in promoting apoptosis and autophagy of target cells**.

We also discuss the site and the mechanism of reactive oxygen species' formation by sulforaphane, the toxicological relevance of sulforaphane-formed reactive oxygen species, and the death pathways triggered by sulforaphane-derived reactive oxygen species.

Plants constitute a primary and large source of various chemical compounds including alkaloids, flavonoids, phenolics, tocopherols, organic acids, triterpenes, and isothiocyanates.

Belonging to the Cruciferae family, broccoli, cauliflower, cabbage, kale, Brussels sprouts, and radish have been linked to the high content of secondary metabolites and multipharmacological functions.

Clinical and preclinical studies have actually reported that cruciferous vegetables exert anticarcinogenic, anti-inflammatory, and antioxidant activities largely attributed to their content of many bioactive components including flavonoids such as quercetin, minerals such as selenium, and vitamins such as vitamin C. (Williamson et al, 1996) (Finley, Davis, Feng, 2000) (Proteggente et al, 2002)

However, glucosinolates are the most studied bioactive compounds in crucifers associated with cancer protection. They are characterized by a basic structure containing a β-D-thioglucose group, a sulfonated oxime group, and a side chain derived from methionine, phenylalanine, tryptophan, or branched-chain amino acids.

Of note, glucosinolates are not bioactive until they have been transformed to a chemically related isothiocyanate (ITC) by a hydrolytic reaction catalyzed by the endogenous enzyme myrosinase. The hydrolytic reaction takes place when myrosinase is released by disruption of the plant cell during harvesting, processing, or chewing of cruciferous vegetables or if the plant myrosinase has been denatured by cooking and by bacterial myrosinase in the human colon.

One of the most promising and characterized anticancer ITCs is sulforaphane (SF), generally found as glucoraphanin in high concentrations in broccoli.

SF is passively absorbed by cells, where it is rapidly conjugated with glutathione (GSH) by glutathione S-transferases (GSTs). Then, it is metabolized sequentially by γ-glutamyl-transpeptidase, cysteinyl-glycinease, and N-acetyltransferase, and the derived conjugates are transported into the systemic circulation.

The major urinary excretion products are mercapturic acid and cysteine conjugate forms. (Egner et al, 2011)

In blood, SF can achieve μmolar concentrations and accumulate in tissues. Rat treatment with a single oral dose of $50\,\mu$mol of SFR leads to a peak plasma concentration of about $20\,\mu$M. (Hu Hebbar et al, 2004)

However, **after dietary consumption, SF levels in humans are lower and closer to $3\,\mu$M**. (Ye et al, 2002)

SF administered orally protects against animal carcinogenesis and induces antiproliferative effects in human tumor cells in xenograft models. Mechanisms of cancer chemoprevention by SF are diversified and include the alterations of carcinogen metabolism through the induction of Nrf2-regulated genes of Phase-II detoxification enzymes (glutathione S-transferase, quinone reductase, glucuronosyltransferase, etc.) and the inhibition of Phase-I enzymes that activate toxic chemical compounds, thus lowering the levels of the carcinogens interacting with DNA.

Of note, the inducer activity was also reported in humans. A placebo-controlled dose escalation study demonstrated that dietary SF-containing broccoli sprout extracts upregulate mRNA levels for Nrf2-dependent enzymes (heme oxygenase 1, NAD(P)H:quinone oxidoreductase-1, and glutathione transferases) in nasal lavage.

The modulation of epigenetic marks is a third mechanism that has been suggested to be involved in the anticancer activity of SF.

Herein, we highlight that SF cytotoxicity derives from complex, concurring, and multiple mechanisms, among which the generation of reactive oxygen species has been identified as playing a central role in promoting apoptosis and autophagy of target cells.

Furthermore, we critically review the scientific knowledge about the site and the mechanism of reactive oxygen species (ROS) formation by SF, the toxicological relevance of SF-formed ROS, and the death pathways triggered by SF-derived ROS.

ROS Signaling in Cancer

Cancer is generally associated with a prooxidative shift in the redox state. Since cancer patients often present reduced glucose clearance capacity, high glycolytic activity, and lactate production, it has been suggested that **the observed prooxidative shift is mediated by an enhanced availability of mitochondrial energy substrate**. (Droge, 2002)

ROS can favor mutagenesis, tumor promotion, and progression. Indeed, they are able to induce DNA and protein damage, damage to tumor suppressor genes, and increased expression of proto-oncogenes. **Damage to DNA by ROS has been widely accepted as a major cause of cancer**. (Ames, 1983)

RMH Note: This refers to the nullified notions of Bruce Ames.

In patients with pathologies associated with a risk of cancer such as Fanconi's anemia, chronic hepatitis, or cystic fibrosis, an increased rate of oxidative DNA damage or deficient DNA repair system has been observed. The ROS-induced mutations include a range of specifically oxidized purines and pyrimidines, alkali labile sites, single-strand breaks, and instability formed directly or by repair processes.

Although all the four DNA bases can be modified by ROS, mutations mainly involve modification of GC base pairs, while AT base pair mutations are rarely observed. In humans, $G \rightarrow T$ transversions are the most frequent mutations observed in the p53 suppressor gene of tumor cells.

High levels of mutated bases observed in neoplastic tissues may be due to the production of large amount of H_2O_2. (Szatrowski, Nathan, 1991)

Also the high incidence of prostatic carcinoma in men aged > 50 years, the paucity of chemicals causally linked to the onset and development of this specific tumor, and the increased ROS production by mitochondria detected in aged tissues led to hypothesizing an association between prostate cancer and endogenously formed genotoxins that accumulate in later life like ROS. (Sikka, 2003)

RMH Note: I believe that EMODs are there as a protective response against cancer, not as a cause of cancer.

The proliferative effects of ROS are related to redox-responsive cell signaling cascades, and sometimes increased proliferation and expression of growth-related genes are observed even in normal cells if exposed to H_2O_2 or O_2^-. Although the role of ROS in cell growth regulation is cell-type specific and dependent upon the form of the oxidant as well as the concentration of the particular ROS, the modification of gene expression by ROS has been found to affect cell proliferation and apoptosis through the activation of transcription factors including MAPK, AP-1, and NF-κB pathways.

Likewise, **ROS can function as second messengers and activate NF-κB by tumor necrosis factor and cytokines**. (Waris, Ahsan, 2006)

Finally, oxidative stress is involved in malignant transformation. Epithelial-mesenchymal transition, characterized by loss of cell-cell junctions, polarity and epithelial markers, and acquisition of mesenchymal features and motility, has been suggested to be involved in cancer progression and metastasis.

Recently, it has been found that **matrix metalloproteinases cause epithelial-mesenchymal transition associated with malignant transformation *via* a pathway dependent upon production of ROS**. (Cichon, Radisky, 2014)

Putative Role of ROS in the Cytotoxic and Anticancer Activity of SF

The term hormesis is used to describe the apparently paradoxical phenomenon in which a specific compound induces biologically opposite effects depending on its concentration:

in particular, there is a stimulatory or beneficial effect at low doses and an inhibitory or toxic effect at higher ones.

Today there is general consensus on the fact that **SF (and some other ITCs) can be considered as a hormetic moiety**; that is, **at low doses it exerts chemopreventive, indirect antioxidant, and cytoprotective effects, while at higher doses it exhibits cytotoxic and antitumor properties.** (Zanichelli et al, 2012) (Zanichelli, Capasso, et al, 2012)

This scenario paves the way to a double exploitation of SFR in cancer, as a chemopreventive agent to reduce the onset of tumors through diets enriched in functional foods, as well as a direct antineoplastic agent at higher dosage regimens more reliably attainable through pharmaceutical delivery of purified SFR. (Fimognari, Hrelia, 2007)

Most of the studies have been aimed at elucidating the chemopreventive activity of SF, which, as above reported, has been attributed to its indirect antioxidant capacity involving the activation of Phase-II detoxification enzymes and the inhibition of Phase-I enzymes: in this light, SF acts by strengthening the cellular defenses against oxidative damage and promoting the removal of carcinogens.

However, increasing attention has been devoted to the cytotoxic and anticancer activity since the discovery of SF antitumor effects in pancreatic carcinoma cells and other tumor cell lines. Notably, **all the studies dealing with SF toxicity report that these effects occur at concentrations above 5–10 μM, that is, levels which can be barely maintained through cruciferous diet intake.** (Fimognari et al, 2014)

SFR cytotoxicity seems to derive from complex, concurring, and multiple mechanisms. Among these mechanisms, **the generation of ROS is important in promoting apoptosis and autophagy of target cells.** (Doudiccan et al, 2012) (Xiao et al, 2009)

Indeed, Singh et al. reported that **high concentrations of SF caused extensive death in prostate cancer cells, an effect which could be prevented by catalase overexpression.** (Singh et al, 2005)

ROS generation in SF-treated cells was accompanied by disruption of mitochondrial membrane potential, cytosolic release of cytochrome C, cleavage of poly-ADP-ribose polymerase, and apoptosis. (Singh et al, 2005)

ROS generation is *per se* a potentially toxic phenomenon, (I disagree!) but it is important noting that **cells treated with high**

doses of SF undergo a situation of increased ROS sensitivity since a peculiar capacity of the isothiocyanate consists in depleting the GSH cellular pool, an effect which is particularly severe with high, supranutritional SFR concentrations. (Liu et al, 2008) (Kim et al, 2003)

Indeed, depletion of GSH deprives cells of a first line, soluble antioxidant defense, giving rise to a "vicious oxidative cycle" (ROS production in cells which at the same time are being depleted in GSH) which is indirectly demonstrated by the fact that **N-acetylcysteine (NAC) supplementation enhanced cell survival opposing to GSH depletion** rather than acting itself as a mere, direct antioxidant.

An important issue arising from the above studies is where and how ROS are formed.

As to the site and the mechanism of ROS formation by SF, it was noted that **mitochondrial respiratory complex inhibitors prevented SF-caused ROS generation, an event which was paralleled by increased cell survival**. (Xiao et al, 2009) (Singh et al, 2005)

Similarly, **cells with respiration deficient phenotype were significantly less sensitive as compared to respiratory proficient, wild-type cells, and they did not produce ROS upon SF treatment**. (Xiao et al, 2009) (Singh et al, 2005)

SF-caused ROS have been detected and visualized in cultured cells by means of specific dyes such as dihydrorhodamine or dihydrodichlorofluorescein which fluoresce upon oxidation by ROS: importantly the conditions described above (i.e., the use of respiratory complexes inhibitors, cells bearing respiratory deficient phenotype) prevented the oxidation of these dyes caused by SF. Thus, **mitochondria are likely to represent the site where SF promotes ROS generation**.

This finding is in keeping with the observation that loss of mitochondrial transmembrane potential, release of cytochrome C, and mitochondrial damage are in effect induced by SF and other ITCs. The molecular interaction of SF with mitochondria has also been studied: **it appeared that SF is capable of inhibiting, probably *via* electrophilic interactions with specific SH residues, mitochondrial respiratory chain Complex I, Complex II, and Complex III**. (Xiao et al, 2009)

However, although confirming Complex I, Complex II, and Complex III inhibition, a more recent study by our group indicated that the major and likely most crucial inhibition affects Complex III. Indeed, using pharmacological inhibitors of respiratory complexes, we showed that

rotenone, but also myxothiazol, prevented ROS formation in SF intoxicated Jurkat leukemia cells.

Rotenone is likely to hamper ROS formation in SF-treated cells because, as a Complex I inhibitor, it impedes at the origin the electron flow to other, possibly pivotal targets located downstream, such as Complex III. Indeed, myxothiazol, which was as effective as rotenone in preventing SF-derived ROS, is a selective Complex III inhibitor, which blocks the electron flow through this complex and, importantly, the accumulation of ubisemiquinone (see below).

Its efficacy indirectly demonstrates that SF (at least up to $30 \mu M$, the highest concentration tested in this study) does not affect electron flow through the respiratory chain upstream to Complex III since, if electrons do not reach this site, myxothiazol would not prevent SF-caused ROS formation. Notably, **chemical inhibition of Complex III by agents acting as antimycin A (i.e., differently from myxothiazol) is known to represent a common and toxicologically relevant mechanism capable of boosting ROS generation within mitochondria**. (Cantoni, Guidarelli, 2008)

Indeed, this latter mode of inhibiting Complex III, which is **likely shared by SF, causes an accumulation of ubisemiquinone which starts serving as an electron donor for molecular oxygen in a reaction producing superoxide anion and its dismutation product H_2O_2**, which undergoes Fenton reaction and finally attacks sensitive cellular targets.

Thus, **SF does not undergo any direct oxidation/reduction reaction leading to ROS or radical species by-products but rather promotes the onset of mitochondrial events culminating in ROS formation through its antimycin-like Complex III inhibitory properties**.

The next important issues refer to the toxicological relevance of mitochondrially formed ROS and to which death pathways are triggered by SF-derived ROS.

One of the most sensitive cellular targets of ROS is nuclear DNA, where ROS cause extensive damage. Evidence of some genotoxic activity of SFR and other ITCs had already emerged, but the first study investigating the DNA damaging activity of SF was that by Sekine-Suzuki et al. reporting that **SF induces DNA double strand breaks in the nuclear DNA of HeLa cervical cancer cells**. (Sekine-Suzuki et al, 2008)

However, these authors did not investigate the mechanism of the DNA damaging effect of SF and they probably detected secondary DNA fragmentation due to the ongoing apoptosis caused by the ITC rather than frank DNA lesions: indeed the exposure times to SF were too long (24 h, i.e., a time conceivable with the onset of apoptosis) as compared to the kinetic of ROS formation in SF intoxicated cells (1–3 h).

In our previously cited study, we specifically addressed the relationship between ROS formation and DNA damage in SF-treated human leukemia and umbilical vein endothelial cells. We found that **SF causes DNA single strand breaks (i.e., the type of lesion typically induced by ROS, unlike double strand breaks which are generated only in the presence of very high ROS concentrations**) with a kinetic (1–3 h) which paralleled that of ROS formation in SF-treated cells. (Sestili et al, 1986)

Furthermore, it was found that **all the conditions blocking the mitochondrial respiratory chain and in particular myxothiazol, or quenching ROS by means of the iron chelator o-phenanthroline, prevented DNA damage**.

These findings clearly indicate that ROS, produced *via* the antimycin-like interaction of SF with mitochondrial respiratory chain at the Complex III level and then diffusing within the nucleus, are responsible for the observed DNA lesions.

Recent observations have extended our knowledge on SFR interactions with DNA homeostasis since, besides its ROS-mediated DNA damaging capacity, **SF was also shown to inhibit DNA repair processes**.

SF sensitized HeLa cells to X-irradiation, and the radiosensitization was ascribed to the capacity of SF of inhibiting the two major processes of DNA double-strand breaks repair (DNA double-strand breaks are a highly toxic DNA lesion typically and efficiently caused by ionizing radiations), namely, homologous recombination repair and non-homologous end joining. Accordingly, other authors found that **high SF concentrations decrease the expression of a number of DNA repair genes and inhibit nuclear excision repair *via* abstraction of zinc from the xeroderma pigmentosum A (XPA) protein**.

The ROS dependence of these effects has not been addressed, but the picture arising from this further notion is indicative of a marked pleiotropism of the SF-DNA interactions since SFR is simultaneously capable of damaging DNA, inhibiting DNA repair, and finally sensitizing cells to established anticancer agents such as X-rays or doxorubicin mostly acting through a DNA damaging action.

DNA damage, depending on its level and persistence, might promote cell death: indeed **DNA lesions are recognized as efficient pro-apoptotic stimuli**. Hence, ROS-dependent DNA breaks are likely to contribute to SF-induced apoptosis which, in fact, is the type of cell death caused by SF.

Many authors have investigated the role of ROS in SF-induced apoptosis and they invariably reported that <u>ROS (EMODs) generated within mitochondria contribute to or are fully responsible for the apoptotic response</u>. (Jo et al, 2014) (Park et al, 2014)

Besides DNA damage, **the proapoptotic events which have been attributed to SF-caused ROS are the collapse of mitochondrial membrane permeability, activation of caspase-3 and caspase-9, downregulation of antiapoptotic Bcl-2 expression, Bax and p53 gene activation, and G2/M phase cell cycle arrest and have been observed in a wide variety of heterogeneous cell lines**.

SF has been shown to induce autophagy in colon and prostate cancer cells and more recently in pancreatic cells: in this cell line, **SF induces autophagy *via* a ROS-dependent mechanism**. SF, at supranutritional and cytotoxic concentrations (20 or 60 μM for 24h), induced a significant increase of autophagosome formation as well as of other reliable markers of autophagy, and **all these effects could be prevented by NAC cotreatment, suggesting that this response is causally related to ROS production or depletion of GSH, that is, two prooxidative events**.

Modulation of autophagy with specific inhibitors (rapamycin or chloroquine) did not affect, however, cell survival in SF-treated cells, suggesting that, at least in this cell system, autophagy does not concur to the actual cytotoxic activity of SF itself. On the contrary, in other cell systems (colon and prostate cancer cells) induction of autophagy by SF seems to exert a cytoprotective effect but, unfortunately, the ROS dependence of the autophagic process had not been investigated in these studies.

Thus, although **the ROS dependence of SF-induced autophagy has been demonstrated by Xiao et al. and Naumann et al.**, the problem of its sensitizing *versus* protective relevance in SF-induced cytotoxicity is not yet clear and needs further investigations. (Xiao et al, 2009) (Naumann et al, 2011)

Taken collectively, **the above reports unequivocally suggest that mitochondrial production of ROS is an important event in high SF concentrations cytotoxicity**.

However, there is not clear consensus on the relative contribution of ROS-dependent mechanisms to SF toxic capacity. Indeed, **some reports show that abrogating ROS production or quenching ROS almost completely protects target cells from SF killing**, while another found that similar conditions granted only a partial protection. (Singh et al, 2005) (Xiao et al, 2009) (Choi et al, 2008)

One possible explanation may relate to cell-type specific effects: indeed different cell lines have been used in these studies. Another possible explanation is that some studies interpreted the full prevention of SF cell killing by NAC as a neat antioxidant effect; that is, acting as an antioxidant NAC quenches ROS-derived SFR thus abrogating SF toxicity. However, it is of worth that **preloading of cells with fairly high doses (2–10 mM) of a –SH-bearing compound such as NAC is likely to prevent also the fall of GSH stores in cells exposed to the comparatively low doses (1–30 μM) of SF used in these studies: in this light, the full protection of NAC would not be solely dependent on the presumed quantitative quenching of SF-caused ROS, but rather it would reflect the cumulative effect of GSH preservation plus that of ROS scavenging**.

Indeed, **another study showed that an established antioxidant which cannot, unlike NAC, serve as GSH repletive, namely, o-phenanthroline, abrogated ROS production and the ensuing DNA damage but did not completely protect cells from SF toxicity**. (Sestili et al, 2010)

Similar results were obtained with inhibitors of mitochondrial respiratory chain. (Sestili et al, 2010)

Interestingly, all these conditions prevented SFR-induced ROS but did not prevent the fall in cellular GSH, an effect which, on the contrary, is likely to be afforded by NAC.

In this light, the catastrophic depletion of cellular GSH caused by high SFR concentrations would represent *per se* another cytotoxically relevant phenomenon. In addition, this same event may act additively or synergistically with ROS with its own contribution to generate oxidatively stressing/sensitizing conditions, that is, the "*vicious oxidative cycle*" described at the beginning of this chapter: notably, Han et al. showed that, **below certain threshold levels, mitochondrial GSH depletion increases ROS production and diffusion under conditions of Complex III inhibition.** (Han et al, 2003)

That ROS are not the only mediators of SF toxicity is also suggested by the finding that SF inhibits protein synthesis in human prostate cancer cells *via* a ROS insensitive mechanism. (Wiczk et al, 2012)

A selective toxicity of SFR to cancer cells has been demonstrated in different experimental models.

As an example, **SF induces cytotoxic and cytostatic effects in different prostate cancer cell lines, but not in their normal counterpart.** (Clarke et al, 2011)

On the basis of different observations, **several studies strongly suggest a role of ROS (EMODs) in the selective toxicity to cancer cells by SF**.

SFR-induced ROS causes membrane lipid peroxidation and generation of 4-hydroxynonenal and **apoptotic signals generated by SF can be abrogated by inhibiting SF-induced lipid peroxidation and accumulation of 4-hydroxynonenal.** This evidence supports the pivotal role that 4-hydroxynonenal plays in the biological activity of SF. (Sharma, Sharma et al, 2010)

4-Hydroxynonenal is an important second messenger involved in signaling for cell proliferation and apoptosis and in regulating gene expression in different cell types.

In particular, it evokes dichotomous effects through the activation of the defense mechanisms against oxidative stress, such as Nrf2 and heat shock factor 1, at low concentrations and the induction of apoptosis at higher, supraphysiologic ones.

Thus, it is possible that similar dichotomous effects of SFN are responsible for its differential effects on normal and cancer cells.

The ability of SFR to generate ROS and oxidative stress in cells leading to the activation of proapoptotic signaling and simultaneously activate defense mechanisms, such as Nrf2, that protect against oxidative stress and its intrinsic toxicity is consistent with the above reported hypothesis. Generation of 4-hydroxynonenal upon cell exposure to SRF could therefore represent an event implicated in its selective effects on cancer cells.

Conclusion

Although further studies are needed to clarify the relative importance of ROS in SF toxicity, **the effects which tie SF to ROS generation are definitely important for the ITC's cytotoxic activity** and may represent the bases for its rationale exploitation in cancer therapy as a single agent or in association with other antineoplastic agents or drugs to potentiate their anticancer efficacy.

SF generates ROS-apoptosis of human leukemia cells

Sulforaphane generates reactive oxygen species leading to mitochondrial perturbation for apoptosis in human leukemia U937 cells.

Abstract

Sulforaphane, an isothiocyanate found in cruciferous vegetables, has been shown to possess growth-inhibiting and apoptosis-inducing activities in cancer cell lines in vitro. In order to further explore the critical events leading to apoptosis in sulforaphane-treated U937 human leukemia cells, the following effects of sulforaphane on components of the mitochondrial apoptotic pathway were examined: generation of reactive oxygen species (ROS), alteration of the mitochondrial membrane potential (MMP), and the expression changes of Bcl-2 family proteins. The cytotoxic effect of sulforaphane was mediated by its induction of apoptosis as characterized by the occurrence of DNA ladders, apoptotic bodies and chromosome condensation in U937 cells. The sulforaphane-induced apoptosis in U937 cells correlated with the generation of intracellular ROS, collapse of MMP, activation of caspase-3, and downregulation of anti-apoptotic Bcl-2 expression. The quenching of ROS generation with antioxidant N-acetyl-L-cysteine conferred significant protection against sulforaphane-elicited ROS generation, disruption of the MMP, caspase-3 activation and apoptosis. In conclusion, the present study reveals that the **cellular ROS generation plays a pivotal role in the initiation of sulforaphane-triggered apoptotic death in U937 cells.** (Choi et al, 2008)

Mitochondrial reactive oxygen species in cell death signaling

Abstract

During apoptosis, mitochondrial membrane permeability (MMP) increases and the release into the cytosol of pro-apoptotic factors (procaspases, caspase activators and caspase-independent factors such as apoptosis-inducing factor (AIF)) leads to the apoptotic phenotype. Apart from this pivotal role of mitochondria during the execution phase of apoptosis (documented in other reviews of this issue), **it appears that reactive oxygen species (ROS) produced by the mitochondria can be involved in cell death.** These toxic compounds are normally detoxified by the cells, failing which oxidative stress occurs. However, ROS are not only dangerous molecules for the cell, but they also display a physiological role, as mediators in signal transduction pathways. **ROS participate in early and late steps of the regulation of apoptosis, according to different possible molecular mechanisms**. In agreement with this role of ROS in apoptosis signaling, inhibition of apoptosis by anti-apoptotic Bcl-2 and Bcl-x(L) is associated with a protection against ROS and/or a shift of the cellular redox potential to a more reduced state.

Furthermore, **the fact that active forms of cell death in yeast and plants also involve ROS suggests the existence of an ancestral redox-sensitive death signaling pathway that has been independent of caspases and Bcl-2**. (Fleury et al, 2002)

SF induction of antioxidant enzymes

Induction of Phase 2 Antioxidant Enzymes by Broccoli Sulforaphane: Perspectives in Maintaining the Antioxidant Activity of Vitamins A, C, and E

(Boddupalli et al, 2012)

Consumption of fruits and vegetables is recognized as an important part of a healthy diet. Increased consumption of cruciferous vegetables in particular has been associated with a decreased risk of several degenerative and chronic diseases, including cardiovascular disease and certain cancers.

Members of the cruciferous vegetable family, which includes broccoli, Brussels sprouts, cauliflower, and cabbage, accumulate significant concentrations of glucosinolates, which are metabolized *in vivo* to biologically active isothiocyanates (ITCs).

The ITC sulforaphane (SF), which is derived from glucoraphanin, has garnered particular interest as an indirect antioxidant due to its extraordinary ability to induce expression of several enzymes via the KEAP1/Nrf2/ARE pathway. Nrf2/ARE gene products are typically characterized as Phase II detoxification enzymes and/or antioxidant (AO) enzymes.

Over the last decade, human clinical studies have begun to provide *in vivo* evidence of both Phase II and AO enzyme induction by SF. Many AO enzymes are redox cycling enzymes that maintain redox homeostasis and activity of free radical scavengers such as vitamins A, C, and E. In this review, we present the existing evidence for induction of PII and AO enzymes by SF, the interactions of SF-induced AO enzymes and proposed maintenance of the essential vitamins A, C, and E, and, finally, the current view of genotypic effects on ITC metabolism and AO enzyme induction and function.

Fruits and vegetables are recognized as being part of a healthy diet with current U.S. dietary guidelines reflecting this relationship (U. S. Department of Agriculture, and U. S. Department of Health, 2010).

While fruits and vegetables represent a nutrient-dense, low-fat, low-calorie food option, evidence also suggests that their consumption may reduce the risk of several degenerative and chronic diseases. In particular, diets rich in cruciferous vegetables have demonstrated potential health benefits for their association with a decreased risk of cardiovascular disease and certain types of cancer. The exact mechanisms and potential bioactives underlying this relationship have been the subject of intense investigation over the last several decades.

Cruciferous vegetables are a rich source of thioglycoside precursors of isothiocyanates (ITCs) called glucosinolates. Upon consumption, glucosinolates are hydrolyzed by myrosinase (β-thioglucoside glucohydrolase, EC 3.2.1.147), which is normally segregated from glucosinolates in plants, to their representative ITCs through the action of physical damage to the plant (i.e., chewing).

There is also evidence that glucosinolates are hydrolyzed in the colon through the actions of gut microorganisms.

Broccoli accumulates significant amounts of 4-methylsulfinylbutyl glucosinolate (4-MSB) or glucoraphanin. SF has been intensively studied not only due to the high concentration of GR in broccoli florets and sprouts but also due to its extraordinary ability to induce antioxidant response element (ARE) gene products.

While out of the scope of this review, evidence for additional mechanisms of action have also been described for SF, namely modulation of P450 enzymes, induction of apoptosis, inhibition of cell proliferation, inhibition of angiogenesis and metastasis, and modulation of histone deacetylase activity. The biological impact of SF, especially in modulating cytoprotective mechanisms, underscores the potential health benefits, and research interest into SF.

Cruciferous vegetables like broccoli are not only important sources of phytonutrients like SF but are also important dietary sources of many essential nutrients like vitamins A, C, and E. The interaction between SF and vitamins A, C, and E may play a significant dietary protective role during times of oxidative stress. This is especially important when the balance of cellular redox status shifts from a reductive to an oxidative environment.

These changes mediate cell signaling cascades through changes in redox tone. (Landar and Darley-Usmar, 2003) (Landar A., Darley-Usmar V. M. (2003). Nitric oxide and cell signaling: modulation of redox tone and protein modification. Amino Acids 25, 313–321 10.1007/s00726-003-0019-7)

The phytonutrient SF affects redox tone by modulating induction of ARE-dependent gene products, namely through phase II detoxification and antioxidant (AO) enzymes, which participate in the recycling and maintenance of vitamins A, C, and E, maintaining cellular redox balance.

Nutrigenomics, Sulforaphane, and Phase II Enzymes

With the advent and use of omics technologies (**genomics, transcriptomics, proteomics, and metabolomics**) there is an increasing awareness and desire to understand the systemic response to nutritional and dietary interventions. Nutrigenomics, which is defined as "the scientific study of the way specific genes and bioactives interact", has been embraced as an approach to help understand the complex and systemic interactions of diet at the individual level. (Trujillo et al., 2006)

While epidemiological studies have demonstrated a relatively consistent relationship between vegetable consumption and human health, this relationship has failed to prove conclusive. (World Cancer Research Fund, and American Institute for Cancer Research, 2007).

Accordingly, efforts have been made to identify genetic factors that may modify the effects of dietary components on disease risk.

Sulforaphane metabolism

The absorption, distribution, metabolism, and excretion characteristics of bioactives influence their ultimate effectiveness on health and wellness. GSTs play an important role in ITC metabolism and disposition in humans.

Upon absorption, ITCs are conjugated to glutathione by GSTs and further metabolized via the mercapturic acid pathway and ultimately excreted as N-acetylcysteine conjugates.

The relationship between GST genotype, SF/ITC metabolism, and human health remains far from clear.

Antioxidant or redox enzymes

Major biological actions of SF are mediated by the induction of antioxidant enzymes regulated by the Nrf2/ARE pathway. Genetic polymorphisms within the ARE family of antioxidant enzymes could have a profound effect on the functional outcomes of cruciferous vegetable intake and impact on health. (Ginsberg et al., 2010)

Polymorphisms within antioxidant enzymes undoubtedly affect their actions, yet whether the interaction occurs at the expression or activity level is unclear. Nonetheless, the influence of polymorphisms within many antioxidant enzymes ultimately affects the metabolism and actions of SF and the recycling and maintenance of vitamins A, C, and E.

There remain significant challenges ahead; yet through the implementation of omics technologies, we can gain further insight into the relationship between SF consumption and health and wellness.

Summary and Conclusion

Evidence continues to accumulate relating the dietary consumption of SF-containing cruciferous vegetables and chronic and degenerative disease reduction. While a number of potential mechanisms have been put forth to help explain this relationship, the strongest evidence, at least in *in vitro* and in animal models, supports SF's role in the induction of PII drug metabolizing and antioxidant enzymes. **However, these findings have not been as clear when extended to functional or clinical outcomes**.

There is evidence of induction of ARE-mediated gene products in humans, yet **translation to disease reduction, especially cancer risk, has proven difficult**. Furthermore, little effort has been done to understand the effects of polymorphisms on potential downstream effectors of ITCs, such as PII and AO enzymes.

In summary, consumption of SF results in the induction of key enzymes involved in the cellular antioxidant network, and many of these same enzymes also appear to play a role in the maintenance and redox recycling of the essential vitamins A, C, and E.

Polymorphisms within many antioxidant enzymes affect the metabolism and actions of SF, which in turn may affect the recycling and maintenance of vitamins A, C, and E. The challenge and opportunity ahead is to provide a direct link between dietary substances that are direct antioxidants and phytonutrients that induce antioxidant enzymes. (Boddupalli, 2012)

http://www.ncbi.nlm.nih.gov/pmc/articles/PMC3264924/

SF inhibits breast cancer stem cells

Sulforaphane, a Dietary Component of Broccoli/Broccoli Sprouts, Inhibits Breast Cancer Stem Cells

(Yanyan et al, 2010)

The existence of cancer stem cells (CSCs) in breast cancer has profound implications for cancer prevention. In this study, we evaluated sulforaphane, a natural compound derived from broccoli/broccoli sprouts, for its efficacy to inhibit breast CSCs and its potential mechanism.

Experimental Design

Aldefluor assay and mammosphere formation assay were used to evaluate the effect of sulforaphane on breast CSCs *in vitro*. A NOD/SCID xenograft model was employed to determine whether sulforaphane could target breast CSCs *in vivo*, as assessed by Aldefluor assay and tumor growth upon cell re-implantation in secondary mice. The potential mechanism was investigated utilizing Western blotting analysis and β-catenin reporter assay.

Results

Sulforaphane (1~5 μM) decreased aldehyde dehydrogenase (ALDH)-positive cell population by 65%~80% in human breast cancer cells (P < 0.01), and reduced the size and number of primary mammospheres by 8~125-fold and 45%~75% (P < 0.01), respectively. Daily injection with 50 mg/kg sulforaphane for two weeks reduced ALDH-positive cells by more than 50% in NOD/SCID xenograft tumors (P = 0.003). **Sulforaphane eliminated breast CSCs *in vivo*, thereby abrogating tumor growth after re-implantation of primary tumor cells into the secondary mice** (P < 0.01). Western blotting analysis and β-catenin reporter assay showed that sulforaphane down-regulated Wnt/β-catenin self-renewal pathway.

Conclusions

Sulforaphane inhibits breast CSCs and down-regulates Wnt/β-catenin self-renewal pathway. These findings support the use of sulforaphane for chemoprevention of breast cancer stem cells and warrant further clinical evaluation.

Sulforaphane was shown to target pancreatic tumor-initiating cells in a very recent report. (Kallifatidis et al, 2009) (Kallifatidis G, Rausch V, Baumann B, et al. Sulforaphane targets pancreatic tumour-initiating cells by NF-kappaB-induced antiapoptotic signalling. Gut. 2009;58:949–63)

On May 18, 2015 Dr. Mercola said: 1) The so-called "broccoli pill" (Sulforadex) consists of a stabilized, synthetic form of sulforaphane. 2) Sulforaphane helps to lower the risk of cancer, slow cancer growth and stop its spread, 3) One of the best ways to maximize sulforaphane in broccoli is to steam it lightly for three to four minutes until it's tough-tender and 4) Broccoli sprouts also offer a particularly concentrated source of phytochemicals, including sulforaphane.

Sulforaphane is found in cruciferous vegetables, including not only broccoli but also Brussels sprouts, cabbage, cauliflower, horseradish, and arugula. Broccoli sprouts are the richest source.

Sulforaphane has anti-microbial properties and kills cancer stem cells, which slows tumor growth. It also normalizes DNA methylation, which plays a role in a number of diseases, including hypertension, kidney function, gut health and cancer.

It has been called "one of the most powerful anticarcinogens found in food" because it increases enzymes in the liver that help destroy cancer-causing chemicals.

Sulforaphane is usually unstable and must be kept at minus 20 degrees Fahrenheit.

Sulforaphane is formed when you chew or chop broccoli and your gut bacteria help release the sulforaphane. However, sulforaphane is attached to a sugar molecule with a sulfur bond and Science Daily reported, "When broccoli enzyme breaks off the sugar to release the sulforaphane, a sulfur-grabbing protein can remove the newly exposed sulfur on the sulforaphane and inactivate it."

A company called Evgen reportedly stabilized the compound. Clinical trials are being conducted on Sulforadex at this time and is also being tested to reduce arthritic joint pain.

Researchers stated in the Journal of Food Science that **frozen broccoli may not contain sulforaphane**.

Another phytochemical in broccoli is diindolylmethane (DIM), which is believed to boost the immune system and help to prevent or treat cancer. Scientists at the Linus Pauling Institute suggest that **DIM may trigger EMOD-induced apoptosis in cancer cells**.

DIM is also found in other cruciferous vegetables but it would require eating 2 pounds a day to get the required amount.

Some argue that this suggests that supplements are better than natural food sources of sulforaphane or DIM.

When phytochemicals like sulforaphane are excluded, watercress may be the most nutrient-dense vegetable available and watercress contains phenylethyl isothiocyanate (PEITC), which may suppress breast cancer cells.

On October 27, 2014, Dr. Mercola said: 1) Sulforaphane can improve your blood pressure and kidney function by normalizing DNA methylation, 2) Preliminary research suggests sulforaphane may also be of benefit in autism, improving verbal communication an decreasing repetitive behaviors, 3) Broccoli has the ability to affect gene expression and promote detoxification of harmful environmental pollutants, 4) Sulforaphane influences bacteria as well and inhibit Helicobacter pylori, 5) Autistic children are known to have higher levels of environmental toxins in their system, as well as fewer health-promoting gut bacteria.

Broccoli and broccoli sprouts contain large amounts of glucosinolates. Numerous studies have substantiated the chemoprevention effect of increasing cruciferous vegetable intake against cancer, which has been attributed to the activity of various isothiocyanates that are enzymatically hydrolyzed from glucosinolates.

Sulforaphane was found to be converted from glucoraphanin, a major glucosinolate in broccoli/broccoli sprouts. The chemoprevention properties of sulforaphane against cancer are through both "blocking" and "suppressing" effects.

Sulforaphane was also shown to suppress angiogenesis and metastasis by down-regulating VEGF, HIF-1α, MMP-2 and MMP-9.

Accumulating evidence has shown that many types of cancer, including breast cancer, are initiated from and maintained by a small population of cancer stem cells (CSCs).

Several dietary compounds, such as **curcumin** (Wang et al, 2006) (Jaiswal et al, 2002), **quercetin and epigallocatechin-gallate** (Pahlke et al, 2006), **were found to be potentially against CSC self-renewal**.

Taken together with the in vivo Aldefluor assay results, these findings suggest that sulforaphane targets breast CSCs with high potency.

The anti-cancer efficacy of sulforaphane, a natural compound derived from broccoli/broccoli sprouts, has been evaluated in various cancers. For instance, **oral or intraperitoneal administration of sulforaphane inhibited the tumor growth in prostate PC-3 and pancreatic Panc-1 xenografts**. (Pham et al, 2004) (Singh et al, 2004)

A very recent study demonstrated the effectiveness of sulforaphane in abrogating pancreatic tumor resistance to TRAIL by interfering with NF-κB induced anti-apoptotic signaling. Another study indicated that **sulforaphane could overcome doxorubicin resistance and restore apoptosis induction in cells**. (Fimognari et al, 2006)

These findings provide a strong rationale for investigating the chemoprevention property of sulforaphane or broccoli/broccoli sprouts in clinical trials.

As a chemoprevention agent, **sulforaphane possesses many advantages, such as high bioavailability and low toxicity.** (Zang, Tang, 2007)

Sulforaphane from broccoli extracts is efficiently and rapidly absorbed in human small intestine, and distributed throughout the body. (Ye et al, 2002)

In conclusion, we have demonstrated that **sulforaphane was able to target breast CSCs as determined by the mammosphere formation assay, Aldefluor assay, and tumor growth upon reimplantation in secondary mice**.

These findings provide a strong rationale for preclinical and clinical evaluation of sulforaphane or broccoli/broccoli sprouts for breast cancer therapies. (Li et al, 2010)

Prostate cancer

Prostate cancer is one of the most common cancers in men and is the second leading cause of male cancer death in the United States. An estimated 220,900 new cases and 28,900 deaths from prostate cancer cells occurred in 2003. However, men in Asia have a much lower incidence and mortality of prostate cancer than do men in

North America and Europe. The differences in the cancer incidence among ethnic groups are believed to be due to different lifestyles and environmental factors. Asians who emigrated from their native countries to the United States and adopted Western lifestyles typically experienced an increasing incidence of hormone-related cancers, suggesting that the diet in their native countries may have a role in protecting against hormone-related cancers. It has been estimated that more than two-thirds of human cancers can be prevented by modification of lifestyle, including dietary modification. The consumption of fruits, soybeans, and vegetables has been associated with reduced risk of several types of cancers. Epidemiological and dietary studies have shown an association between high dietary intake of vegetables and decreased prostate cancer risk. Indole-3-carbinol (I3C), a phytochemical common in cruciferous vegetables, inhibits carcinogenesis in animal experiments and growth of various cancer cells in culture.

The following was adapted, modified or excerpted from: https://empiricalnutrition.wordpress.com/2013/10/31/the-magic-of-broccoli-2/ This entry was posted on October 31, 2013 by Jacob Libby.

The Magic of Broccoli

Sulforaphane Isothiocyanate

Conditions of the Mouth, Throat, & Stomach

Abstract

Regular consumption of broccoli is clearly associated with lower instance of multiple forms of cancer.

Broccoli contains multiple well-studied compounds that explain this phenomenon. Foremost among these is a substance called sulforaphane. **Sulforaphane cannot be obtained from a pill or from cooked or canned vegetables, but must be ingested in the form of raw broccoli, or better yet, from raw Broccoli sprouts, which are 10 to 100 times stronger**.

Raw broccoli contains large quantities of glucoraphanin and a delicate enzyme called myrosinase. **When you chew it, a chemical interaction takes place that converts glucoraphanin into sulforaphane**.

This small change is necessary to unleash the powerful effects of sulforaphane. There is no better way to access this healing agent than by ingesting well-chewed raw broccoli sprouts.

H. pylori is a spiral-shaped bacteria that digs into the lining of the stomach and small intestine. There, the bacteria damage tissues, stimulate inflammation, contribute to the formation of ulcers, block the stomach's nature defense against bacterial infestation, and increase pH levels.

These changes contribute to the development of gastritis and its progression into a more severe form called chronic atrophic gastritis (CAG). In CAG, permanent changes occur to the structure of the gastric acid secreting ducts, resulting in decreased secretion of gastric acid and vitamin C. **These changes greatly increase the risk of cancers of the stomach and its glandular ducts**.

Multiple strains of H. pylori, including antibiotic-resistant strains, stop reproducing and die off when cultured with relatively low levels of sulforaphane.

When human cells are present, sulforaphane moves into them, builds up to very high concentrations, and for this reason shows even stronger bacteria-killing effects inside the cells. **These antibacterial effects were shown on human stomach cells implanted in mice, on mice infected with H. pylori, and inferred from tests conducted on a small sample of humans.**

Studies show that **these protective effects are associated with sulforaphane's ability to deactivate an enzyme called urease**, which is key to both the bacteria's survival and its disease promotion.

Protective effects in chronic gastritis are also associated with the activation of a protein called Nrf2, which induces the expression of a host of antioxidants as well as detoxifying, anti-cancer, and anti-inflammatory molecules collectively called Phase 2 enzymes.

RMH Note: Nrf2 has been shown to be a prooxidant.

Phase 2 enzymes were examined in the context of chronic periodontal disease, where it was shown that sulforaphane protects against inflammation of the gums through the stimulation of this protein. **They also play a big role in the the anti-cancer properties of sulforaphane, particularly due to increased synthesis of glutathione and an antioxidant called NQO1, which together help to regenerate vitamins A, C, and E**.

In addition to Phase 2 enzyme induction and interrupting the progression of chronic gastritis, sulforaphane acts against cancer via a number of other mechanisms.

Sulforaphane plays a role in blocking cancer's ability to survive without oxygen by altering its metabolism and blocking the formation of blood vessels.

It kills cancer cells by halting cell division and activating programmed pathways for automatic cell death.

RMH Note: Apoptotic induction is predominantly due to prooxidants.

It modulates important pro-inflammatory signaling molecules that have been implicated in the development of cancer. So far the research seems to suggest that in combination, these mechanisms allow sulforaphane to reduce tumor size while protecting adjacent healthy cells from carcinogenesis.

Sulforaphane has shown anti-cancer effects against cancer cells of the liver, prostate, colon, rectum, pancreas, bone, skin, ovaries, cervix, bladder, lung, and breast.

Sulforaphane may be especially therapeutic in conditions of the mouth, throat, and stomach due to its high level of access to these tissues following oral ingestion. With this in mind, **this paper reviews studies on Barret Esophogeal Adenocarcinoma, Oral Squamous Cell Carcinoma, Tongue Cancer, Mucosa-Associated Lymphoid Lymphoma, and Gastric Cancer**.

In addition, sulforaphane has been shown to enhance effects of chemotherapy drugs, perhaps by slowing the excretion of these drugs from the cancer cells. The results are so promising one team of researchers attempted to produce a novel anti-cancer drug based on the basic biochemistry sulforaphane.

Preparation, Ingestion, and Absorption

Broccoli is a member of the *brassica* genus, which comprises the cruciferous category of vegetables as well as several species of turnip and mustard.

It is a cultivated line of the species *Brassica oleracea,* the species to which cruciferous vegetables such kale, collards, cabbage, cauliflower, and brussels sprouts belong.

Hundreds of peer edited research articles have been published linking cruciferous vegetables consumption and the unique phytonutrients they contain to decreased risk of cancer. (Tang et al, 2010) (Bonnesen et al, 2001)

Specifically, the following chemicals have been isolated and studied in the context of cancer prevention and treatment:

1. Benzyl isothiocyanates
2. Phenethyl isothiocyanates
3. 3,3'-diindolylmethane (DIM)
4. Indole-3-carbinol (I3C), including Phase I human trials
5. Ascorbigen, a product of I3C and ascorbic acid
6. Indolo[3,2-b]carbazole
7. Sulforaphane isothiocyanate (hereafter: sulforaphane)

PEITC and EMOD induced apoptosis

The following abstract illustrates that the mechanism for PEITC induction of apoptosis is via prooxidants, as I have said all along. **Translational implication of these findings is that cancer chemopreventive efficacy of PEITC may be compromised in the presence of antioxidants.**

Among various sites of mitochondrial ROS production, complex I (site IQ) and complex III (site IIIQo) have the greatest capacities to produce ROS. Whereas complex I produces superoxide in the mitochondrial matrix, ROS production by the complex III is now believed to be directed toward both matrix and intermembrane space at about equal rates under de-energized conditions.

Phenethyl isothiocyanate (PEITC), a constituent of edible cruciferous vegetables such as watercress, not only affords significant protection against chemically induced cancer in experimental rodents but also inhibits growth of human cancer cells by causing apoptotic and autophagic cell death. However, the underlying mechanism of PEITC-induced cell death is not fully understood. Using LNCaP and PC-3 human prostate cancer cells as a model, we demonstrate that the PEITC-induced cell death is initiated by production of reactive oxygen species (ROS, EMODs) **resulting from inhibition of oxidative phosphorylation (OXPHOS).**

In conclusion, the present study provides novel insight into the molecular circuitry of PEITC-induced cell death involving ROS production due to inhibition of complex III and OXPHOS. (Xiao et al, 2010)

Beta-Phenylethyl isothiocyanate (PEITC) is a promising chemoprotective compound that is routinely consumed in the diet as its glucosinolate precursor. Furthermore, we also demonstrate **a concentration- and time-dependant burst of superoxide (O_2^-) in PEITC-treated cells**.

However, pre- and co-treatment with the free radical scavengers Trolox, ascorbate, mannitol, uric acid and the superoxide mimetic manganese (III) tetrakis (N-methyl-2-pyridyl) porphyrin failed to prevent PEITC-mediated apoptosis. Taken together, these results suggest that PEITC potently induces apoptosis and cell cycle arrest in HepG2 cells and that the generation of reactive oxygen species appears to be a secondary effect. (Rose et al, 2003)

Phenethyl isothiocyanate (PEITC) is a natural isothiocyanate with anticancer activity against many drug-resistant cancer cells. **A body of evidence suggests that PEITC enhances oxidative stress leading to cancer cell death**. PEITC rapidly kills KKU-100 CCA cells with concurrent induction of cellular glutathione depletion, superoxide formation, and loss of mitochondrial transmembrane potential. The loss was associated with increased Bax and decreased Bcl-xl proteins followed by the release of cytochrome c and the activation of caspase-9 and -3. Although TEMPOL could prevent superoxide formation, it did not prevent the disruption of glutathione (GSH) redox, mitochondrial dysfunction, and cell death.

On the other hand, N-acetylcysteine could prevent the events and cell death. Curiously, it was concluded that disruption of GSH redox but not superoxide formation may be an initial step leading to mitochondrial injury. PEITC could be a promising chemopreventive agent for CCA. (Tusskom et al, 2013)

Still, others continue to find prooxidants responsible for induction of apoptosis as follows: Benzyl isothiocyanate–induced apoptosis in human breast cancer cells is initiated by reactive oxygen species and regulated by Bax and Bak. It is possible that **the ROS (EMOD) generation by BITC in cancer cells is transient and serves to trigger the apoptosis signaling cascade.** (Xiao et al, 2006)

Studies have linked the consumption of broccoli and other cruciferous vegetables to a reduced risk of breast cancer. The phytochemical indole-3-carbinol (I3C), present in cruciferous vegetables, and its major acid-catalyzed reaction product 3,3'-diindolylmethane (DIM) have bioactivities relevant to the inhibition of carcinogenesis.

Indole-3-carbinol (I3C) is a phytochemical (derived from broccoli, cabbage, and other cruciferous vegetables) with proven anticancer efficacy including the reduction of cervical intraepithelial neoplasia (CIN) and its progression to cervical cancer.

Cruciferous vegetables and specific compounds they contain have been shown to modulate carcinogenesis in animals and humans (1-10). Among these compounds is glucobrassicin (3-indolylmethyl glucosinolate). Indole-3-carbinol (I3C) is a potent inducer of cytochrome P450 enzymes in many species, including humans.

Ascorbigen (ABG) belongs to the glucosinolate family and occurs mainly in *Brassica* vegetables. It is formed by its precursor glucobrassicin. Glucobrassicin is enzymatically hydrolyzed to indole-3-carbinol, which in turn reacts with l-ascorbic acid to ABG. The degradation of glucobrassicin is induced by plant tissue disruption. ABG may partly mediate the known anticarcinogenic effect of diets rich in *Brassicacae*. Furthermore, ABG is able to induce phase I and II enzymes that are centrally involved in the detoxification of xenobiotics. Cosmeceuticals containing ABG as an active principle are becoming increasingly popular.

Indole-3-carbinol (I3C) is a naturally occurring substance that shows anti-carcinogenic properties in animal models. Besides its clear anti-carcinogenic effects, some studies indicate that I3C may sometimes act as a tumor promoter.

Cytochrome P450 (CYP) is a family of enzymes involved in the oxidative metabolism of both synthetic and natural compounds. Humans are exposed to many CYP inducers from eating plant chemicals such as indolo(3,2-b)carbazole (ICZ), from broccoli and other cruciferous vegetables, and also from environmental contaminants such as 2,3,7,8-tetrachlorodibenzo-p-dioxin (TCDD).

https://empiricalnutrition.wordpress.com/2013/10/31/the-magic-of-broccoli-2/

Sulforaphane-induced apoptosis and EMODs

Investigators examined the molecular mechanisms by which sulforaphane enhances the therapeutic potential of tumor necrosis factor-related apoptosis-inducing ligand (TRAIL) in prostate cancer. Sulforaphane enhanced the therapeutic potential of TRAIL in PC-3 cells and sensitized TRAIL-resistant LNCaP cells. **Sulforaphane-induced apoptosis in PC-3 cells correlated with the generation of intracellular reactive oxygen species (ROS),** collapse of mitochondrial membrane potential, activation of caspase-3 and caspase-9, and up-regulation of DR4 and DR5. Sulforaphane induced the expression of Bax, Bak, Bim, and Noxa and inhibited the expression of Bcl-2, Bcl-X(L), and Mcl-1.

The quenching of ROS generation with antioxidant N-acetyl-L-cysteine conferred significant protection against sulforaphane-induced ROS generation, mitochondrial membrane potential disruption, caspase-3 activation, and apoptosis. Sulforaphane alone or in combination with TRAIL can be used for the management of prostate cancer. (Shankar et al, 2008)

In general, such capacities are studied via *in vitro* analysis of sulforaphane on isolated cancerous cell lines, with further tests attempting to derive mechanism of action (**apoptosis**, cell cycle arrest, antioxidant protection, detoxification) through the presence and concentration of various chemical markers.

Some studies go further and use human tissue grafts in immune-suppressed mice for elementary *in vivo* analysis. Such studies leave out the question of ideal modes of delivery.

In 2013, however, Veernaki *et al* undertook a study to determine which organs were most exposed to sulforaphane following oral ingestion.

Highest concentrations developed in the stomach and bladder, while "very low" levels were found in the prostate and colon.

This paper discusses the health benefits of sulforaphane consumption on cancers and inflammatory diseases of the mouth, esophagus, and stomach.

While DIM and I3C have received a good deal of attention in the popular press in recent years, and both available over-the-counter in pill form, **sulforaphane is an extremely delicate bioactive compound which in isolated form is stable only when maintained at -20°C**.

Alternatively, glucoraphanin—which can be isolated at room temperature from dried broccoli powder and is available over-the-counter—can be incubated in solution with an enzyme from broccoli called myrosinase to produce sulforaphane. However, chemically isolated myrosinase must also be maintained at -20°C and in depth knowledge is required for its proper use.

Sulforaphane and myrosinase can be purchased from biochemical tech companies such as Sigma-Aldrich, but only to those with institutional privileges and for rather high prices.

Luckily there are two other ways to acquire biologically active sulforaphane. Although the human body cannot itself produce myrosinase, researchers have determined that intestinal bacteria can do so.

When cooked watercress juice was anaerobically incubated with fresh human feces for two hours, 17% of the glucosinolates were hydrolyzed to ITC. Following consumption of fully cooked broccoli or dried broccoli powders containing glucoraphanin, urinary output of ITC conjugates was measured. Researchers concluded that a significant presence of active ITC develops in human tissues following the activation of glucosinolates in the small and large intestines. Sulforaphane would be amongst these.

The absorption of isothiocyanates from cooked *brassica*, however, has been estimated at between three and ten times less efficient than as from consumption of the raw vegetable.

Fresh, raw broccoli and broccoli sprouts contain glucoraphanin as well as the active enzyme myrosinase. Mastication of broccoli or broccoli sprouts releases myrosinase and glucoraphanin from their partitioned state within the normal structure of the plant, causing sulforaphane to then be produced via the myrosinase-dependent hydrolysis of glucoraphanin.

Broccoli sprouts, in particular, were found to contain 10 – 100x higher concentrations of glucoraphanin then the mature broccoli floret, as well as ample quantities of myrosinase.

One study attempted to determine if consumption of extra glucoraphanin in the form of a supplemental broccoli-powder, ingested along with fresh broccoli sprouts, would increase the absorption of active sulforaphane, but the results only supported the high bioavailability of isothiocyanates from raw sprouts.

Two studies identified the biokinetic half-life of sulforaphane at approximately 2 hours. Maximum serum levels were attained at one hour after ingestion of broccoli or broccoli sprouts, while after 8 hours approximately 60% of the total dose had been excreted.

These studies suggest that the simplest and most efficient way to include sulforaphane in the human diet is through the ingestion of fresh, thoroughly blended or chewed broccoli sprouts every few hours throughout the day.

H Pylori, Gastritis, & Chronic Atrophic Gastritis

H pylori infection is a risk factor in the development of gastritis, duodenal ulcer, peptic ulcer, and gastric cancer.

At least 90% of duodenal ulcers and 60% of gastric ulcers occur in the presence of infection, while eradication of the bacteria reduces recurrence rates to 0% and 10%, respectively.

The World Health Organization categorizes H pylori as a Class I carcinogen.

The U.S. National Cancer Institute does not recommend widespread H pylori eradication, but recommends testing and eradication in the case of gastric and duodenal ulcers and testing as a concomitant to gastric cancer treatment.

H pylori secretes protease and lipase, which breakdown the protective mucosa and phospholipid barrier protecting the epithelium from gastric acids.

Through expression of vacuolating cytotoxins, the bacteria produces pathological vacuoles in epithelial cells which lead to ulceration of the gastrointestinal epithelium.

By far the most important compound secreted by *H pylori* is the enzyme urease. Urease lowers acidity in the immediate proximity of the biofilm by converting urea to carbon dioxide and ammonia, decreasing the bacteriocidal effect of the gastric acid.

One of the components of gastric acid is peroxynitrate (ONOO-), a metabolite of nitric oxide and superoxide with bacteriocidal effects against *H pylori*. Carbon dioxide deactivates the bacteriocidal effects of ONOO-, while ammonia produces cytotoxic effects on gastric cells through derivative compounds such as monochloramine.

Chemotaxis in *H pylori*, which allows the bacterium to guide itself via the pH gradient into the more alkaline environment of the gastric mucosa, has been shown to be dependent upon the production of urease. The urease-inhibiting drugs flurofamide and acetohydroxamic acid suppressed chemotaxis *in vitro*, while a urease-deficient strain of *H pylori* was unable to swarm up the chemical gradient.

H pylori is also able to induce the pro-inflammatory tumor necrosis factor-alpha (TNF-α) protein through its injection of a certain Tipα molecule into the nucleus of an host cell, as well as trigger the increased secretion of pro-inflammatory cytokines and the breakdown of cell-to-cell junctions in the gastric epithelium.

The bacteria can modulate eukaryote immune processes, inducing inflammation, affecting the differentiation of macrophages, activating phagocytes, and increasing the infiltration of T cells.

***H pylori* also stimulates oxidative burst in neutrophils, which is a contributing factor in mucosal cell injury**.

The above mechanisms contribute to the exacerbation of gastritis and the development of gastric cancer. **The common pattern is the development of gastritis into chronic atrophic gastritis, intestinal metaplasia, and finally cancer**.

One direct consequence of such metaplasia is damage to gastric glands resulting in chronic gastric acid hyposecretion.

The resultant hypochlorhydria or achlorhydria decreases the survival of H pylori itself, but rapidly increases the colonization rates of other bacteria.

Similar concerns of bacterial overgrowth have been raised over the chronic use of proton-pump inhibitors, which eradicate H pylori by decreasing gastric acid secretion.

One often overlooked sequelae of decreased gastric secretions is decreased gastric levels of ascorbic acid, which is actively secreted into the stomach along with hydrochloric acid.

Low gastric ascorbic acid levels may be directly associated with the development of gastric cancer due to the inhibitory effect that ascorbic acid has on carcinogenic N-nitroso compounds.

In sum, H pylori contributes to the development of cancer by upregulating inflammatory pathways (increased TNF-α, increased cytokines, leukocyte infiltration), diminishing bacteriocidal properties of host defense (decreased ONOO- decreased pH), directly damaging epithelial cells (vacuolating cytotoxin, protease, lipase, monochloramine), and finally contributing to the development of decreased gastric acid secretion in chronic atrophic gastritis (increased N-nitroso compounds, bacterial overgrowth).

In 2002, a team of researchers at John Hopkins undertook to determine the effects of sulforaphane on the growth of H pylori bacteria. They noted that **infection with this bacteria increases the risk of gastric cancer and mucosa-associated lymphoid tissue (MAST) lymphoma by a factor of three to six times,** yet its eradication is often difficult due to its prevalence in underserved populations, its resistance to multiple conventional antibiotics, and its unique adaptation to human physiology. *In vitro,* **at concentrations between 1/20th ppm and 8 ppm, sulforaphane demonstrated bacteriostatic activity against 48 of 48 strains of H pylori.**

This means that at rather low concentrations, sulforaphane stopped the bacteria from reproducing. Amoxicillin proved equally powerful, while metronidazole worked against 40 strains and clarithromycin only 37. **There was no relationship between the resistance of the strains to the antibiotic drugs and the concentration of sulforaphane needed to provide bacteriostatic effect.**

The researchers went on to determine the bacteriocidal effects of sulforaphane on extracellular and intracellular bacteria *in vitro*. Outside of the cells, concentrations as high as 10 and 20 ppm were needed to impact the strains tested, but for bacteria inside liver cells, concentrations as low as 2 to 4 ppm eradicated *H pylori* within 24 hours. This difference could be explained in part by the tendency of sulforaphane to accumulate within cells to levels up to 100 times higher than extracellular concentrations. These bacteriostatic and bacteriocidal effects were consistent throughout the range of pH levels typical of the *H pylori* gastric habitat.

In 2003, a French team published a smaller study testing the effects of sulforaphane on the growth of *H pylori*. The researchers engrafted human embryonic stomachs into the peritoneal cavities of immune suppressed "nude" mice. After eight weeks gestation, *H pylori* was introduced into the human gastric cells via a surgically implanted catheter, and three week later biopsies were taken to determine infection level.

1.33mg sulforaphane—equivalent to 100mg for an adult human—was then administered via catheter daily for five days. In 72% of mice (8/11), histological and culture analysis showed complete eradication of *H pylori* growth. **Cultures from the remaining three mice demonstrated a fourfold increase in minimum inhibitory concentration—meaning that these bacteria were somewhat resistant to sulforaphane**.

Just like the John Hopkins study, sulforaphane was found to accumulate in the infected cells—though in this case to a level just five times that of the extracellular concentration.

The production of urease by *H pylori* enhances the bacteria's survival while directly damaging surrounding host tissues by multiple synergistic mechanisms. This explains why treatment with pharmaceutical urease inhibitors was found to decrease both bacterial load and gastric lesions.

In 2013, John Hopkins University researchers identified a specific mechanism by means of which sulforaphane bonds with urease and thereby inactivates it. While sulforaphane is not unique among isothiocyanate in this ability, it is unique in being both an urease inactivator and also a bacteriocidal agent against *H pylori*.

In 2009, researchers at the Tokyo University of Science evaluated the effects on *H pylori* infection of oral sulforaphane intake by mice and humans. **H pylori infection was attenuated in mice fed sulfora- phane-rich broccoli sprouts, and for forty-eight H pylori-infect- ed patients fed 70 g/day broccoli sprouts for eight weeks, urea breath test and stool antigen tests showed decreased pres- ence of H pylori as compared to a control group fed an equal serving of isothiocyanate-free alfalfa sprouts**.

Additionally, multiple markers of inflammation were reduced, includ- ing mucosal expression of TNFα and interleukin-1β. Interestingly, these protective effects were not demonstrated on a mouse clone with its *NFE2L2* gene removed.

Reporting in a subsequent paper in 2011, the same Japanese research- ers drew connections between the basic science of Nrf2, the clinical effects of sulforaphane on the gastric mucosa, and indications in the research that **sulforaphane stimulates expression of nrf2 gene- dependent antioxidants**.

Via the transcription factor, Nrf2, *NFE2L2*induces the transcription of over 200 genes expressing proteins with a wide range of cytoprotec- tive effects, including metabolism of drugs and toxins, stabilization of proteins, removal of damaged proteins, antioxidant scavenging of free radicals, and interaction with key molecules involved in regulation of the cell cycle and protection against cancer.

The anti-inflammatory and bacteriocidal effects of sulforaphane provide important preventative and palliative action against conditions of the stomach and mouth.

Sulforaphane's ability to treat *H pylori* infection through multiple mecha- nisms (bacteriocidal, urease-inhibiting, anti-inflammatory) may be sig- nificant enough to stall pathogenesis of gastritis, to stop its progression into chronic atrophic gastritis, and perhaps even to aid in the preven- tion of subsequent carcinogenesis.

Indeed, **one epidemiological study connected cruciferous veg- etable consumption with decreased risk of lung, stomach, co- lon, and rectal cancers, as well as to a lower incidence of death from cancer in general**.

While another research team found no association between broccoli consumption and decreased risk of chronic atro- phic gastritis in Japanese men, raw vegetable consumption is unusual in Japanese culture, and the researchers did not consider this variable.

Meanwhile, as elaborated above, *H pylori* infection is highly correlated with the development of gastritis and gastric cancer, and sulforaphane from raw broccoli or broccoli sprouts showed strong bacteriocidal effects against the bacterium *in vitro,* in animal models, as well as in one human trial. There is direct evidence that sulforaphane consumption directly fights gastric, tongue, oral, and esophageal cancers.

Phase Two Antioxidant Synthesis, Inflammation, & Cancer

There is convincing evidence that broccoli and broccoli-sprout consumption plays a role in the prevention of multiple cancers; however, large scale meta-analysis and human trials have not yet been conducted on the effects of sulforaphane as a chemotherapeutic agent.

Nevertheless, biochemical mechanisms are beginning to be identified. These include induction of powerful antioxidants and detoxification molecules; **stimulation of apoptosis** and cell cycle arrest; inhibition of pro-cancer, pro-inflammatory molecules such as TNFα and COX-2; and inhibition of tumor-promoting changes to cancer cell metabolism.

By 1991, it was already known that sulforaphane induces the Phase 2 enzyme cascade while curbing Phase 1 enzyme expression.

Phase I and Phase 2 enzymes both play a role in detoxification by modifying xenobiotic molecules in different ways. Phase I enzymes add or subtract molecules in order to add functional groups to and thereby increase the biological activity of foreign substances.

Phase II enzymes react with these intermediary products, typically increasing their water solubility through conjugation so as to enhance their excretion from the body.

Phase 2 enzyme induction has been widely assumed to explain sulforaphane's powerful effects against multiple cell lines of cancer.

Since the late nineties, **sulforaphane has been shown to induce the Phase 2 cascade in human prostate cells *in vitro,* as well as in mouse gastric cells, human airway epithelial cells, rat** cardiac muscle cells, human nasal cells, and human skin (all *in vivo*), with chemotherapeutic effects noted in multiple cases.

It is now known that the Phase 2 enzyme cascade is mediated via a transcription factor called Nrf2, transcribed by the *NFE2L2* gene, via its interaction with the Antioxidant Response Element (ARE) of the human genome, so named for its direct induction of a host of antioxidant products.

When Nrf2 is not needed—while the cell maintains good antioxidant tone—a protein called Keap1 holds Nrf2 tightly in place in a complex outside of the nucleus designed to facilitate its destruction.

However, **when reactive oxygen species (ROS; e.g., oxidants, free radicals, EMODs) are present in high cytoplasmic levels, they are likely to react with a sulfur-containing amino acid on the Keap1 protein.** This reaction causes Keap1 to uncouple from Nrf2, allowing the latter to translocate into the nucleus. Here it joins with transcription factor sMaf to activate ARE, inducing the biosynthesis of a wide array of powerful antioxidants and detoxifying agents— including GST and NQO1, as well as glutathione peroxidase (GPX), heme-oxygenase 1 (HMOX1), thioredoxin (TXN), and others.

In 2013, Irundika *et al* from the UK subjected these Nrf2-related effects to thorough analysis in the context of sulforaphane's ameliorative effects on the progression of periodontal disease.

Superoxide is allegedly a toxic ROS produced during respiratory burst by neutrophils. Neutrophils are white blood cells, and their production of ROS (EMODs) is thought to contribute to the bacteriocidal effects of the immune system.

In chronic inflammatory periodontal disease, however, persistent infection leads to hyperactive neutrophil activity, which is not resolved by mechanical removal of the microbial biofilm. **Excessive superoxide levels increase, causing cellular damage to the gums and inducing further inflammation.**

Under normal, healthy conditions, this dynamic is mediated by the body's most prevalent antioxidant, glutathione.

The ratio between the antioxidizing and oxygenated forms of glutathione (glutathione s-transferase [GST] and GSSG, respectively) is a standard measure for the level of antioxidant activity within a cell, as well as of the cell's overall health.

When the GST:GSSG ratio is low within the neutrophil, a special cell structure called an NADPH oxidase lipid raft forms in the cell membrane. Lipid rafts float on the outside of the membrane while anchoring themselves deep within it and in this way allow certain types of molecules safe passage out of the cell. In this particular lipid raft, **NADPH oxidase shuttles free radicals from the inside to the outside of the cell**.

Free radicals are highly reactive bits of molecules that are allegedly toxic to the cell.

Once outside, they react with extracellular oxygen to form the ROS superoxide molecules. **These may contribute to the bacteriocidal effects of neutrophil activity**, but they also damages healthy tissues and induces inflammation. Low cytoplasmic GST:GSSG ratio also induces the Keap1/Nsf1/ARE cascade, increasing glutathione and NQO1 levels. NQO1 deactivates NADPH oxidase, directly inhibiting the formation of these lipid rafts, while glutathione deactivates free radicals, thereby slowing lipid rafts formation and decreasing the flow of free radicals through those that remain. Extracellular superoxide remains low, and chronic inflammation does not develop.

In the case of chronic inflammatory periodontal disease, this protective mechanism fails and even when bacterial residues are cleared away, inflammation persists. In this context, sulforaphane promises a preventative and palliative role. When it enters neutrophil cells in the oral cavity, sulforaphane attaches to the same binding site on the Keap1 protein as reacts with ROS, where it directly promotes the translocation of Nrf2, causing the transcription of antioxidant and detoxification ARE gene products.

In Irundika's study, sulforaphane administration increased GSH: GSSG ratio but NQO1 expression was—unexpectedly—found not to change. Saliva levels of superoxide and periodontal inflammation decrease, but NADPH oxidase lipid raft formation was assumed to persist. The researchers concluded that in the case of chronic periodontal disease a permanent alteration in the Nrf2 signaling pathway must cause persistent inflammation, and that sulforaphane treatment ought to help to ameliorate the disease.

They do not raise the question as to whether this permanent pro-inflammatory change might be avoided through preventative consumption of raw broccoli, although poor diet (no vegetables, low potassium) is associated with the development of periodontal disease.

Increased expression of Phase 2 detoxification and antioxidant enzymes plays a big role in sulforaphane's anti-cancer properties. Through the Keap1/Nrf1/ARE biochemical pathway, powerful antioxidants like glutathione (GST) and NOQ1 are expressed. **Not only do these gene products directly reduce (deactivate) toxic free radicals, but they also reduce (regenerate) the oxidized forms of retinal/retinol, L-ascorbate, and α-tocopherol (vitamins A, C, and E, respectively)**.

It has been shown that sulforaphane treatment reduces oxidative damage to the delicate retinal tissues of the eye through a Keap1-dependent process.

When L-ascorbate scavenges free radicals, it changes into semi-dehydroascorbate and dehydroascorbate, which are recycled back to L-ascorbate by GST and its metabolites. L-ascorbate—along with GST itself—in turn recycles the oxidation products of α-tocopherol. Moreover, NOQ1 reduces α-tocopherylquinone (TQ), the primarily oxidation product of α-tocopherol, into α-tocopheryl-hydroquinone (TQH2), an antioxidant that some research suggests is at least as potent an antioxidant as α-tocopherol itself.

Against this background of basic biochemistry, let us recall that sulforaphane has shown anti-cancer effects against cells of the liver, prostate, colon, rectum, pancreas, bone, skin, ovaries, cervix, bladder, lung, and breast. Due to the nutrient's high penetration in stomach and bladder tissues following oral ingestion, considering its obvious access to oral and esophageal tissues, and because of its synergistic effects in the context of the gastric disease progression, I have chosen to highlight research connecting sulforaphane to cancer protection in tissues of the stomach, throat, and mouth only. A review of this research shows the central role of Phase 2 enzyme induction but also reveals additional mechanisms—such as activation of apoptosis pathways, stimulation of cell cycle arrest, inhibition of cancer cell adhesion, improved detoxification of carcinogenic chemicals, enhancement of chemotherapy drugs, and selective blocking of COX2.

It should be kept in mind that the broader research into sulforaphane cancer-fighting properties has revealed still further possible anti-carcinogenic mechanisms, including inhibition of angiogenesis and metastasis, and modulation of molecules such as NFκB, MAPK, and HDAC.

Earlier, I described a John Hopkins team's research into sulforaphane's antibacterial effects against H pylori growth. This team went on to test for anti-tumor effects in a mouse model for gastric cancer.

In this model, cancer is induced by forcing mice to consume benzo[a] pyrene, a powerful carcinogen from coal tar. Further, wild type mice were compared with a special mouse line genetically engineered with the Nrf2-expressing gene (*NFE2L2*) deleted.

Approximately 1.33 grams (7.5 μmol) per day sulforaphane was delivered through oral ingestion for seven days preceding carcinogen administration and for two days following. **Twenty weeks later, the wild sulforaphane-fed mice had developed an average of 39% fewer tumors, while for the*NFE2L2*-deleted line no statistical improvement was observed. Sulforaphane had significantly decreased tumor formation at least partially via the Nrf2 pathway**.

In 2008, researchers in Korea tested the effects of sulforaphane *in vitro* on multiple cell lines of oral squamous cell carcinoma. They reported selectively decreased COX-2 expression—a different anti-inflammatory mechanism from that established by Irundika *et al* that is associated with oral squamous cancer—coupled with downregulation of a downstream product of COX-2 called Bcl2, which has been shown elsewhere to act as an inhibitor on the mitochondrial apoptosis pathway. By decreasing expression of Bcl2 and COX2, sulforaphane was able to encourage the self-destruction of these cancer cells.

One year later, some of the same researchers published a new study, this time describing sulforaphane inhibiting two cell lines of oral carcinoma by 46% and 58%, respectively. Not surprisingly, there was a correlation between the phases of the cell cycle in which cancer cells had been arrested (G2 and Mitosis) and the signaling proteins that control cell growth. In short, the cell reproduction cycle occurs via the following steps:

G1 Phase: mRNA and proteins needed for DNA synthesis are transcribed.

Synthesis Phase: DNA are exactingly replicated in duplicate in preparation for mitosis.

G2 Phase: protein and mRNA in preparation for mitosis and cell division are synthesized.

M Phase: Chromosomes are collated into two separate but identical sets, each with its own nucleus, and then the cell divides.

Progression through these stages is guided by a family of proteins called cyclins that activate members of a corresponding family of kinase enzymes (CDK's). CDK's serve as switches that coordinate stage changes through selective phosphorylation. Phosphorylation is the transfer of high energy phosphate groups derived from the metabolism of glucose to molecules that need the phosphate groups to power anabolic chemical reactions. Through phosphorylation the CDK enzymes activate signalling proteins and transcription factors that guide cell activities during cell division.

Now back to the Korean research on oral cancer.

Sulforaphane's effect was to decrease concentrations of cyclin B, the coordinating protein most active during the transition between the G2 and M phases, while also increasing a protein called p21—a generalized CDK inhibitor protein normally induced in the context of DNA damage, which triggers cell cycle arrest to inhibit tumor growth. Thus, a mechanism was revealed whereby sulforaphane disrupted the growth cycle of oral carcinoma cells.

Barret's Esophageal Adenocarcinoma (BEAC) is an increasingly common form of esophageal cancer that progresses from Barret's (precancerous) esophagus. It is a condition marked by precancerous metaplastic cell changes induced by chronic gastric reflux and is linked to inflammatory cytokines, obesity, and carcinogens from tobacco smoke.

In 2010, Aamer *et al* published work examining sulforaphane's effects on BEAC by inoculating immunodeficient mice with BEAC cell lines.

In vitro, sulforaphane produced total die-off of BEAC cells at low concentrations over a two to five day period, while no changes in cell viability or quality were observed in normal esophageal and fibroblast cells after 72 hour treatment. Of four mice subcutaneously inoculated with BEAC cells, 25 mg/kg SFN per day for two weeks attenuated increase in tumor size in three mice. For all four mice, average tumor size was approximately one third less than that of the controls.

As with oral carcinoma, the researches observed increased expression of p21, the generalized inhibitor of the CDK enzymes, which regulate cell growth and reproduction. This corresponds with their observation that a majority of sulforaphane-treated cancer cells arrested in the G1 phase. It has been shown elsewhere that G1 cell cycle arrest can be induced when p21 binds to and thus inhibits CDK2 from complexing with cyclin E, a critical mediator of G1 phase regulation.

They also found a dose-dependent expression of caspase 8, a cysteine-rich protease (protein catabolizing molecule) directly involved in the non-mitochondrial apoptosis pathway. Researches also discovered sulforaphane to produce a dose-dependent inhibition of multidrug resistance protein (MRP), which is involved in the extrusion of drugs from the cell. This capacity to increase intracellular concentration of xenobiotic chemicals might explain the remarkable synergistic effects observed when sulforaphane was added to a chemotherapeutic agent.

In sum, **Aamer's examination of sulforaphane found multifactorial chemotherapeutic effects against an increasingly prevalent esophageal cancer**.

One final study, from 2008, investigating tongue and prostate cancer cell lines, explored sulforaphane's ability to modify cancer cell metabolism via interaction with a transcription factor called hypoxia-inducible factor-1 (HIF-1). Under conditions of normal cell oxygenation, HIF-1 is sequestered within a ligase complex where it is marked for proteasomal disintegration. Because of this destructive mechanism, the transcription factor is virtually undetectable in healthy, oxygenated tissues. In hypoxia, however, HIF-1 stabilizes, becomes active, and influences expression of as many as 2% of all human genes.

Over 100 of these genes have been identified, and their functions have been related not only to angiogenesis but also to increased glucose metabolism via oxygen-independent glycolysis, increased red blood cell formation, encouragement of cell growth and survival via stimulation of growth factor, and stimulation of caspase 3, caspase 9, and p21 apoptotic pathways.

HIF-1 is closely associated with tumor development, with increased concentrations found in more malignant tumors, and many known carcinogenic gene alterations inducing its expression. HIF-1 helps to stabilize hypoxic tumor regions through oxygen-independent metabolism and encourages subsequent tumor oxygenation through angiogenesis (blood vessel formation). Treatment of cancer with HIF-1-inhibiting drugs has been studied in multiple contexts.

In their investigation of human tongue squamous cell carcinoma, The 2008 study found sulforaphane to decrease HIF-1 expression by blocking its phosphorylation by JNK and ERK pathways. This anti-angiogenic effect was further verified by decreased expression of vascular endothelial growth factor, the signal protein involved in the final step of this pathway.

Afterward: Big Pharma

It is common practice for pharmaceutical companies to attempt modifications of biologically active substances for the development of patentable drugs. In 1997, Gerhäuser *et al* synthesized a compound formed by conjoining sulforaphane and an indole-based compound extracted from cabbage called brassinin. While sulforaphane induces Phase 2 enzymes while inhibiting Phase 2 enzymes, brassinin is known to induce the expression of both Phase I and Phase II enzymes. Gerhäuser's team expressed concern over research that showed that while Phase I enzymes stimulate the detoxification of xenobiotic toxins, the intermediary products thus created are highly biologically reactive and therefore potentially more toxic than their precursors.

Therefore, to synthesize their novel drug, they first removed from brassinin the Phase I enzyme-inducing component, and then attached it to a modified sulforaphane molecule. The sulforaphane molecule was modified by the removal of the isothiocyanate component. The resultant product, which they called sulforamate, was then tested against sulforaphane. It produced nearly identical or slightly better or worse results in a every category tested—including expression of the antioxidants NQO1, catalase, and glutathione and inhibition of cancer lesions in a mouse model.

To justify the removal of the isothiocyanate component from sulforaphane, Gerhäuser's team referred to research demonstrating that isothiocynates could under certain conditions increase the cytotoxicity of xenobiotic agents.

The original researchers showed, however, that these effects are reversed by increased cellular glutathione—recall that sulforaphane induces glutathione synthesis—and they concluded that the isothiocyanate component likely plays a role in the transport of toxins out of the cell.

The Gerhäuser article also references a paper by Yang, *et al,* whose Rutgers University team wrote a research review in 1994 that illustrates the complex picture regarding isothiocyanates and Phase I enzyme inhibition. Sulforaphane—as well as flavanoids, isothiocyanates, and sulfides from fruits, other cruciferous vegetables, and garlic—all modify cytochrome P450 enzymes (particularly 2E1, 3A, and 1A2) involved in the induction of the Phase I cascade. Though complex, these effects tends toward inhibition of Phase I enzymes, thus blocking activation of toxins.

The researchers conclude that **p450 inhibition may be therapeutic under specific, limited conditions, but urged caution because inhibition of the activation of these enzymes in the liver could arrest the metabolism and excretion of cytotoxins, causing them to pass through the liver and travel throughout the body in the blood.**

The **paradox** is that **Gerhäuser's team questioned sulforaphane** for its inhibition of the Phase I enzyme cascade (via its isothiocyanate moiety), while simultaneously questioning brassinin for its induction of the same chemical pathways (via its indole moiety). In the first case the concern is that xenobiotic toxins will not be metabolized, while in the second case the concern is that in the process of being metabolized, they will become more toxic through biological activation. Ironically, indole-containing compounds like brassinin and indole-3-carbonyl and isothiocyanates such as sulforaphane (and others) *coexist* in unadulterated raw broccoli. I do not know of any research that attempts to determine whether the Phase-1-inhibiting and Phase-1-inducing aspects of these broccoli compounds balance out or operate through some kind of complex synergy.

Certainly, sulforaphane's ability to stimulate Phase 2 enzyme antioxidants while promoting the regeneration of retinal, l-ascorbate, and α-tocopherol should reduce our caution. Gerhäuser's reductive attempt to bypass questions of natural balance surely advanced our knowledge of sulforaphane. As for the sulforamate, however, aside from a review written by of the one of the same authors nine years later, I could find no further published research on the synthetic drug, while in the meantime subsequent research on the natural compound sulforaphane continues to accumulate.

My conclusions on broccoli (sulforaphane) are as follows:

Broccoli

In test tube and animal studies, sulforaphane exhibits properties that suggest it could, indeed, help prevent many forms of cancer.

Numerous observational studies have found that a high consumption of vegetables in the cabbage family is associated with a reduced risk of cancer, especially breast, prostate, lung,

stomach, colon, and rectal cancer. However, it is a long way from such studies to reliable evidence of benefit.

Sulforaphane Induces Cell Cycle Arrest and Apoptosis in Acute Lymphoblastic Leukemia Cells

This is the first report on the anti-leukemic property of SF in hematological malignancies, supporting its use as an adjunctive chemotherapy in ALL.

Sulforaphane cytotoxicity derives from complex, concurring, and multiple mechanisms, among which **the generation of reactive oxygen species has been identified as playing a central role in promoting apoptosis and autophagy of target cells**.

Notably, **all the studies dealing with SF toxicity report that these effects occur at concentrations above 5–10 μM, that is, levels which can be barely maintained through cruciferous diet intake**.

Many authors have investigated the role of ROS in SF-induced apoptosis and they invariably reported that <u>ROS (EMODs) generated within mitochondria contribute to or are fully responsible for the apoptotic response</u>.

Mitochondrial production of ROS is an important event in high SF concentrations cytotoxicity.

I am particularly encouraged about SF because its tumoricidal action is prooxidative, just as I have found to be the case with all other effective tumoricidal agents. Hope spring eternal for sulforaphane.

SECTION FOUR

CURCUMIN

Curcumin [1,7-bis (4-hydroxy-3-methoxyphenyl)-1,6-heptadiene-3,5-dione] (diferuloylmethane, CUR), the main component of the yellow extract from the plant Curcuma longa (turmeric, a popular Indian spice), is a main bioactive **polyphenol**, which has been used widely as a spice, food additive, and a herbal medicine in Asia. Tetrahydrocurcumin (THC) is an active metabolite of CUR. Orally ingested CUR is metabolized into THC by a reductase found in the intestinal epithelium.

THC possesses extremely strong antioxidant activity compared to other curcuminoids. The antioxidant role of THC has been implicated in recovery from renal injury in mice and in anti-inflammatory responses.

But, please keep in mind the following: **Contradictory to the commonly-mentioned antioxidant effect, curcumin has significant prooxidant activity**. Studies **indicate a role of ROS (EMODs) in curcumin-induced cell death.** (Woo et al, 2003)

Turmeric

Turmeric is a bright yellow spice that has been used in cooking for 4,000 years in India.

Referred to as **"Indian saffron"** in Southeast Asia, it's has long been used by healing practitioners of Ayurveda, a traditional Indian medical practice. Turmeric has gained popularity among Western practitioners for its alleged healing properties over the last 25 years.

Turmeric is a South Asian tropical plant with tall, green spade-like leaves and trumpet-shaped white flowers. The plant reproduces by growing a part of its stem (called rhizome) underground. The rhizome's flesh is bright yellow-orange. The spice you see for sale in the grocery store is the rhizome that's been boiled, dried, and ground into powder.

Traditional Indian healing practices use turmeric to treat many ailments, including arthritis, stomach problems, poor circulation, and skin diseases. Turmeric is mixed with liquids, made into a paste or ointment, or burned for the patient to inhale.

Turmeric contains about 100 different properties that account for its long-lived success.

Turmeric blocks certain enzymes and cytokines that lead to inflammation. It seems to have an immune system-modifying effect too. It prevents the body from making an antibody called tumor necrosis factor (TNF).

A small 2012 study of rheumatoid arthritis (RA) patients showed that **a curcumin product worked better on joint pain and swelling than a non-steroidal anti-inflammatory drug (NSAID) called diclofenac**.

Another study showed that turmeric seems to be better at preventing joint inflammation than reducing it.

Turmeric speculation

None of the following uses for turmeric have been conclusively proven yet—studies remain ongoing. However, there is some evidence that turmeric may:

- prevent or slow the spread of cancer
- help prevent blood clots
- help prevent or slow the loss of cognitive function
- treat some digestive problems
- lower blood cholesterol
- treat viral infections
- treat uveitis (eye inflammation)

Turmeric is used as a spice or for coloring in foods like cheese and mustard. It's considered safe by the Food and Drug Administration (FDA), but **possible side effects from large doses include stomach upset and diarrhea**.

Dosage

In large doses, tumeric may interact with some prescription drugs. It might also have a bad effect on your health if you have certain conditions. Check with your doctor before taking turmeric if you take medicine for:

- diabetes
- inflammation
- cholesterol
- blood thinners

http://www.healthline.com/health-slideshow/8-essential-everyday-exercises-for-ra-pain

----

http://www.ncbi.nlm.nih.gov/pmc/articles/PMC3535097/

Therapeutic Roles of Curcumin: Lessons Learned from Clinical Trials

The following has been adapted, excerpted or modified from: (Gupta, Patchva and Aggrarwal, 2013)

Extensive research over the past half century has shown that curcumin (diferuloylmethane), a component of the golden spice turmeric (*Curcuma longa*), can modulate multiple cell signaling pathways. Extensive clinical trials over the past quarter century have addressed the pharmacokinetics, safety, and efficacy of this nutraceutical against numerous diseases in humans.

Some promising effects have been observed in patients with various pro-inflammatory diseases including cancer, cardiovascular disease, arthritis, uveitis, ulcerative proctitis, Crohn's disease, ulcerative colitis, irritable bowel disease, tropical pancreatitis, peptic ulcer, gastric ulcer, idiopathic orbital inflammatory pseudotumor, oral lichen planus, gastric inflammation, vitiligo, psoriasis, acute coronary syndrome, atherosclerosis, diabetes, diabetic nephropathy, diabetic microangiopathy,

lupus nephritis, renal conditions, acquired immunodeficiency syndrome, ß-thalassemia, biliary dyskinesia, Dejerine-Sottas disease, cholecystitis, and chronic bacterial prostatitis.

Curcumin has also shown protection against hepatic conditions, chronic arsenic exposure, and alcohol intoxication.

Dose-escalating studies have indicated the safety of curcumin at doses as high as 12 g/day over 3 months.

Curcumin's pleiotropic activities emanate from its ability to modulate numerous signaling molecules such as pro-inflammatory cytokines, apoptotic proteins, NF–κB, cyclooxygenase-2, 5-LOX, STAT3, C-reactive protein, prostaglandin E_2, prostate-specific antigen, adhesion molecules, phosphorylase kinase, transforming growth factor-β, triglyceride, ET-1, creatinine, HO-1, AST, and ALT in human participants.

In clinical trials, curcumin has been used either alone or in combination with other agents. Various formulations of curcumin, including nanoparticles, liposomal encapsulation, emulsions, capsules, tablets, and powder, have been examined.

Curcumin is one such widely studied nutraceutical that was first discovered about two centuries ago by Harvard College laboratory scientists Vogel and Pelletier from the rhizomes of *Curcuma longa* (turmeric). (Vogel, Pelletier, 1815)

Curcumin is a highly pleiotropic molecule that was first shown to exhibit antibacterial activity in 1949. (Schraufstatter, Bernt, 1949)

Since then, **this polyphenol** has been shown to possess anti-inflammatory, hypoglycemic, **antioxidant**, wound-healing, and antimicrobial activities. (Aggarwal, Sung, 2009)

Extensive preclinical studies over the past three decades have indicated curcumin's therapeutic potential against a wide range of human diseases. (Aggarwal, Haikumar, 2009)

In addition, **curcumin has been shown to directly interact with numerous signaling molecules**. These preclinical studies have formed a solid basis for evaluating curcumin's efficacy in clinical trials.

Although the therapeutic use of *Curcuma* was recorded as early as 1748, the first article referring to the use of curcumin in human disease was published in 1937 by Oppenheimer. (Oppenheimer, 1937)

In this study, the author examined the effects of "curcumin" or "curcunat" containing 0.1 g to 0.25 g sodium curcumin and 0.1 g calcium cholate in human biliary diseases. An intravenous injection of 5% sodium curcumin solution in healthy persons was associated with rapid emptying of the gallbladder. The author treated 67 patients with subacute, recurrent, or chronic cholecystitis. **Oral administration of curcunat for 3 weeks showed remarkably good results against cholecystitis.** All but one patient were completely cured of the disease throughout periods of observation lasting from 3 months to more than 3 years.

No ill effects were observed or reported, even when the medication was continued for many consecutive months. (Oppenheimer, 1937)

Since this initial identification, interest in curcumin research in human participants has increased remarkably.

As of July 2012, observations from almost 67 clinical trials have been published, whereas another 35 clinical trials are in progress.

The safety, tolerability, and nontoxicity of curcumin at high doses are well established by human clinical trials. (Vogel, Pelletier, 1815) (Gupta et al, 2012)

Gupta's own group found that curcumin at 8 g/day in combination with gemcitabine was safe and well-tolerated in patients with pancreatic cancer. (Kanai et al, 2011) (Dhillon et al, 2008)

The clinical trials conducted thus far have indicated the therapeutic potential of curcumin against a wide range of human diseases. **It has also shown protection against hepatic conditions, chronic arsenic exposure, and alcohol intoxication.** In these clinical trials, curcumin has been used either alone or in combination with other agents such as quercetin, gemcitabine, piperine, docetaxel, soy isoflavones, bioperine, sulfasalazine, mesalamine, prednisone, lactoferrin, N-acetylcysteine, and pantoprazole.

How a single agent can possess these diverse effects has been an enigma over the years, both for basic scientists and clinicians. However, numerous lines of evidence have indicated curcumin's ability in human participants to modulate multiple cell signaling molecules such as pro-inflammatory cytokines (tumor necrosis factor [TNF]-α, interleukin [IL]-1β, IL-6), apoptotic proteins, NF–κB, cyclooxygenase (COX)-2, STAT3, IKKβ, endothelin-1, malondialdehyde (MDA), C-reactive protein (CRP), prostaglandin E$_2$, GST, PSA, VCAM1, glutathione (GSH), pepsinogen, phosphorylase kinase (PhK), transferrin receptor, total cholesterol, transforming growth factor (TGF)-β, triglyceride, creatinine, HO-1, antioxidants, AST, and ALT.

Poor bioavailability

Although curcumin has shown efficacy against numerous human ailments, **poor bioavailability due to poor absorption, rapid metabolism, and rapid systemic elimination have been shown to limit its therapeutic efficacy**. (Anand et al, 2007)

As a result, numerous efforts have been made to improve curcumin's bioavailability by altering these features. **The use of adjuvants that can block the metabolic pathway of curcumin is the most common strategy for increasing the bioavailability of curcumin**.

The effect of combining piperine, a known inhibitor of hepatic and intestinal glucuronidation, was evaluated on the bioavailability of curcumin in healthy human volunteers. (Shoba et al, 1998)

In humans receiving a dose of 2 g of curcumin alone, serum levels of curcumin were either undetectable or very low. Concomitant administration of 20 mg of piperine with curcumin, however, produced much higher concentrations within 30 min to 1 h after drug treatment; **piperine increased the bioavailability of curcumin by 2,000%.**

Other promising approaches to increase the bioavailability of curcumin in humans include the use of nanoparticles, liposomes, phospholipid complexes, and structural analogues.

Meriva is a patented phytosome complex of curcumin with soy phosphatidylcholine that has better bioavailability than curcumin. The absorption of a curcuminoid mixture and Meriva was examined in a randomized, double-blind, crossover human study. (Cuomo et al, 2011)

Total curcuminoid absorption was about 29-fold higher for the Meriva mixture than it was for the corresponding unformulated curcuminoid mixture.

Interestingly, the phospholipid formulation increased the absorption of demethoxylated curcuminoids much more than that of curcumin. (Cuomo et al, 2011)

The bioavailability of curcumin has also been shown to be greatly enhanced by reconstituting curcumin with the non-curcuminoid components of turmeric. (Antony et al, 2008)

Most of the curcumin's clinical studies have been focused mainly on people with health problems. A recent study, however, evaluated the health-promoting efficacy of lipidated curcumin in healthy middle aged participants (40–60 years old). In this study, the participants were given either lipidated curcumin (80 mg/day) or placebo for 4 weeks.

Curcumin, but not placebo, produced decrease in salivary amylase and in the plasma levels of triglycerides, beta amyloid, alanine amino transferase, and sICAM.

Furthermore, curcumin administration in these participants increased salivary radical scavenging capacities and activities in plasma catalase, myeloperoxidase, and nitric oxide production.

Overall, these results demonstrated the health-promoting effects of lipidated curcumin in healthy middle aged people. (Disilvestro et al, 2012)

Although relatively pure curcumin has been used in some human studies, most studies have used either a mixture of curcuminoids or even **turmeric, from which curcuminoids are derived. Approximately 2%–6% (w/w) of turmeric is curcuminoids.** The latter contains 80% curcumin, 18% demethoxycurcumin, and 2% bisdemethoxycurcumin.

The United States Food and Drug Administration has approved curcumin as being GRAS (generally recognized as safe), and the polyphenol is now being used as a supplement in several countries. (Goel et al, 2008)

It is marketed in several forms, including capsules, tablets, ointments, energy drinks, soaps, and cosmetics. In the following sections, the authors summarize the studies documenting the activities of curcumin against numerous diseases in human participants and its mechanisms of action.

Completed clinical trials

Cancer therapy

Cancer is a multistage process involving a series of events and resulting from the dysregulation of more than 500 genes at multiple steps in cell signaling pathways.

Although currently available monotargeted cancer therapeutics have had some effect, these drugs are associated with numerous adverse effects and are expensive. The current paradigm for cancer treatment is either to combine several monotargeted drugs or to design drugs that modulate multiple targets. **Because of its multitargeting activities, curcumin has exhibited activities against numerous cancer types in human clinical trials.**

Probably the first indication of curcumin's anticancer activities in human participants was shown in 1987 by Kuttan and co-workers, who conducted a clinical trial involving 62 patients with external cancerous lesions. **Topical curcumin was found to produce remarkable symptomatic relief as evidenced by reductions in smell, itching, lesion size, and pain.** Although the effect continued for several months in many patients, only one patient had an adverse reaction. (Kuttan et al, 1987) (Kuttan R, Sudheeran PC, Josph CD. Turmeric and curcumin as topical agents in cancer therapy. Tumori. 1987;73(1):29–31)

Since then, **curcumin, either alone or in combination with other agents, has demonstrated potential against colorectal cancer, pancreatic cancer, breast cancer, prostate cancer, multiple myeloma, lung cancer, oral cancer, and head and neck squamous cell carcinoma (HNSCC).**

Colorectal cancer

Colorectal cancer (CRC) is the second leading cause of cancer deaths in the United States, with 143,460 new cases and 51,690 deaths expected in 2012. Currently, there is no effective treatment except resection at a very early stage with or without chemotherapy. Thus, new strategies are needed to replace or complement current therapies. Curcumin has demonstrated potential against CRC in numerous clinical trials.

A dose-escalation pilot study evaluated the pharmacokinetics and pharmacodynamics of a standardized *Curcuma* extract in proprietary capsule form at doses between 440 and 2,200 mg/day, containing 36–180 mg of curcumin. (Sharma et al, 2007)

Fifteen patients with advanced **colorectal cancer (CRC)** refractory to standard chemotherapies received *Curcuma* extract daily for up to 4 months. Activity of glutathione S-transferase and levels of M_1G, a marker of DNA adduct formation, were measured in patients' blood cells. Oral *Curcuma* extract was well-tolerated, and dose-limiting toxicity was not observed. Neither curcumin nor its metabolites were detected in blood or urine, but curcumin was recovered from feces.

Curcumin sulfate was identified in the feces of one patient. Ingestion of 440 mg of *Curcuma* extract containing 36 mg of curcumin for 29 days was accompanied by a 59% decrease in lymphocytic glutathione S-transferase activity. At higher dose levels, however, the effect was not observed. Leukocytic M_1G levels were constant within each patient and unaffected by treatment. (Sharma et al, 2007)

In another study, patients were given curcumin capsules at three different doses (3.6, 1.8, and 0.45 g/day) for 7 days. However, **levels of COX-2 were unaffected by curcumin**. The study concluded that a daily dose of 3.6 g of curcumin is pharmacologically efficacious in CRC patients. (Garcea et al, 2005)

Curcumin has also demonstrated potential for the prevention and treatment of CRC in combination with other agents. Familial adenomatous polyposis (FAP) is an autosomal-dominant disorder characterized by hundreds of colorectal adenomas that eventually develop into CRC. The number and size of polyps had decreased after 6 months of combination treatment without any appreciable toxicity in the five patients. Although the combinations seemed to reduce the adenomas, randomized controlled trials are needed to further validate these findings. (Cruz-Correa et al, 2006)

In a nonrandomized, open-label clinical trial in smokers, polyphenol reduced the formation of aberrant crypt foci (ACF), the precursor of colorectal polyps. (Carroll et al, 2011)

In this study, 44 smokers were given curcumin orally at two different doses (2 or 4 g/day) for 30 days. The levels of procarcinogenic eicosanoids, prostaglandin E_2, and 5-hydroxyeicosatetraenoic acid in ACF or normal flat mucosa were unaffected by the curcumin treatment at lower doses. Curcumin at 4 g/day, however, significantly reduced ACF formation. The reduction in ACF formation by curcumin was associated with a significant fivefold increase in post-treatment plasma curcumin/conjugate levels. Curcumin was well-tolerated at both concentrations. These findings demonstrated the effect of curcumin against ACF formation in smokers. (Carroll et al, 2011)

In another recent study, curcumin was administered to patients with CRC after diagnosis and before surgery. Curcumin (360 mg in a capsule form) was given three times a day for 10–30 days. Curcumin administration increased body weight, decreased serum TNF-α level, increased the number of apoptotic cells, and enhanced the expression of p53 in tumor tissue. **The authors of this study concluded that curcumin treatment can improve the general health of CRC patients via the mechanism of increased p53 expression in tumor cells**. (He et al, 2011)

Pancreatic cancer

Because oxidative stress is believed to be one of the causes of tropical pancreatitis, use of antioxidants may improve this condition. A single-blind, randomized, placebo-controlled study from India was conducted to evaluate the effects of oral curcumin with piperine on the pain and markers associated with oxidative stress in patients with tropical pancreatitis. Twenty patients with tropical pancreatitis were randomly assigned to receive 500 mg of curcumin with 5 mg of piperine or to receive placebo for 6 weeks, and the effects on the pattern of pain and on red blood cell (RBC) levels of MDA and GSH were assessed.

The results indicated a significant reduction in the erythrocyte MDA levels compared with placebo after curcumin therapy, with a significant increase in GSH levels. **The pain, however, was not improved by curcumin administration.** The authors of this study concluded that **oral curcumin with piperine may reverse lipid peroxidation in patients with tropical pancreatitis**. (Durgaprasad et al, 2005)

Curcumin was found safe and well-tolerated in a phase II clinical trial of patients with advanced pancreatic cancer. Of the 25 patients enrolled in the study, 21 were evaluable for response. Patients were given 8 g of curcumin per day orally until disease progression, with restaging every 2 months. Circulating curcumin was detectable as the glucuronide and sulfate conjugate forms, albeit at low steady-state levels, suggesting poor oral bioavailability. Two patients showed clinical biological activity, and one had ongoing stable disease for more than 18 months. Interestingly, one additional patient had a brief, but marked, tumor regression accompanied by significant increases in serum cytokine levels (IL-6, IL-8, IL-10, and IL-1 receptor antagonists).

No toxicities associated with curcumin administration were noted in the patients. A downregulation in the expression of NF–κB, COX-2, and pSTAT3 in peripheral blood mononuclear cells of patients was observed after curcumin intake. There was considerable interpatient variation in plasma curcumin levels, and drug levels peaked at 22 to 41 ng/ml and remained relatively constant over the first 4 weeks. The study concluded that **the oral curcumin is well-tolerated and, despite limited absorption, has biological activity in some patients with pancreatic cancer**. (Dhillon et al, 2008)

An open-label phase II trial evaluated the efficacy of curcumin in combination with gemcitabine against advanced pancreatic cancer. The authors of this study concluded that a curcumin dose of 8 g/day is above the maximum tolerated dose when taken with gemcitabine and that the efficacy of the combinations seemed modest. A large number of patients are needed to draw a solid conclusion. (Epelbaum et al, 2010)

Kanai *et al.* recently evaluated the safety and feasibility of combinations of curcumin and gemcitabine in 21 patients with gemcitabine-resistant pancreatic cancer. **Curcumin at 8 g/day in combination with gemcitabine was safe and well-tolerated**. (Kanai et al, 2011)

Breast cancer

Breast cancer is the second most common cause of cancer death in women and is very rare in men. According to one estimate, almost 226,870 new cases of invasive breast cancer are expected to occur among women in the United States during 2012. Docetaxel, a microtubule inhibitor, has been commonly used either as a single agent in metastatic disease or in combination with other chemotherapeutic agents in early stages of breast cancer. The feasibility and tolerability of the combination of docetaxel and curcumin in patients with advanced and metastatic breast cancer were evaluated in an open-label phase I trial. (Bauet-Robert et al, 2010)

Prostate cancer

Prostate cancer is the most common malignancy of men. According to the American Cancer Society's most recent estimates, 241,740 new cases of prostate cancer will occur in the United States during 2012. The disease is normally monitored by the prostate-specific antigen (PSA) test. An elevated level of PSA *per se* reflects the risk of developing prostate cancer. Thus, intervention to improve the PSA level may help prevent prostate cancer. A **randomized, double-blind, controlled study** evaluated the effects of soy isoflavones and curcumin on serum PSA levels in men who underwent prostate biopsies because of increased PSA but who had negative findings for prostate cancer. (Ide et al, 2010)

Eighty-five participants were randomly assigned to take a supplement containing isoflavones and curcumin or placebo daily. Participants were subdivided by the cut-off of their baseline PSA value at 10 ng/ml. Forty-three participants were given a combination of 100 mg of curcumin and 40 mg of isoflavones, and 42 were given placebo for 6 months. PSA values were evaluated before and 6 months after treatment. PSA levels decreased in the patient group, with PSA values greater than 10 ng/ml among those who received supplementation containing isoflavones and curcumin (Fig. 3a). These results indicated that **isoflavones and curcumin could modulate serum PSA levels**. The authors of this study concluded that **curcumin presumably synergizes with isoflavones to suppress PSA production**. (Ide et al, 2010)

Multiple Myeloma

Multiple myeloma, also known as plasma cell myeloma, is a generalized malignancy of plasma cells associated with diverse clinical features, including bone lesions, hypercalcemia, anemia, and renal failure. It is the second most common hematological cancer in the United States after non-Hodgkin lymphoma. **While advances in treatment, including the use of bortezomib (Velcade), thalidomide, and lenalidomide (Revlimid), have improved patient outcomes, multiple myeloma remains an incurable disease for most patients**.

Monoclonal gammopathy of undetermined significance (MGUS) is a common premalignant plasma cell proliferative disorder with a lifelong risk of progression to multiple myeloma.

Curcumin decreased the paraprotein load in the ten patients with paraprotein >20 g/L, and five of these ten had a 12% to 30% reduction in paraprotein levels while receiving curcumin therapy. In addition, 27% of patients receiving curcumin had a >25% decrease in urinary N-telopeptide of type I collagen. (Golombick et al, 2009)

The study suggested the therapeutic potential of curcumin against monoclonal gammopathy of undetermined significance (MGUS).

Lung cancer

Smokers excrete significant amounts of mutagens in the urine and are at high risk of developing lung cancer. Whereas smoking increases the risk for mutagenicity and lung cancer, dietary factors including turmeric reduce the risk. One study assessed the anti-mutagenic effects of turmeric in 16 chronic smokers and six non-smokers who served as a control. When given at 1.5 g/day for 30 days, turmeric significantly reduced the urinary excretion of mutagens in the smokers, **but in the control group, no changes in the urinary excretion of mutagens were observed**. Furthermore, **turmeric had no significant effect on serum aspartate aminotransferase and alanine aminotransferase, blood glucose, creatinine, or lipid profile**. (Polasa et al, 1992)

Authors of this study suggested that dietary turmeric can act as an effective anti-mutagen in smokers and can reduce the risk of lung cancer.

Cancer lesions

Oral cancer is one of the leading cancers of the Indian subcontinent and is associated mostly with tobacco chewing. The most common precancerous oral lesions such as oral submucous fibrosis, oral leukoplakia, and oral lichen planus are associated with tobacco chewing.

One study evaluated the effects of alcoholic extracts of turmeric oil and turmeric oleoresin on the number of micronuclei in healthy participants and in patients with submucous fibrosis. (Hastak et al, 1997)

None of the extracts had any effects on the number of micronuclei in lymphocytes from healthy participants. All three extracts, however, offered protection against benzo[a]pyrene-induced increase in micronuclei in patients circulating lymphocytes. In another set of experiments, patients with submucous fibrosis were given a daily oral dose of turmeric oil (600 mg) plus turmeric (3 g), turmeric oleoresin (600 mg) plus turmeric (3 g), or turmeric alone (3 g) for 3 months. Results indicated that all three treatment modalities decreased the number of micronucleated cells both in exfoliated oral mucosal cells and in circulating lymphocytes.

Another phase I study evaluated the toxicology, pharmacokinetics, and biologically effective dose of curcumin in patients with resected urinary bladder cancer, arsenic-associated Bowen disease of the skin, uterine cervical intraepithelial neoplasm (CIN), oral leucoplakia, and intestinal metaplasia of the stomach. A total of 25 patients were enrolled in this study. Curcumin was given orally for 3 months, and biopsy of the lesion sites was done immediately before and 3 months after initiation of curcumin treatment. No treatment-related toxicity occurred with doses up to 8 g/day. At doses higher than 8 g/day, however, the bulky volume of the drug was unacceptable to the patients. The serum concentration of curcumin usually peaked at 1 to 2 h after curcumin intake and gradually declined within 12 h.

However, urinary excretion of curcumin was undetectable. One of four patients with CIN and one of seven with oral leucoplakia developed frank malignancies in spite of curcumin treatment. In contrast, histologic improvement of precancerous lesions was seen in one of two patients with resected bladder cancer, two of seven patients of oral leucoplakia, one of six patients of intestinal metaplasia of the stomach, one of four patients with CIN, and two of six patients with Bowen disease. (Cheng et al, 2001)

These data demonstrate the safety of curcumin at doses up to 8 g/day taken orally for 3 months. The study also suggested the chemopreventive potential of curcumin against cancerous lesions.

A randomized, double-blind, placebo-controlled trial was conducted in 100 patients with oral lichen planus to evaluate the efficacy of curcuminoids. (Chainani-Wu et al, 2007)

The trial included two interim analyses, and the participants were randomly assigned to receive either placebo or curcuminoids at 2 g/day for 7 weeks. In addition, all participants received prednisone at 60 mg/day for the first week. The primary outcome was a change in symptoms from baseline, and secondary outcomes were changes in clinical signs and occurrence of any side effects. **The results of the first interim analysis using data from 33 participants did not show any significant difference between the placebo and curcuminoid groups.** Conditional power calculations suggested that the likelihood of the curcuminoid group having significantly better outcome than that of the placebo group if the trial were to be completed was less than 2%. Therefore, the study was ended before completion. However, curcuminoids were well-tolerated. For future studies of efficacy, the authors suggested the use of a larger sample size and a higher dose and/or longer duration of curcuminoids without an initial course of prednisone. (Chainani-Wu et al, 2007)

Since the earlier studies had examined the effects of alcoholic extracts of turmeric, turmeric oil, and turmeric oleoresin in patients with submucous fibrosis but the later study used curcumin, **it remains unclear whether differences in the preparations accounted for the differences in results**.

Head and neck squamous cell carcinoma (HNSCC)

HNSCC is the sixth most common cancer worldwide, with approximately 600,000 cases diagnosed per year. HNSCC is a heterogeneous disease that includes oral, laryngeal, and pharyngeal malignancies, with about 40% of these arising in the oral cavity. Despite medical advancements, the 5-year survival rate for patients with HNSCC remains in the range of 40% to 50%. Studies over the past several years have indicated the role of NF–κB and inflammatory molecules such as IL-6, IL-8, and VEGF in the pathogenesis of this disease (86). Therefore, targeting these signaling molecules might prove useful against HNSCC. Whether curcumin can inhibit IκB kinase β (IKKβ) kinase activity, an enzyme involved in NF–κB activation that suppresses expression of inflammatory cytokines in patients with HNSCC, was investigated. A total of 39 patients (13 with dental caries, 21 with HNSCC, and 5 healthy volunteers) participated in this study. Saliva was collected before and 1 h after participants chewed two curcumin tablets for 5 min. Curcumin treatment led to a reduction in IKKβ kinase activity in the salivary cells of patients with HNSCC. Treatment of UM-SCC1 cell lines with curcumin as well as with post-curcumin salivary supernatant showed a reduction of IKKβ kinase activity. Significant reduction in IL-8 levels was seen in post-curcumin samples from patients with dental caries.

Although IL-8 expression was reduced in 8 of 21 post-curcumin samples of patients with HNSCC, **the data did not reach statistical significance**. The authors of this study concluded that IKKβ kinase could be used as a biomarker for detecting the effect of curcumin in HNSCC. (Kim et al, 2011)

Inflammatory bowel disease

Patients with IBD have a significantly higher risk of developing colon cancer than the general population has.

One open-label study evaluated the efficacy of curcumin in five patients with ulcerative proctitis and in five patients with Crohn disease. (Holt et al, 2005)

The patients with ulcerative proctitis were given 550 mg of curcumin twice daily for 1 month and then 550 mg three times daily for another month. In the patients with Crohn disease, curcumin was administered at a dose of 360 mg three times a day for 1 month and then 360 mg four times a day for another 2 months. Significant decrease in symptoms as well as in inflammatory indices (erythrocyte sedimentation rate and CRP) were observed in all patients with proctitis. Only four of the five patients with Crohn disease, however, completed the study. There was a mean reduction of 55 points in the Crohn disease activity index, and reductions in erythrocyte sedimentation rate and CRP were observed in these patients. **Although this study suggests the efficacy of curcumin against IBD, large double-blind, placebo-controlled studies are required for confirmation**.

Another study evaluated the efficacy of curcumin as maintenance therapy in 89 patients with quiescent ulcerative colitis. (Hanai et al, 2006)

For this randomized, double-blind, multicenter trial, 45 patients received curcumin, 1 g after breakfast and 1 g after the evening meal, plus sulfasalazine or mesalamine, and 44 patients received placebo plus sulfasalazine or mesalamine for 6 months. **The relapse rates were 4.65% in the curcumin-treated group and 20.51% in the placebo group.**

Irritable bowel syndrome

Irritable bowel syndrome (IrBS) is a chronic problem of the large intestine. The most common symptoms of IrBS are cramping, abdominal pain, bloating, gas, diarrhea, and constipation. The causes of IrBS are unclear, and there is no commonly accepted cure. A partially blinded, randomized, two-dose, pilot study assessed the effects of turmeric extract on IrBS symptoms in healthy adults.

Turmeric was given to the volunteers in tablet form: 102 patients were given one tablet containing 72 mg of standardized turmeric extract, and 105 patients were given two tablets a day, both for 8 weeks. The prevalence of IrBS was reduced by 53% and 60% in the one-tablet and two-tablet groups, respectively, and was associated with a marked decrease in IrBS symptoms. (Bundy et al, 2004)

Although these results suggest that turmeric may help reduce IrBS symptoms, placebo-controlled trials are needed to confirm these findings. **Another study conducted with eight healthy participants reported that turmeric has the potential to increase bowel motility and to activate hydrogen-producing bacterial flora in the colon**. (Shimouchi et al, 2009)

Arthritis

Arthritis is a chronic disease that results from the inflammation of one or more joints. It usually results from dysregulation of pro-inflammatory cytokines (e.g., TNF, IL-1β) and pro-inflammatory enzymes that mediate the production of prostaglandins (e.g., COX-2) and leukotrienes (e.g., lipoxygenase), together with the expression of adhesion molecules and matrix metalloproteinases.

Although more than 100 different kinds of arthritis have been reported, the three most common forms are osteoarthritis, rheumatoid arthritis, and gout. Typically, a combination of exercise, modifications in lifestyle factors, and NSAIDs are used for the treatment of osteoarthritis. The use of NSAIDs, however, is associated with numerous adverse effects.

The potential of curcumin against arthritis was first reported in 1980 in a short-term, double-blind, crossover study involving 18 young patients with rheumatoid arthritis. (Deodhar et al, 1980)

In this study, curcumin's efficacy was compared with that of the prescription drug phenylbutazone. Patients were randomly assigned to receive either curcumin (1.2 g/day) or phenylbutazone (0.3 g/day) for 2 weeks. **Curcumin was well-tolerated, had no adverse effects, and exerted an anti-rheumatic activity identical to that of phenylbutazone as shown by improvement in joint swelling, morning stiffness, and walking time.** However, one of the major drawbacks of this study was the lack of a control or placebo group (38). Further well-controlled studies are therefore required to examine the long-term effects of curcumin against rheumatoid arthritis.

In another recent study, **curcumin alone (0.5 g) and in combination with diclofenac sodium (0.05 g) was found to be safe and effective in 45 patients with rheumatoid arthritis**. (Chandran, Goel, 2012)

Furthermore, the level of CRP was suppressed in these patients after curcumin administration.

Another study in 50 patients with osteoarthritis evaluated the efficacy of Meriva at a dose that corresponded to 200 mg of curcumin per day. (Belcaro et al, 2010)

The signs and symptoms of osteoarthritis were evaluated with use of WOMAC scores, an indicator of pain level. The mobility was assessed by walking performance (treadmill), and inflammatory status was assessed by measuring the levels of CRP. **After 3 months of treatment, the global WOMAC score was decreased by 58%; walking distance was increased from 76 m to 332 m, and CRP levels were significantly decreased**. In comparison, only modest improvement in these measurements was observed in the control group. Overall, these results suggested the efficacy of Meriva in the management of osteoarthritis. (Belcaro et al, 2010)

In a subsequent study, this group investigated the long-term efficacy and safety of Meriva in a longer (8-month) study involving 100 patients with osteoarthritis. (Belcaro, Cesarone et al, 2010)

The patients were divided into the control group (50 patients) and the curcumin group (50 patients), in which patients received 1 g/day of Meriva for 8 months. The WOMAC score was decreased by more than 50%, whereas treadmill walking performance was increased almost threefold compared with the control. Serum inflammatory biomarkers such as IL-1β, IL-6, soluble CD40 ligand, soluble vascular cell adhesion molecule-1, and erythrocyte sedimentation rate were also significantly decreased in the treatment group.

In addition, remarkable decreases in gastrointestinal complications, distal edema, and the use of NSAIDs/painkillers by the patients were also noted after Meriva treatment. The need for hospital admissions, consultations, and tests by the patients was also decreased after Meriva treatment. The authors of this study concluded that Meriva is worth considering for the long-term complementary management of osteoarthritis. (Belcaro et al, 2010)

Uveitis

Uveitis is an inflammation of the uvea, the middle layer of the eye. Uveitis is a major cause of visual impairment and has been estimated to account for 10% to 15% of all cases of total blindness in the United States.

One study evaluated the efficacy of curcumin against chronic anterior uveitis. (Lal et al, 1999)

Curcumin was administered orally to patients with chronic anterior uveitis at a dose of 375 mg three times a day for 12 weeks. Of 53 patients enrolled, 32 completed the 12-week study and were divided into two groups. One group of 18 patients received curcumin alone, whereas the other group of 14 patients, who had a strong reaction to tuberculin purified protein derivative, also received anti-tubercular treatment. After 2 weeks of treatment, both groups showed significant improvement in the disease.

Whereas all patients who received curcumin alone exhibited improvement, the group receiving anti-tubercular therapy along with curcumin had a response rate of 86%. Furthermore, follow-up of all patients for the next 3 years found recurrence rates of 55% for the first group and 36% for the second group. However, 22% of patients in the first group and 21% of patients in the second group lost their vision in the follow-up period due to various complications in the eyes.

The efficacy of curcumin on recurrences after treatment was comparable to that of corticosteroid therapy. Furthermore, lack of any adverse effects with curcumin was an advantage over corticosteroid therapy. (Lal et al, 1999)

One nonplacebo-controlled study evaluated the efficacy of Meriva against recurrent anterior uveitis. (Allegri et al, 2010)

The study group consisted of 106 patients divided into three main groups of different uveitis origin: group 1 (autoimmune uveitis, 56 patients), group 2 (herpetic uveitis, 28 patients), and group 3 (various etiologies of uveitis, 22 patients). All patients were given Norflo containing 600 mg of Meriva twice daily during the follow-up period (about 12–18 months). The primary end point was relapse frequency in all treated patients, before and after Meriva treatment, followed by the number of relapses in the three etiological groups. The secondary end points were relapse severity and overall quality of life. **A total of 106 and 19 patients, respectively, had relapses before and after treatment with Norflo. Furthermore, the total number of relapses was reduced from 275 to 36 after the 1-year treatment with Norflo**. Meriva was well-tolerated and reduced eye discomfort after a few weeks of treatment in more than 80% of patients. Thus, the study demonstrated the therapeutic role of curcumin and its efficacy against recurrent anterior uveitis. (Allegri et al, 2010)

Postoperative inflammation

In a study of curcumin's anti-inflammatory properties, Satoskar *et al.* evaluated the effects of this polyphenol on spermatic cord edema and tenderness in 46 men (15–68 years old) who had just undergone surgical repair of an inguinal hernia and/or hydrocele. After surgery, patients were randomly assigned to receive curcumin (400 mg), placebo (250 mg lactose powder), or phenylbutazone (100 mg) three times a day for 6 days. Spermatic cord edema, spermatic cord tenderness, operative site pain, and operative site tenderness reflected by intensity score (TIS) were measured. TIS on day 6 decreased by 84.2% in the curcumin group, by 61.8% in placebo group, and by 86% in phenylbutazone group. Although TIS values for the curcumin and phenylbutazone groups were similar on day 6, curcumin proved to be superior by reducing all four measures of inflammation. (Satoskar et al, 1986)

Peptic ulcer

Peptic ulcers are the most common ulcer of the gastrointestinal tract and can be extremely painful. These ulcers are usually open sores that develop on the inner lining of the esophagus, stomach, and the upper portion of the small intestine. If the peptic ulcer is located in the stomach, it is called a gastric ulcer. According to one estimate, 5% to 10% of adults globally are affected by peptic ulcers at least once in their lifetime. The preferred medications for peptic ulcers include proton pump inhibitors, histamine receptor blockers, and antibiotics to kill a *Helicobacter pylori* infection. A randomized controlled clinical trial from Thailand compared the efficacy of turmeric and liquid antacid (containing 333 g of aluminum hydroxide and 33.3 g of magnesium hydroxide per 1,000 ml) against benign gastric ulcers (45). Of the 60 patients who participated in the study, 30 received turmeric (250 mg, four times per day), and the other 30 received antacid (30 ml, four times per day).

The treatment was continued for 6 to 12 weeks. **Although both antacid and turmeric improved gastric ulcers in patients, the former was better in reducing the ulcers**. (Kositchaiwat et al, 1993)

A phase II clinical trial from Thailand evaluated the safety and efficacy of curcumin in patients with peptic ulcers. Forty-five patients (24 men and 21 women, aged 16–60 years) were included in the study. Twenty-five patients (18 men and 7 women) underwent endoscopy, and their ulcers were found in the duodenal bulb and gastric (angulus) region. The remaining 20 patients did not have ulcers but appeared to have erosions, gastritis, and dyspepsia. Two capsules (300 mg each) of turmeric were given orally five times daily over a period of 4 weeks.

Results after 4 weeks of treatment showed that ulcers were absent in 12 patients; after 8 weeks of treatment, ulcers were absent in 18 patients; and after 12 weeks of treatment, ulcers were absent in 19 patients. The remaining patients had symptomatic relief after turmeric treatment. (Prucksunand et al, 2001)

Alzheimer's disease

Alzheimer's disease is a progressive neurodegenerative disorder, usually affecting people older than age 65 years. The pathogenesis of Alzheimer's disease involves aggregation of Aβ (especially $A\beta_{1-42}$) into fibrils, formation of amyloid plaques, and deposition of these plaques into the brain.

A total of 33 patients who were enrolled in the study were randomly assigned to a placebo group, low-dose curcumin group (2 g/day), or high-dose curcumin group (4 g/day). After 24 weeks, the patients who were receiving curcumin continued the treatment at their assigned dose, whereas those who were receiving the placebo were given one of the two doses of curcumin. The study examined the safety, tolerability, pharmacokinetics, and efficacy of curcumin in patients with Alzheimer's disease, as well as the effects of curcumin on biomarkers associated with the pathology of this disease. Although the study has been completed, the observations have yet to be published. (Ringman et al, 2005)

Baum *et al.* conducted a randomized, double-blind, placebo-controlled study in 34 patients with Alzheimer's disease. The study participants were randomly assigned to receive curcumin at two different doses (1 or 4 g) or placebo (4 g). The Mini-Mental State Examination (MMSE) score that assesses mental status was not improved after curcumin treatment. Similarly, the level of serum Aβ40 was not affected by curcumin treatment. However, curcumin administration was associated with an increase in vitamin E level, and curcumin did not cause any adverse effects.

These authors concluded **that the anti-oxidant activity of curcuminoids might decrease the need for anti-oxidant vitamin E**. (Baum et al, 2008)

These observations support the opening of a clinical trial of curcumin against Alzheimer's disease using large numbers of patients.

Acute coronary syndrome (ACS)

A randomized, double-blind, controlled trial from Jakarta evaluated the effects of curcumin on total cholesterol, LDL cholesterol, HDL cholesterol, and triglyceride levels in patients with ACS (56). A total of 70 patients were assigned to four different groups: placebo, low-dose (45 mg/day), moderate-dose (90 mg/day), and high-dose (180 mg/day) curcumin. The curcumin was administered orally to the patients for 2 months.

Low-dose curcumin was highly effective, compared with high-dose curcumin, in reducing total cholesterol and LDL

cholesterol in patients. Conversely, low-dose curcumin increased HDL cholesterol to a greater extent than did the high-dose. The increase in triglyceride content by curcumin was greatest at the moderate dose. These studies suggest the beneficial effects of curcumin in improving lipid profiles in patients with ACS. (Alwi et al, 2008)

However, **improving the lipid profile does not necessarily mean that curcumin is effective against ACS**.

Atherosclerosis

One study evaluated the effects of curcumin in reducing the serum levels of cholesterol and lipid peroxides in ten healthy human volunteers (57). Curcumin (at 0.5 g/day) administered to the volunteers for 7 days reduced serum lipid peroxides by 33% and total serum cholesterol levels by 11.63%, and increased HDL cholesterol by 29%.

Diabetes

Type 1 result from the body's failure to produce insulin, whereas in type 2 diabetes (T2DM) the body fails to use insulin properly. **Extensive research over the past several years has indicated that pro-inflammatory cytokines and oxidative stress play a role in the pathogenesis of T2DM**. Because of its anti-inflammatory property, curcumin represents a promising therapeutic option for T2DM.

A randomized, double-blind, placebo-controlled clinical trial assessed the efficacy of curcumin in delaying development of T2DM in the pre-diabetes population. A total of 240 participants were randomly assigned to receive either curcumin (1.5 g/day) or placebo capsules, and changes in β cell functions (homeostasis model assessment [HOMA]-β, C-peptide, and proinsulin/insulin), insulin resistance (HOMA-IR), and anti-inflammatory cytokine (adiponectin) levels were monitored at the baseline and at 3, 6, and 9 months of treatment. **After 9 months of treatment, 16.4% of participants in the placebo group were diagnosed with T2DM, whereas none were diagnosed with T2DM in the curcumin-treated group**. In addition, the participants of curcumin-treated group showed a better overall function of β cells, with higher HOMA-β and lower C-peptide levels. The curcumin-treated participants also exhibited a lower level of HOMA-IR and higher adiponectin when compared with the placebo group. The authors of this study concluded that the **curcumin may be beneficial in a prediabetes population**. (Chuengsmarn et al, 2012)

Diabetic microangiopathy

One study evaluated the potential of Meriva in improving diabetic microangiopathy. In these patients, the disease was associated with microcirculatory alteration that was managed without insulin for at least 5 years. All patients were treated with what could be considered the best treatment protocol for the disease. In the treatment group, Meriva (1 g/day) was added as a supplement to the standard treatment for 4 weeks and was well-tolerated, with no dropouts reported, and all participants in the treatment and control group completed the study. In the treatment group, at 4 weeks, microcirculatory and clinical evaluations indicated a decrease in skin flux at the surface of the foot, an indicator of an improvement in microangiopathy. Also, a significant decrease in the edema score and a corresponding improvement in the venoarteriolar response were observed. **An increase in PO_2, possibly due to better oxygen diffusion into the skin and decreased edema, was observed**. These features were observed in all participants using Meriva, whereas no clinical or microcirculatory effects were observed in the control group. (Appendino et al, 2011)

Renal transplantation

Curcumin and quercetin can improve early outcomes in cadaveric renal transplantation, possibly through induction of HO-1. (Shoskes et al, 2005)

Acquired Immunodeficiency syndrome (AIDS)

A clinical trial from New England examined the effectiveness of curcumin as an anti-viral agent in 40 AIDS patients. Two participants dropped out due to adverse events unrelated to the curcumin study. Of the remaining 38 patients, 23 were randomly assigned to a high-dose group (2.5 g/d) and 15 to a low-dose group. The treatment was continued for 8 weeks. No evidence of curcumin-associated reduction in viral load was observed. CD4 cells showed a slight increase in the high-dose group and a consistent decrease in the low-dose group. However, none of the results was statistically significant. **Despite the lack of apparent anti-viral or CD4 effects, most participants liked taking curcumin because they felt better.** (James, 1996)

It is likely that curcumin could provide benefits in unknown ways.

ß-Thalassemia

β-Thalassemia is an inherited blood disorder in which the body makes an abnormal form of β-chains of hemoglobin (Hb). The disorder results in excessive destruction of RBCs, which leads to anemia. In Southeast Asians, HbE, a common Hb variant, is normally associated with the β-thalassemia phenotype. Disturbances in oxidative stress and in the anti-oxidant defense system are commonly reported in patients with β-thalassemia. (Fibach, Rachmilewitz, 2008)

One study examined whether measures of oxidative stress can be ameliorated after treatment with curcumin in patients with β-thalassemia. (Kalpravidh et al, 2010)

Twenty-one patients were given curcuminoids (500 mg/d) for 12 months. Blood was collected every 2 months during treatment and 3 months after withdrawal and was analyzed for MDA, superoxide dismutase, glutathione peroxidase (GSH-Px), and reduced GSH in RBCs, as well as non-transferrin-bound iron in serum.

An increase in oxidative stress was reported, as indicated by higher levels of MDA, superoxide dismutase, and GSH-Px in RBCs, higher non-transferrin-bound iron in serum, and lower levels of RBC GSH in patients. Curcuminoid administration was associated with improvement in these measures. Furthermore, 3 months after withdrawal of curcuminoid treatment, all measures returned close to baseline levels. The authors of this study concluded that **curcuminoids may be used to ameliorate oxidative damage in patients with β-thalassemia**.

Gallbladder contraction

A randomized, double-blind, crossover study compared the effect of 20 mg of curcumin or placebo on the gallbladder volume of 12 healthy volunteers. Ultrasonographic examination was carried out serially to measure the gallbladder volume. The gallbladder volume was reduced within the period after curcumin administration. The percentages of gallbladder volume reduction at 0.5, 1, 1.5, and 2 h after curcumin administration were 11.8%, 16.8%, 22%, and 29.3%, respectively. **These results suggest the ability of curcumin in stimulating gallbladder contraction and reducing the risk of gallstones formation.** (Rasyid, Lelo, 1999)

Recurrent respiratory tract infections

One study examined the clinical and immunologic effects of lactoferrin and curcumin (LC) oral supplementation in healthy children with RRTIs. Ten children with RRTIs received LC orally at 1 g (900 mg lactoferrin plus 100 mg curcumin) every 8 h for 4 weeks. Administration of LC was associated with reduction in RRTIs and beneficial immune-modulatory effects in children. (Zuccotti et al, 2009)

Chronic arsenic exposure

Groundwater arsenic contamination is a global threat to human health and is associated with carcinogenic effects. The biggest cases of groundwater arsenic contamination can be found in Bangladesh and in West Bengal in India. **The carcinogenic effects of arsenic are likely mediated through oxidative DNA damage. Therefore, agents with antioxidant capacity may have potential against arsenic-induced genotoxic effects.**

A field trial from West Bengal evaluated the role of curcumin against the genotoxic effects of arsenic. A total of 286 volunteers exposed to groundwater arsenic were recruited into the study. The participants were randomly assigned to a placebo group (143 persons) and a curcumin-treated group (143 persons). Curcumin was given at a dose of 500 mg twice daily for 3 months in combination with piperine. DNA damage in lymphocytes was assessed by the comet assay and fluorescence-activated DNA unwinding assay. Curcumin was analyzed in blood by high-performance liquid chromatography. Arsenic-induced oxidative stress and curcumin's antagonistic role were evaluated by measuring reactive oxygen species (ROS) generation, lipid peroxidation, and protein carbonyl contents. The blood samples from this arsenic-exposed population showed severe DNA damage with increased levels of ROS and lipid peroxidation.

Three months of curcumin intervention reduced the DNA damage and retarded ROS generation and lipid peroxidation. Curcumin treatment was also associated with significant enhancement in the levels of such anti-oxidants as catalase, superoxide dismutase, glutathione peroxidase, and glutathione. The authors of this study concluded that curcumin may have some protective role against arsenic-induced DNA damage. (Biswas et al, 2010)

Adverse events associated with curcumin

Although curcumin has been shown to exhibit beneficial activities in a plethora of human diseases with minimal toxicities, **some investigators have reported undesired adverse effects associated with this polyphenol**.

Lao *et al.* conducted a dose-escalation study to determine the maximum tolerable dose and safety of a single oral dose of curcumin in 34 healthy volunteers. (Lao et al, 2006)

The volunteers were given escalating doses of curcumin ranging from 500 to 12,000 mg, and safety was assessed for 72 h after administration. Twenty-four participants completed the trial, seven of whom experienced minimal toxicity that did not appear to be dose-related. **More specifically, these seven participants experienced diarrhea, headache, rash, and yellow stool.**

In another study, curcumin at doses ranging from 0.45 to 3.6 g/day for 1 to 4 months was associated with nausea and diarrhea and caused an increase in serum alkaline phosphatase and lactate dehydrogenase contents in human participants. In patients with high-risk or premalignant lesions, doses of curcumin above 8 g/day were unacceptable to patients because of the bulky volume of the tablets. In one study of patients with advanced pancreatic cancer, 5 of the 17 patients receiving curcumin (8 g/day) in combination with gemcitabine reported intractable abdominal pain after a few days to 2 weeks of curcumin intake. Thus, more studies are required to evaluate the long-term toxicity associated with curcumin before it can be approved for human use.

Conclusions

Subsequent to the first seminal paper published in 1949 in *Nature*, numerous preclinical studies have provided a solid basis for examining curcumin's efficacy against human diseases. Curcumin has shown therapeutic potential against a number of human diseases. **Common to all of these studies have been the safety, tolerability, and non-toxicity of this polyphenol, even at doses up to 8 g per day.** The underlying mechanism for curcumin's clinical efficacy seems to be modulation of numerous signaling molecules. However, because of the complex nature of the diseases, the underlying mechanism in many cases remains unclear.

From the findings of the completed clinical trials, it may seem that curcumin's clinical efficacy is too good to be true. However, **this polyphenol has not yet been approved for human use**.

Poor bioavailability and limited adverse effects reported by some investigators are a major limitation to the therapeutic utility of curcumin. We hope that the results from ongoing clinical trials will provide a deeper understanding of curcumin's therapeutic potential and will help to place this fascinating molecule at the fore front of novel therapeutics. (Gupta, Patchva and Aggrarwal, 2013)

RMH Note: My interpretation of the Gupta paper illustrates the wide application of curcumin in disease conditions which is associated with rather weak clinical data. I am not convinced of the magical nature of curcumin, at this point.

Turmeric and curcumin: Biological actions and medicinal applications

(Chattopadhyay et al, 2004)

http://repository.ias.ac.in/5196/1/306.pdf

Antioxidant effect

The antioxidant activity of curcumin was reported as early as 1975. It acts as a scavenger of oxygen free radicals. (Sharma, 1976) (Subramanian et al, 1994)

RMH Note: It can protect hemoglobin from oxidation. But, **please do not forget about its prooxidant activity as well**.

In vitro, **curcumin can significantly inhibit the generation of reactive oxygen species (ROS, EMODs) like superoxide anions, H_2O_2 and nitrite radical** generation by activated macrophages, which play an important role in inflammation. (Joe et al, 1994)

Curcumin also lowers the production of EMODs in vivo. (Joe et al, 1994)

Its derivatives, demethoxycurcumin and bis-demethoxycurcumin also have antioxidant effect.

Curcumin exerts powerful inhibitory effect against H_2O_2-induced damage in human keratinocytes and fibroblasts and in NG 108-15 cells. (Mahakunakorn et al, 2003)

Curcumin reduces oxidized proteins in amyloid pathology in Alzheimer transgenic mice. (Lim et al, 2001)

It also decreases lipid peroxidation in rat liver microsomes, erythrocyte membranes and brain homogenates. This is brought about by maintaining the activities of antioxidant enzymes like superoxide dismutase, catalase and glutathione peroxidase. (Pulla, Reddy, 1992)

Recently, we have observed that curcumin prevents oxidative damage during indomethacin-induced gastric lesion not only by blocking inactivation of gastric peroxidase, but also by direct scavenging of H_2O_2 and ·OH (unpublished observation).

Since ROS (EMODs) have been implicated in the development of various pathological conditions, curcumin has the potential to control these diseases through its potent antioxidant activity. (Bandyopadhyay et al, 1999) (Halliwell, 1998) (Halliwell 1990)

Contradictory to the above-mentioned antioxidant effect, curcumin has prooxidant activity.

Kelly et al. reported that **curcumin not only failed to prevent single-strand DNA breaks by H_2O_2, but also caused DNA damage.** (Kelly et al, 2001)

As this damage was prevented by antioxidant a-tocopherol, **the prooxidant role of curcumin has been proved.**

Curcumin also causes oxidative damage of rat hepatocytes by oxidizing glutathione and of human erythrocyte by oxidizing oxyhemoglobin, thereby causing hemolysis. (Galati et al, 2002)

The prooxidant activity appears to be mediated through generation of phenoxyl radical of curcumin by peroxidase–H_2O_2 system, which co-oxidizes cellular glutathione or NADH, accompanied by O_2 uptake to form EMODs. (Galati et al, 2002)

Mechanism of apoptosis:

The mechanism of curcumin-induced apoptosis has also been studied in Caki cells, where curcumin causes apoptosis through down-regulation of Bcl-XL and IAP, release of cytochrome c and inhibition of Akt, which are markedly blocked by N-acetylcysteine, indicating a role of ROS (EMODs) in curcumin-induced cell death. (Woo et al, 2003)

Curcumin induces apoptosis in human leukaemia HL-60 cells, which is blocked by some antioxidants. (Kuo et al, 1996)

Pro/antimutagenic activity

Curcumin exerts both pro- and antimutagenic effects. At 100 and 200 mg/kg body wt doses, curcumin has been shown to reduce the number of aberrant cells in cyclophosphamide-induced chromosomal aberration in Wistar rats. (Shukla et al, 2002)

Turmeric also prevents mutation in urethane (a powerful mutagen) models. (el Hamss et al, 1999)

Contradictory reports also exist. Curcumin and turmeric enhance g-radiation-induced chromosome aberration in Chinese hamster ovary. (Araujo et al, 1999)

Curcumin has also been shown to be non-protective against hexavalent chromium-induced DNA strand break. In fact, the total effect of chromium and curcumin is additive in causing DNA breaks in human lymphocytes and gastric mucosal cells. (Blasiak et al, 1999)

Dietary curcumin does not protect kidney in glycerol-induced acute renal failure

Generation of reactive oxygen species significantly contribute to the pathogenesis of renal injury induced by myoglobin release. The present study was performed to investigate the effects of dietary curcumin, a natural antioxidant isolated from plant *Curcuma longa*, in an experimental model of myoglobinuric acute renal failure. Rats received curcumin at an oral dose of 100 mg/kg/day for 30 days. Renal injury was induced with injection of hypertonic glycerol (10 ml/kg 50% solution) in hind limb muscle with blood urea of 57.8 ± 7.2 vs. 7.72 ± 1.03 mmol/l and serum creatinine of 444.4 ± 61.3 vs. 51.8 ± 10.6 µmol/l, in glycerol-induced acute renal failure (ARF) vs. control rats, respectively. After 48 h rats were sacrificed and thiobarbituric acid reactive substance (TBARS), glutathione, carbonyl content and kidney cortex brush border peptidase activities were determined in serum, kidney and liver. **Rats that received curcumin in addition to glycerol had significantly lower TBARS in serum but not in kidney and liver.** Carbonyl content in kidney and liver was significantly elevated in curcumin and glycerol treated rats and improved in animals treated with curcumin and glycerol together. The activities of kidney cortex enzymes, aminopeptidase N, angiotensinase A and dipeptidyl peptidase IV, were reduced in glycerol as well as in curcumin treated rats. **The results obtained in this study provided additional evidence that despite its limited antioxidant activity curcumin did not protect kidney in myoglobinuric model of ARF.**

(Vlahovic et al, 2007)

Benefits of Adding Turmeric to Your Diet

Adapted from an article by Jeannie R. Boylan

Turmeric is a dark yellow root of the curcuma longa plant, which is native to south Asia.

Turmeric is a relative of the ginger family. The root can be used fresh or be boiled, dried and ground into a powder.

Turmeric is used to flavor food, very popular in curries. Turmeric is also used as a food colorant in foods such as mustard and cheese. **Because of its antibacterial properties, turmeric is also used as a food preservative.**

Turmeric is made up of many vitamins (including several B vitamins and Vitamin C, among others) and minerals (such as calcium, iron and manganese). **It is also made up of plant chemicals, the most common being the curcuminoids.**

Curcumin is the curcuminoid most commonly studied. **Curcumin makes up about 3 to 5% of most powdered turmeric.**

Turmeric has been most commonly studied for its anti-inflammatory, antibacterial, antioxidant, anti-carcinogenic and detoxifying properties. Curcumin has been researched and shows promise in its use in many diseases such as cancer, Alzheimer's disease and arthritis. As shown on ClinicalTrials.gov, there are many ongoing and completed trials with turmeric/curcumin. (*http://clinicaltrials.gov/ct2/results?term= turmeric&Search=Search*)

Dementia is on the rise worldwide; however, India has been shown to have one of the lowest prevalence in the world. (*Prevalence of dementia in Latin America, India, and China: a population-based cross-sectional survey http://www.sciencedirect.com/science/article/pii/ S0140673608610028*)

It has been suggested that this may be due to the Indian diet and their high intake of turmeric. A study in a non-demented elderly Asian population showed that people who ate curry dishes often to very often did better on the Mini-Mental State Examination than did people who consumed curry rarely or never. (*Curry Consumption and*

Cognitive Function in the Elderlyhttp://aje.oxfordjournals.org/content/ 164/9/898.long)

One animal study showed that curcumin suppresses inflammation and oxidative damage in the brain of mice with Alzheimer's disease pathogenesis. In the same study, curcumin also decreased the amyloid plaques in many affected brain regions of mice. (*The Curry Spice Curcumin Reduces Oxidative Damage and Amyloid Pathology in an Alzheimer Transgenic Mouse http://www.jneurosci.org/content/21/21/8370.long*)

Hishikaw et al also described three case studies in patients with Alzheimer's disease with Behavioral and Psychological Symptoms of Dementia. **After taking Turmeric 764 mg/day for 12 weeks, behavior and psychological symptoms greatly improved**. (Effects of turmeric on Alzheimer's disease with behavioral and psychological symptoms of dementia *http://www.ncbi.nlm.nih.gov/pmc/articles/ PMC3665200/?report=classic*)

There is some limited research done in depressive disorders and curcumin. A recent study compared the antidepressant fluoxetine, curcumin supplement and fluoxetine + curcumin supplement combination. The combination group showed the best results at 77.8% improvement, and the antidepressant 64.7% improvement and the curcumin supplement 62.5% improvement. However, **this data did not reach level of significance**. (*Sanmukhani, J., Satodia, V., Trivedi, J., Patel, T., Tiwari, D., Panchal, B., Goel, A. and Tripathi, C. B. (2013), Efficacy and Safety of Curcumin in Major Depressive Disorder: A Randomized Controlled Trial. Phytother. Res.. doi: 10.1002/ptr.5025http://onlinelibrary.wiley.com/doi/10.1002/ptr.5025/ abstract*)

A pilot study tested the efficacy and safety of curcumin in patients with rheumatoid arthritis. This study compared the use of curcumin, diclofenac sodium and curcumin + diclofenac sodium combination. The study showed a 44.5% change in the Disease Activity Score (DAS) (a test used to measure disease activity in rheumatoid arthritis). This result was comparable to diclofenac sodium, which had a 42.1% change in DAS. The group which took both curcumin + diclofenac sodium had a 44.4% change in DAS.

In a recently published in vitro study, it was shown that curcumin can sensitize colon cancer cells to the chemotherapeutic agent 5 Fluoruracil (5FU). The authors concluded that "our data suggests that a combination of the plant chemical together with 5FU have the potential to benefit in the treatment of cancer". (Curcumin

Chemosensitizes 5-Fluorouracil Resistant MMR-Deficient Human Colon Cancer Cells in High Density Cultures*http://www.plosone.org/article/info%3Adoi%2F10.1371%2Fjournal.pone.0085397*)

It is of note that the German Commission E (the German version of the Food and Drug Administration in the United States (*http://en.wikipedia.org/wiki/Commission_E*), **has approved Turmeric for its use in some digestion conditions**. (*Turmeric - University of Maryland Medical Centerhttp://umm.edu/health/medical/altmed/herb/turmeric*)

So, is it better, therefore, to take turmeric or curcumin as a supplement in one's diet?

In an animal study, completed at the University of Louisville School of Medicine, the investigators showed that **taking turmeric may exert it's effect in increasing the bioavailability of curcumin** and/or it may exert an effect directly on the proinflammatory genes. (*Effect on pro-inflammatory and antioxidant genes and bioavailable distribution of whole turmeric vs curcumin: Similar root but different effects; Robert C.G. Martin, Harini S. Aiyer, Daniel Malik, Yan Li. http://www.sciencedirect.com/science/article/pii/S0278691511005783*)

It may be possible that the minerals, vitamins and phytochemicals that turmeric contains will help our bodies absorb the nutrients much more readily than if you take a curcumin supplement.

Adding turmeric to our diet is a great way to enjoy the benefits without having to take a supplement. We can incorporate turmeric into your diet using powder or fresh root.

There are many recipes online for different dishes (like curries) and drinks such as turmeric tea. Be sure to use pure organic turmeric to ensure you are getting a good source of turmeric without any fillers and chemicals.

Safety

Turmeric, taken in large doses or taking a curcumin supplement, may have adverse effects such as blood thinning effects, stimulating the uterus or promoting menstruation, increasing bile production and gastrointestinal upset (*Turmeric Side Effects & Safety http://*

www.webmd.com/vitamins-supplements/ingredientmono-662-TURMERIC.aspx? activeIngredientId=662&activeIngredientName=TURMERIC).

Always be sure to consult your healthcare professional before starting a supplement regime, as some supplements may not benefit you and your health needs or may interact with medications.

Curcumin is also a powerful antioxidant. Antioxidants scavenge molecules in the body known as free radicals, which **allegedly** damage cell membranes, tamper with DNA, and even cause cell death. Antioxidants can **allegedly** fight free radicals and may reduce or even help prevent some of the damage they cause.

The roots, or rhizomes and bulbs, are used in medicine and food. They are generally boiled and then dried, turning into the familiar yellow powder. Curcumin, the active ingredient, has antioxidant properties. Other substances in this herb have antioxidant properties as well.

In addition, curcumin lowers the levels of two enzymes in the body that cause inflammation. It also stops platelets from clumping together to form blood clots.

Available Forms

Turmeric is available in the following forms:

- Capsules containing powder
- Fluid extract
- Tincture

Because bromelain increases the absorption and anti-inflammatory effects of curcumin, it is often combined with turmeric products.

How to Take It

Pediatric

Turmeric supplements haven't been studied in children, so there is no recommended dose.

Adult

The following are doses recommended for adults:

- Cut root: 1.5 - 3 g per day
- Dried, powdered root: 1 - 3 g per day
- Standardized powder (curcumin): 400 - 600 mg, 3 times per day
- Fluid extract (1:1) 30 - 90 drops a day
- Tincture (1:2): 15 - 30 drops, 4 times per day

Source: Turmeric | University of Maryland Medical Center http://umm.edu/health/medical/altmed/herb/turmeric#ixzz3V3Itzlah

University of Maryland Medical Center

Possible Interactions

If you are being treated with any of the following medications, you should not use turmeric or curcumin in medicinal forms without first talking to your health care provider.

Blood-thinning Medications -- Turmeric may make the effects of these drugs stronger, raising the risk of bleeding. Blood-thinners include warfarin (Coumadin), clopidogrel (Plavix), and aspirin, among others.

Drugs that reduce stomach acid -- Turmeric may interfere with the action of these drugs, increasing the production of stomach acid:

- Cimetidine (Tagamet)
- Famotidine (Pepcid)
- Ranitidine (Zantac)
- Esomeprazole (Nexium)
- Omeprazole
- Lansoprazole (Prevacid)

Diabetes Medications -- Turmeric may make the effects of these drugs stronger, increasing the risk of hypoglycemia (low blood sugar).

Antioxidant Therapy: Current Status and Future Prospects

(Firuzi et al, 2011)

Reactive oxygen species (ROS, EMODs) are widely believed to cause or aggravate several human pathologies such as neurodegenerative diseases, cancer, stroke and many other ailments. Antioxidants are assumed to counteract the harmful effects of ROS and therefore prevent or treat oxidative stress-related diseases. In this report, recent human studies exploring the efficiency of antioxidants in prevention and treatment of various diseases are reviewed.

Few antioxidants including edaravone (for ischemic stroke in Japan), N-acetylcysteine (for acetaminophen toxicity), alfa-lipoic acid (for diabetic neuropathy) and some flavonoids (polyphenolic compounds present in dietary plants), such as micronized purified flavonoid fraction (diosmin and hesperidin) and oxerutins (for chronic venous insufficiency) as well as baicalein and catechins (for osteoarthritis) have found accepted clinical use.

However, **despite much enthusiasm in the 1980s and 1990s, many well-known agents such as antioxidant vitamins and also more recently developed compounds such as nitrones have not successfully passed the scrutiny of clinical trials for prevention and treatment of various diseases.**

This has given rise to a pessimistic view of antioxidant therapy, however, the evidence from human epidemiological studies about the beneficial effects of dietary antioxidants and preclinical in vitro and animal data are compelling. We have probably wasted too much time on agents like antioxidant vitamins instead of focusing on more disease specific, target-directed, highly bioavailable antioxidants.

Arguably, there is growing scientific agreement that antioxidants, particularly the polyphenolic forms, may help lower the incidence of disease, such as certain cancers, cardiovascular and neurodegenerative diseases, DNA damage, or even have anti-aging properties. On the other hand, **questions remain as to whether some antioxidants or phytochemicals potentially could do more harm than good, as an increase in glycation-mediated protein damage (carbonyl stress) and some risk has been reported.** (Obrenovich et al, 2011)

Numerous natural compounds have been extensively investigated for their potential for cancer prevention over the decades.

Curcumin, from *Curcuma longa*, is a natural compound that can be potentially used for chemoprevention of multiple cancers. Curcumin modulates multiple molecular pathways involved in the lengthy carcinogenesis process to exert its chemopreventive effects through several mechanisms: promoting apoptosis, inhibiting survival signals, scavenging reactive oxidative species (ROS), and reducing the inflammatory cancer microenvironment. Curcumin fulfills the characteristics for an ideal chemopreventive agent with its low toxicity, affordability, and easy accessibility. Nonetheless, **the clinical application of curcumin is currently compromised by its poor bioavailability**. (Shin et al, 2013)

The natural product curcumin has gained considerable attention in recent years for its multiple pharmacological activities, but more efforts are needed to understand how curcumin can have these pharmacological effects **considering its low bioavailability**.

In addition, it is unclear how curcumin exerts inhibitory effects against numerous enzymes, especially those that cannot accommodate curcumin within recognized binding pockets.

By analyzing the similarities between the biological activities of curcumin and its degradation products against diseases such as Alzheimer's disease and cancer, as well as the preferential inhibition of some enzymes by degradation products, **it appears that the bioactive degradation products may contribute to the pharmacological effects of curcumin.** This possibility should be given full attention when elucidating the pharmacology of this promising natural product for various diseases. (Shen, Ji, 2012)

Questions still remain as to whether some antioxidants could be potentially harmful to health, because an increase in glycation-mediated protein damage (carbonyl stress) has been reported in some cases.

Curcumin possesses therapeutic potential in the amelioration of a host of neurodegenerative ailments as evidenced by its antioxidant, anti-inflammatory and anti-protein aggregation effects. However, **issues such as limited bioavailability and a paucity of clinical studies examining its therapeutic effectiveness in illnesses such as Alzheimer's disease (AD) and Parkinson's disease (PD) currently limit its therapeutic outreach**.

Turmeric: Does It Have Antiseizure Activity?

Gayle Nicholas Scott, PharmD. January 27, 2015

Is turmeric or curcumin useful as an antiepileptic agent?

Turmeric (*Curcuma longa*) is in the same botanical family as ginger (Zingiberaceae). The rhizome is used as a coloring agent and a spice in such foods as curries, and as a medicinal agent in India and China.

Curcumin, a constituent of the turmeric rhizome, is a bright-yellow polyphenolic compound, chemically diferuloylmethane. Preliminary research suggests that turmeric and curcumin have a variety of pharmacologic properties, including anti-inflammatory, antitumor, and antimicrobial activities.

Clinical research in small numbers of patients has been conducted on curcumin for a diverse group of medical conditions, such as osteoarthritis; inflammatory bowel disease; pancreatitis; gastric ulcer; psoriasis; and cancer, including breast, colorectal, pancreatic, and others. (Fan, et al, 2013)

Although a search of curcumin on PubMed yields more than 7,000 citations, most articles report bench research; no commercial interest has applied for a drug license for any curcumin preparation.

Curcumin is poorly bioavailable, but it is a low-molecular-weight, lipophilic compound, which allows it to be absorbed and penetrate the blood/brain barrier. (Noorfshan, Ashkani-Esfahani et al, 2013)

Some research suggests that curcumin might have neuroprotective and antioxidant activity, which might be useful for treatment of seizures. **Studies in several animal models have shown that curcumin can reduce seizures that have been induced chemically or electrically.** (Kaur et al, 2014) (Du et al, 2012)

To date, no clinical trials of curcumin or turmeric for seizures have been published.

Turmeric and curcumin are available in the United States as dietary supplements. Both appear to be safe for most people, although no studies demonstrating safety in patients with epilepsy are available. Curcumin did not adversely affect rats concurrently given conventional antiepileptic drugs.

Preliminary clinical research suggests that curcumin might inhibit cytochrome P450 (CYP)1A2 and enhance CYP2A6. (Chen et al, 2010)

In summary, research on induced seizures in animals suggests that **turmeric or its constituent, curcumin, might have antiseizure effects**. However, neither agent has been studied in patients with epilepsy.

Capsaicin - pepper; curcumin - turmeric; pycnogenol - proanthocyanidin

pyc nog e nol - natural antioxidant: a powerful antioxidant containing proanthocyanidin, extracted from pine bark and used in dietary supplements

Some of the following was excerpted or modified from: **Tumeric (Curcuma longa): An Overview of the Research and Clinical Indications**.
By Lise Alschuler, ND. 2012. http://www.drlise.net/attachments/tumeric.pdf

The information presented has been obtained from research of reference books, clinical and scientific published papers, and other published works. The lay reader is advised to consult a licensed health care practitioner regarding the information contained herein.

Turmeric is a mild spice that enhances the flavor of other spices and foods and is the base of most Indian curries. Traditionally, turmeric has been used topically to heal and reduce bleeding associated with bruises, sprains, leech bites and inflamed joints. It has also been used internally for liver and digestive complaints, menstrual insufficiency and cramping, jaundice, and as an anti-inflammatory agent.

In the Ayurvedic tradition, turmeric, or "haldi" as it is known in Hindi, works well with all doshas, with its main action being to reduce mucus from the system.

Turmeric is considered to be one of the most important herbs in the Ayurvedic tradition. The medical use of turmeric goes back more than 5000 years. Turmeric is ubiquitous in India, and can be found in the turmeric plantations, herbal medicine preparations, spice bazaars, dyes, and in food.

In the United States of America, Turmeric has been granted "Generally Recognized as Safe" (GRAS) status by the FDA.

Turmeric has been used traditionally for almost every human ailment and many of these historic uses have been scientifically validated with application in modern times.

The rhizome, or root, of Turmeric is the part used medicinally.

Curcumin is the most well studied constituent. Turmeric also contains: sesquiterpenes (turmerone, atlantone, zingiberone, turmeronol, ger-macrone, and bisabolene), carbohydrates, protein, resins, and caffeic acid.

There are over 3,000 preclinical studies on turmeric and its constituents. Curcumin is considered to be the most active constituent in Curcuma longa.

When administered orally, curcumin inhibits neutrophil function, inhibits platelet aggregation, **inhibits lymphocyte activity**, promotes fibrinolysis, and stabilizes lysosomal membranes.

As of 2012, curcumin has been the subject of over 20 clinical trials in the context of cancer.

Pancreatic Cancer

A phase I/II clinical trial enrolled 21 gemcitabine (Gemzar) resistant patients with **advanced pancreatic cancer**. (Kanai et al, 2011)

The median survival after initiation of curcumin was 161 days (95% CI 109-223). The one-year survival rate was 19% (95% CI 4.4% – 41.4%). However, median survival after failure of first-line gemcitabine is 70 days, which makes the results of this study significant. **Of note, a prior clinical study failed to demonstrate clinical response in 17**

patients with advanced pancreatic cancer with an 8,000mg dose of curcumin concurrent with gemcitabine. (Epelbaum et al, 2010)

Colorectal Cancer

A placebo-controlled clinical trial randomized 126 patients with **colorectal cancer** to either receive curcumin or placebo. (He et al, 2011)

The body weight of Curcumin patients increased (approx. 4%) vs. weight loss of 6% in placebo group (p<0.05). Furthermore, in the resected colon tissue, curcumin increased the prevalence of apoptosis (associated with increased Bax and inhibited Bcl-2) and p53 expression (major tumor suppressor gene) over tissue from placebo group.

Another phase IIa clinical trial assessed the impact of two different doses of curcumin on the prevention of **colorectal neoplasia**. (Carroll et al, 2011)

There was a 40% reduction in aberrant crypt foci number in the 4g group (P<0.005), **whereas no significant reduction was observed in the 2g dose group.**

Multiple Myeloma

Monoclonal Gammopathy of Undetermined Significance (MGUS) and Smoldering Multiple Myeloma (SMM) are asymptomatic plasma cell disorders which can progress to multiple myeloma (MM) over a long period (up to 20 years). A randomized, double-blinded placebo-controlled cross-over trial with curcumin enrolled 19 patients with MGUS and 17 patients with SMM. (Golombick et al, 2012)

Both 4 and 8g daily doses reduced the serum-free light chain ratio (35% and 36% respectively) and reduced total serum protein (P=0.04) in the urine in both MGUS and SMM patients. **Patients with abnormal serum free light chain ratios at study onset had the greatest response.** Curcumin also decreased markers of bone turnover (urinary DPYD) and excretion of crosslinked N-telopeptides by more than 25%.

Cardiovascular disease

Age-related cardiovascular decline in postmenopausal women is characterized, in part, by **increased left ventricular afterload, an indication of vascular dysfunction and hypertension**. An 8 week pilot study randomized 45 postmenopausal women to one of four interventions: placebo, 150mg curcumin, exercise training plus placebo or exercise training plus curcumin. (Sugawara et al, 2012)

Only in the exercise and curcumin group did the aortic brachial systolic pressure, a measure of left ventricular afterload, decrease significantly (p<0.05).

Arthritis

Based upon earlier studies demonstrating the potential benefit of curcumin in improving joint function, the long-term efficacy and safety of curcuminoid and phosphatidylcholine extract was investigated in an 8 month long pilot study involving 100 osteoarthritis patients. (Belcaro et al, 2010) (Belcaro G, Cesarone MR, Dugall M, Pellegrini L, Ledda A, Grossi MG, Togni S, Appendino G. Efficacy and safety of Meriva®, a curcumin-phosphatidylcholine complex, during extended administration in osteoarthritis patients. Altern Med Rev. 2010 Dec;15(4):337-44)

At the conclusion of the study, all subjective and objective parameters were improved in the treatment group over the control group (p<0.05). **The curcumin group had improved scores for joint pain and stiffness, physical function, and social and emotional function**.

Diabetes

A **randomized, parallel-group, placebo-controlled 8-week study** randomized 72 patients with **type 2 diabetes** to receive either 300mg curcumin twice daily, atorvastatin 10mg daily or placebo. (Usharani et al, 2008)

Compared with baseline, **there was significant and comparable improvement in endothelial function in both the atorvastatin and the curcumin groups.**Additionally all biomarkers decreased in both treatment groups, whereas no improvements were seen in the placebo group.

Contraindications

Having been granted "Generally Recognized as Safe" (GRAS) status in the United States of America by the Food and Drug Administration (FDA), turmeric is well tolerated by most people. **Whole herb curcuma might alter the pharmacokinetics of coadministrated drugs** by up-regulating the function and expression levels of intestinal Pgp, a protein involved in drug efflux from the cell. However, curcumin extract does not upregulate P-gp. (Hou et al, 2008

Curcumin inhibits multiple enzymes

Curcumin inhibits CYP3A4 and CYP2C9 and is itself metabolized by CYP1A1 and CYP2B1. (Volak et al, 2008)

Therefore, there is the theoretical possibility of interference with drugs metabolized through 3A4. However, it is possible that curcumin lacks clinically significant (in vivo) CYP3A4 activity.

Toxicity

No significant toxicity has been reported following short or long-term administration of turmeric extracts at standard doses.

Conclusion

Both as a culinary spice and as a medicinal agent, turmeric may thwart the course of chronic illnesses such as uveitis, cancer, osteoarthritis, diabetes, dyspepsia and cardiovascular disease.

Dr. Joseph Mercola speaks of curcumin

Dr. Joseph Mercola says: Curcumin (turmeric) in particular has been shown to be effective against both acute and chronic pain. Curcumin is most known for its potent anti-inflammatory properties. It has been shown to influence more than 700 genes, and can inhibit both the excessive activity and the synthesis of cyclooxygenase-2 (COX2) and 5-lipoxygenase (5-LOX), as well as other enzymes that have been implicated in inflammation. In experiments on rats, turmeric appeared to block inflammatory pathways associated with rheumatoid arthritis.

A study published in April 2012 revealed that a highly bioavailable form of curcumin was more effective in alleviating RA symptoms, including tenderness and swelling of joints, than the NSAID drug Voltaren. Not only that, those who were taking the curcumin only actually experienced the most improvement across the board. (Phytotherapy Research March 9, 2012)

The investigation of dietary constituents should follow a structured design, incorporating parallel preclinical studies of the food source and the isolated agent in terms of efficacy, toxicity, biological mechanisms, and pharmacokinetics.

Either the food source or the isolated agent should be selected for further development on the basis of dose-efficacy and toxicity data. Pilot clinical trials on the pharmacokinetics and mechanism-based markers of efficacy of the selected intervention should precede phase I–III development in suitable populations.

There is the need to utilize alternative concepts or approaches to the prevention of cancer. Many natural products that have been implicated in cancer prevention but many have been met with disappointing results and with recognizable side effects. These molecules originate from vegetables, fruits, plant extracts, and herbs.

There has been a failure of antioxidant therapy in preventing cardiovascular morbidity and mortality in major clinical trials.

However, lipid-soluble quercetin, not water-soluble dihydroquercetin, protects human red blood cells against oxidative damage. This study compared three lipid-soluble polyphenols, muscadine, curcumin and quercetin, and three lipid- (α-tocopherol and α-tocotrienol) or water-soluble (ascorbic acid) vitamins.

Among the tested polyphenols, **muscadine was the most potent in inhibiting superoxide** and 2,2-azobis(2-amidinopropane) dihydrochloride (AAPH)-generated peroxyl radicals, **whereas ascorbic acid was the most potent inhibitor of hydrogen peroxide**.

Activities of the polyphenols after lipid extractions showed that **curcumin inhibited superoxide production to a greater extent than quercetin and muscadine**.

All blood cells were tested 20 min after incubation with the selected compounds. All the polyphenols caused inhibition of N-formyl-l-methionyl-l-leucyl-l-phenylalanine-induced neutrophil oxidative bursts. Quercetin, but not other polyphenols, significantly reduced AAPH-induced oxidative hemolysis. **No significant effect on neutrophil oxidative burst or oxidative hemolysis was found with any of the tested vitamins**.

These results suggest that quercetin enhances the resistance of membrane to destruction by free radicals. **This effect of quercetin is not directly mediated through antioxidative or anti-inflammatory actions. Antioxidant or anti-inflammatory potency may not be used as a simple criterion to select polyphenols for cell protection benefits**. (Christopher et al, 2010)

Traditional agents derived from ancient Hindu medicine, such as curcumin, have been shown to have biological activity at physiologically relevant concentrations in preclinical studies. **Dozens of medicinal properties of curcumin have been described that have been reviewed recently**. (Strimpakos, Sharma, 2008) (Goel et al, 2008) (Goel et al, 2008. Bio Pharma)

The most studied beneficial properties of curcumin are perhaps its anti-oxidant, anticarcinogenic, anti-inflammatory and immunomodulatory activities, among others. However, the pharmacological hepatoprotective properties of curcumin known to Indians in the traditional medicine hundreds of years ago, and tested recently on the basis of modern scientific methods, have not been reviewed in depth.

Curcumin, a polyphenol (diferuloylmethane), is the main active compound found in the perennial plant *Curcuma longa* (commonly known as turmeric).

Polyphenols are naturally occurring compounds found largely in the fruits, vegetables, cereals and beverages. Fruits like grapes, apple, pear, cherries and berries contains up to 200–300 mg polyphenols per 100 grams fresh weight. The products manufactured from these fruits, also contain polyphenols in significant amounts.

Typically a glass of red wine or a cup of tea or coffee contains about 100 mg polyphenols. Cereals, dry legumes and chocolate also contribute to the polyphenolic intake.

Polyphenols are secondary metabolites of plants and are generally involved in defense against ultraviolet radiation or aggression by pathogens. **In food, polyphenols may contribute to the bitterness, astringency, color, flavor, odor and oxidative stability**.

Polyphenols and other food phenolics are the subject of increasing scientific interest because of their possible beneficial effects on human health.

More than 8,000 polyphenolic compounds have been identified in various plant species. All plant phenolic compounds arise from a common intermediate, phenylalanine, or a close precursor, shikimic acid.

Bioavailability is the proportion of the nutrient that is digested, absorbed and metabolized through normal pathways. **Bioavailability of each and every polyphenol differs however there is no relation between the quantity of polyphenols in food and their bioavailability in human body**.

Curcumin, demethoxycurcumin, bisdemethoxycurcumin and cyclocurcumin are the four principal curcuminoids obtained from the colored extracts of dried roots from turmeric.

Whether all four analogues exhibit equal activity is not clear. Although in most systems curcumin was found to be the most potent, in some systems bisdemethoxycurcumin was found to exhibit higher activity. There are also suggestions that the mixture of all three is more potent than either one alone.

India is the main producer of turmeric and consumes about 90% of it and exports the remainder. *Curcuma longa* and its constituents have been used in Asian cookery and traditional medicine for thousands of years: at present, they are used by the food industry as additives, like curry in England, flavorings, preservatives and coloring agents, in soft drinks, mustard and margarine.

Safety

One of the most prominent features of curcumin is its extremely good tolerance and its very low toxicity and side effects. However, although turmeric and curcumin are natural products used in the diet, the doses used in clinical trials exceed those consumed in the diet; therefore, systematic toxicity studies are needed. Curcumin is Generally Recognized As Safe by the Food and Drug Administration, and this compound has been granted an Acceptable Daily Intake level of up to 3 mg/kg by the Joint FAO and WHO Expert Committee on Food Additives, 1996. **No studies in either animals or humans have found any toxicity associated with the consumption of curcumin even at very high doses**. (Rivera-Espinoza, Muriel, 2009)

Curcumin has shown beneficial properties in diverse experimental models of liver damage. It prevents liver damage induced by aflatoxins, iron overdose, erythromycin estolate, ethanol, TAA acute and chronic intoxication, cholestasis (BDL) and acute, subacute and chronic CCl_4intoxication; moreover, it reverses CCl_4 cirrhosis to some extent. Curcumin may act at several molecular targets, but two have been utilized the most to explain its pharmacological properties: one is its anti-oxidant effect and the other is its ability to inhibit NF-κB factors. **However, there is only one report supporting the ability of the compound to reverse the disease**. (Rivera-Espinoza, Muriel, 2009)

Dr. Mercola says that turmeric is a "universal" cancer treatment and much more.

May 4, 2015 http://www.mercola.com/Citations/index.htm

Mercola says:

- Curcumin, a bioactive ingredient in turmeric, exhibits over 150 potentially therapeutic activities, including anti-inflammatory and antimicrobial activity, and anti-cancer properties that have been intensely studied.

- Its benefits are related to its ability to modulate 700 genes; positively modulate more than 160 different physiological pathways; make your cell membranes more orderly; and affect signaling molecules.

- Curcumin can help you maintain a healthy digestive system and be may be useful against Heliobacter pylori (H. pylori) infections, such as gastritis, peptic ulcer and gastric cancer. (Antimicrobial Agents and Chemotherapy. February 9, 2009: 53(4); 1592-1597)

Curcumin is capable of crossing your blood-brain barrier, which has created interest in studying its effect on neurological diseases such as Alzheimer's, Parkinson's and dementia.

Mercola says curcumin actually has the most evidence-based literature supporting its use against cancer of any other nutrient, including vitamin D. Moreover, it does not affect normal cells. (Greenmedinfo.com, Curcumin)

Effects of curcumin and capsaicin on murine oral mucosa

Effects of Curcumin and Capsaicin Irradiated with Visible Light on Murine Oral Mucosa

Abstract

The purpose of this study was to evaluate the histopathological effects of curcumin and capsaicin, with or without visible light (VL) irradiation for 5 min, on the oral mucous membrane in mice. **Capsaicin-treated, but not curcumin-treated, buccal epithelium exhibited slight tissue damage**; VL irradiation caused excessive tissue damage, particularly when combined with the former treatment. The TdT-mediated dUTP-biotin nick end-labeling (TUNEL) method demonstrated that both capsaicin and curcumin induced apoptosis, with the apoptotic effect of capsaicin appearing at an early stage of application. VL irradiation increased the number of apoptotic cells, particularly those upon in the capsaicin-treated area.

Capsaicin and curcumin acted as photosensitizers exposure to VL, in the presence of oxygen. Curcumin and capsaicin with VL irradiation could thus be used for photodynamic therapy in the clinical setting, especially in precancerous oral diseases. **This means that both capsaicin and curcumin have prooxidant activity.** http:// iv.iiarjournals.org/content/26/5/759.full (Okada et al, 2012)

Prooxidant activity of curcumin

Abstract

Curcumin, a well-known antioxidant and a principal ingredient of turmeric, acted as a prooxidant causing a copper-dependent DNA damage and the induction of apoptosis.

Treatment of DNA from plasmid pBR322 and calf thymus with curcumin plus copper ion caused strand scission and the formation of 8-hydroxy-2'-deoxyguanosine in DNA. Addition of catalase protected DNA from the curcumin-dependent injuries, indicating that hydroxyl radical may participate in the DNA damage. Flow cytometry analysis showed that curcumin caused an apoptotic cell death of HL60 cells in a dose- and time-dependent manner.

Curcumin-mediated apoptosis was closely related to the increase in intracellular reactive oxygen species (EMODs). On the contrary, capsaicinoids, which have a ortho-methoxy phenolic structure without β-diketone in the side chain, did not produce 8-hydroxy-2'-deoxyguanosine. **Capsaicin further did not induce apoptosis of HL60 cells, but rather protected cells from prooxidant-induced apoptosis.**

Curcumin can generate reactive oxygen species (EMODs) as a prooxidant in the presence of transition metals in cells, resulting in DNA injuries and apoptotic cell death. The prooxidant action of curcumin may be related to the conjugated β-diketone structure of this compound. (Yoshino et al, 2004)

Prooxidant activity of phenoxyl radicals and polyphenolics

Prooxidant activity and cellular effects of the phenoxyl radicals of dietary flavonoids and other polyphenolics

Abstract

Dietary polyphenolics in fruits, vegetables, wines, spices and herbal medicines have beneficial antioxidant, anti-inflammatory and anticancer effects. However, **we have observed that dietary polyphenolics**

with phenol rings were metabolized by peroxidase to form prooxidant phenoxyl radicals which, in some cases were sufficiently reactive to cooxidize GSH or NADH accompanied by extensive oxygen uptake and ROS, EMOD formation. The order of catalytic effectiveness found for oxygen activation when polyphenolics were metabolized by peroxidase in the presence of GSH was phloretin>phloridzin>4,2'-dihydroxy chalcone>*p*-coumaric acid>naringenin>apigenin>curcumin>resveratrol>isoliquiritigenin>capsaicin>kaempferol.

Ascorbate was also cooxidized by the phenoxyl radicals but without oxygen activation. Polyphenolics with catechol rings also cooxidized ascorbate, likely mediated by semiquinone radicals.

The order of catalytic effectiveness found for ascorbate cooxidation was fisetin luteolin, quercetin, >eriodictyol, caffeic acid, nordihydroguaiaretic acid>catechin>taxifolin, catechol. NADH was stoichiometrically oxidized without oxygen uptake which, suggests that *o*-quinone metabolites were responsible. GSH was not cooxidized and GSH conjugates were formed, likely mediated by the *o*-quinone metabolites. Incubation of hepatocytes with dietary polyphenolics containing phenol rings was found to partially oxidize hepatocyte GSH to GSSG while polyphenolics with a catechol ring were found to deplete GSH through formation of GSH conjugates.

Dietary polyphenolics with phenol rings also oxidized human erythrocyte oxyhemoglobin and caused erythrocyte hemolysis more readily than polyphenolics with catechol rings. It is concluded that **polyphenolics containing a phenol ring are generally more prooxidant than polyphenolics containing a catechol ring**. (Galati et al, 2002)

Eating Spicy Food Linked to a Longer Life

By

Nicholas Bakalar

August 4, 2015

Eating spicy food is associated with a reduced risk for death, an analysis of dietary data on more than 485,000 people found.

Study participants were enrolled between 2004 and 2008 in a large Chinese health study, and researchers followed them for an average of more than seven years, recording 20,224 deaths. The study is in the British Medical Journal.

After controlling for family medical history, age, education, diabetes, smoking and many other variables, the researchers found that **compared with eating hot food, mainly chili peppers, less than once a week, having it once or twice a week resulted in a 10 percent reduced overall risk for death. Consuming spicy food six to seven times a week reduced the risk by 14 percent**.

Rates of ischemic heart disease, respiratory diseases and cancers were all lower in hot-food eaters. The authors drew no conclusions about cause and effect, but they noted that capsaicin, the main ingredient in chili peppers, had been found in other studies to have antioxidant and anti-inflammatory effects.

"We need more evidence, especially from clinical trials, to further verify these findings," said a co-author, Dr. Lu Qi, an associate professor of nutrition at the Harvard T.H. Chan School of Public Health, "and we are looking forward to seeing data from other populations."

Common cooking spice can increase drug effectiveness in head and neck cancer, study finds

Last updated: Friday 5 June 2015 at 6am PST

A new study by UCLA scientists has shown that a synthetic version of a spice commonly used in Southeast Asian cuisine **called curcumin (also known as turmeric) significantly reduced resistance to the well-known chemotherapy drug Cisplatin in head and neck cancer cells**.

Researchers used a first-of-its-kind liposome (a type of vehicle to deliver encapsulated synthetic curcumin) to target-resistant head and neck squamous cell carcinoma (HNSCC). Drs. Marilene Wang and Eri Srivatsan, both UCLA Jonsson Comprehensive Cancer Center members, led the **two-year study which found that the synthetic curcumin was effective in killing Cisplatin-resistant HNSCC**.

"Cisplatin goes through the p16 and p53 pathways, while the curcumin uses an alternate pathway, said Wang, director of the Nasal and Sinus Center at UCLA. **"The resistant cell lines don't respond to the** typical pathway that **Cisplatin would go through; that's why curcumin is able to kill the resistant cancer cells.''**

Head and neck cancers currently affect 600,000 people worldwide each year, including 42,000 in the United States. The five-year survival rate for all head and neck cancer patients is 57 percent, and for patients with stage III and IV oral cancers the survival rate is 10 to 20 percent.

Researchers hope the results will lead to human clinical trials and the development of new therapies for head and neck cancer patients.

The full study is available online in the journal *Oncotarget*. (Basak et al, 2015)

Danger of DNP advertised as tumeric

Global police forces are working together to try to prevent the supply of so-called "diet pills" which can be deadly.

In April 21-year-old Eloise Aimee Parry, from Shrewsbury, died in hospital on April 12, 2015 after becoming unwell after she took a substance she had bought on the internet.

An inquest found that she had consumed four times the fatal amount of **Dinitrophenol, known as DNP, which is a toxic pesticide.**

The International Criminal Police Organisation (Interpol) has now raised an alert with forces in 190 countries.

They declared an "imminent threat" to consumers of DNP, which has also been used in explosives.

One Newsbeat listener who has taken DNP in the past shared some of their experiences.

'I felt like I was on fire'

Gill from Northern Ireland told us that she "thought she was going to die".

"You start to feel a bit of energy off them, but when you expect the energy to wear off it doesn't and that is when my body started to over-heat, she explained.

"I felt like I was on fire, I felt like I was boiling in my skin.

"It was just terrible. My heart was beating so fast. It was the worst feeling ever."

Interpol said that some online distributors have tried to mask its supply from customs and police officers by labelling it as the yellow spice, turmeric.

Police said there were "intrinsic dangers of DNP" and the risks are magnified because it is made in illegal manufacturing conditions.

A study last year warned the drug, sometimes used as a weight-loss or bodybuilding aid, could be linked to five more deaths in the UK between 2007 and 2013.

It also warned that it could cause breathing difficulties, fast heart rates, fever, nausea and vomiting.

More from Mercola on curcumin

On May 16, 2012, Dr Mercola said, 1) the antioxidant resveratrol and **curcumin** (the active substance of the spice turmeric) both show promise as natural chemosensitizers - substances that can help overcome resistance to chemotherapy drugs, 2) Both nutrients have a wide spectrum of anti-cancer actions and functions, 3) By modulating inflammatory pathways and inflammatory molecules, resveratrol may also help alleviate man of the debilitating side effects of conventional cancer treatment, such as wasting, fatigue, depression, neuropathic pain, cognitive impairment and sleep disorders, and 4) **Among all nutrients, curcumin has the most evidence-based literature supporting its use against cancer**. Researchers have found that curcumin can affect more than 100 different pathways, once it gets into a cell.

According to an NPR paper, "The molecular basis of a disease is related to dysregulation of an array of signaling molecules. With the advent of advanced molecular tools, we now know that **over 500 different genes of the signaling pathways control any given disease**. However, most currently available treatments are based on the modulation of a specific single target. Curcumin is a functionally labile molecule with the potential to modulate the biological activity of a number of signaling molecules either indirectly or directly…"

RMH Note: Please remember that curcumin is poorly absorbed.

On Feb 9, 2015, Dr Mercola said, 1) Chronic inflammation is associated with metabolic syndrome, 2) Curcumin is one of the most potent anti-inflammatories in nature, and 3) After taking curcumin for eight weeks, people with metabolic syndrome had lower levels of inflammation and blood sugar.

About 34 percent of Americans have metabolic syndrome, which describes a cluster of symptoms that increases your risk of heart disease, diabetes, stroke and other chronic disease. Those symptoms include a large waistline, high blood pressure, high blood sugar, low levels of HDL cholesterol, and high levels of triglycerides. The common thread linking them is "inflammation."

Then, it makes sense that curcumin would help lower inflammation with this disorder.

A research study found that **after eight weeks of curcumin powder administration, the curcumin group had lower levels of three blood markers of inflammation, including C-reactive protein (CRP), along with lower fasting blood sugar and hemoglobin A1c (a measure of longer term blood sugar levels).**

They concluded that short-term supplementation with bioavailable curcumin significantly improves oxidative and inflammatory status in people with metabolic syndrome, and **could be regarded as a "natural, safe and effective CRP-lowering agent."**

As for its anti-inflammatory properties, curcumin can inhibit both the activity and the synthesis of cyclooxygenase-2 (COX2) and 5-lipooxygenase (5-LOX), as well as other enzymes that have been implicated in inflammation.

A 2006 study found that a turmeric extract composed of curcuminoids blocked inflammatory pathways, effectively preventing the launch of a protein that triggers swelling and pain.

Prof Randolph M. Howes MD, PhD

Turmeric has been referred to as "the spice of life."

Curcumin in turmeric has the ability to modulate genetic activity and expression in destroying cancerous cells. Eastern cultural traditions, including traditional Chinese medicine and Ayurveda, have valued turmeric for it medicinal properties and flavor for more that 5,000 years.

Turmeric powder goes well with a variety of foods but supplements may be necessary to achieve therapeutic levels of curcumin. The turmeric root itself contains only about 3% curcumin concentration.

Mercola says that it is difficult to find supplemental curcumin that has increased bioavailability and a turmeric extract with at least 95% curcuminoids.

Cures and curcumin for oral cancers

Cures and curcumin -- turmeric offers potential therapy for oral cancers

Apr 28, 2015

Curry ingredient slows HPV virus in oral cancer cells

Turmeric - the familiar yellow spice common in Indian and Asian cooking - may play a therapeutic role in oral cancers associated with human papillomavirus, according to new research published in *ecancermedicalscience*.

One of the herb's key active ingredients - **an antioxidant called curcumin - appears to have a quelling effect on the activity of human papillomavirus (HPV).**

HPV is a virus that promotes the development of cervical and oral cancer. There is no cure, but curcumin may offer a means of future control.

"Turmeric has established antiviral and anti-cancer properties," says corresponding author Dr Alok Mishra of Emory University, Atlanta, USA. "And according to our new findings, we could say that it's good for oral health too."

Dr Mishra's research group first noted the effect of curcumin on HPV and cervical cancer cells in 2005. **The antioxidant slowed the expression of HPV, suggesting that curcumin could control the extent of HPV infection.**

"Since HPV-related oral cancer cases are on the rise, we tested the same hypothesis on oral cancer," Dr Mishra says.

"They turned out to be some very interesting findings."

The new research indicates that **curcumin turns down the expression of HPV in infected oral cancer cells by downregulating the levels of cellular transcription factors AP-1 and NF-kB**.

These findings could suggest a new therapeutic role for cucurmin in cancer control.

While Dr Mishra cannot comment on the therapeutic benefits of turmeric in cooking, he says that the use of turmeric and other anti-oxidants may be good for health in general, and HPV-related oral cancers in particular.

Curcumin and lycopene lack of effect on rat prostate cancer

Lack of chemopreventative effects of lycopene and curcumin on experimental rat prostate carcinogenesis

The chemopreventive efficacy of lycopene and curcumin with regard to prostate carcinogenesis was investigated using 3,2′-dimethyl-4-aminobiphenol (DMAB)- and 2-amino-1-methylimidazo[4,5-b]pyridine (PhIP)-induced rat ventral prostate cancer models. Three 60 week experiments with male F344 rats were carried out. In the first DMAB was given for the first 20 weeks and lycopene or curcumin were administered concomitantly or subsequently at dietary doses of 15 and 500 p.p.m., respectively. In the second experiment lycopene and curcumin were given to rats pretreated with DMAB at doses of 5, 15 or 45 p.p.m. or 100 or 500 p.p.m. In the third PhIP was selected as an initiator for prostate carcinogenesis and administered for 20 weeks. Rats were then fed a diet containing lycopene at a dose of 45 p.p.m. or curcumin at a dose of 500 p.p.m. or both together. Chemopreventive effects of lyco-pene and curcumin on development of DMAB-induced ventral prostate carcinomas were observed only in the first experiment and no con-firmation of inhibition potential was obtained in the following studies. Neither summational nor synergistic chemoprevention was evident. It is concluded from the present data that, **overall, neither lycopene nor curcumin can consistently prevent rat prostate carcino-genesis.** (Imaida et al, 2001)

Turmeric general information

http://umm.edu/health/medical/altmed/herb/turmeric

Turmeric *(Curcuma longa)* has been used for thousands of years to treat a variety of conditions. Studies show that turmeric may help fight infec-tions and some cancers, reduce inflammation, and treat digestive prob-lems, and it has gotten a lot of press lately.

But remember several facts when you hear news reports about tur-meric. First, many studies have taken place in test tubes and animals, and turmeric may not work as well in humans. Second, **some studies have used an injectable form of curcumin, the active substance in turmeric**.

Finally, **some of the studies show conflicting evidence**.

Turmeric is widely used in cooking and gives Indian curry its flavor and yellow color. It is also used in mustard and to color butter and cheese. Turmeric has been used in both Ayurvedic and Chinese medicine as an anti-inflammatory, to treat digestive and liver problems, skin diseases, and wounds. (Aggarwal et al, 2007) **"Curcumin: the Indian solid gold."**

Curcumin is also a powerful antioxidant. Antioxidants scavenge mole-cules in the body known as free radicals, which damage cell membranes, tamper with DNA, and even cause cell death. Antioxidants can allegedly fight free radicals and may reduce or even help prevent some of the damage they cause.

RMH Note: Please remember that curcumin also has prooxidant activity.

In addition, curcumin lowers the levels of two enzymes in the body that cause inflammation. It also stops platelets from clumping together to form blood clots.

Research suggests that turmeric may be helpful for the following conditions:

Indigestion or Dyspepsia

Curcumin stimulates the gallbladder to produce bile, which some people think may help improve digestion. The German Commission E, which determines which herbs can be safely prescribed in Germany, has approved turmeric for digestive problems. And **one double-blind, placebo-controlled study found that turmeric reduced symptoms of bloating and gas in people suffering from indigestion**.

Ulcerative colitis

Turmeric may help people with ulcerative colitis stay in remission. Ulcerative colitis is a chronic disease of the digestive tract where symptoms tend to come and go. **In one double-blind, placebo-controlled study, people whose ulcerative colitis was in remission took either curcumin or placebo, along with conventional medical treatment, for 6 months. Those who took curcumin had a relapse rate much lower than those who took placebo**.

Stomach Ulcers

Caution! Turmeric does not seem to help treat stomach ulcers. In fact, there is some evidence that it may increase stomach acid, making existing ulcers worse.

Osteoarthritis

Because of its ability to reduce inflammation, researchers have wondered if turmeric may help relieve osteoarthritis pain. One study found that people using an Ayurvedic formula of herbs and minerals with turmeric, winter cherry (*Withinia somnifera*), boswellia *(Boswellia serrata)*, and zinc had less pain and disability. But **it's impossible to know whether it was turmeric or one of the other supplements -- or all of them together -- that was responsible.** (Funk et al, 2006)

Heart Disease

Early studies suggested that turmeric may help prevent atherosclerosis, the buildup of plaque that can block arteries and lead to heart attack or stroke. In animal studies, an extract of turmeric lowered cholesterol levels and kept LDL "bad" cholesterol from building up in blood vessels. Because it stops platelets from clumping together, turmeric may also prevent blood clots from building up along the walls of arteries. But **a double-blind, placebo-controlled study found that taking curcumin, the active ingredient in turmeric, at a dose of up to 4 g per day did not improve cholesterol levels.**

Cancer

There has been a great deal of research on turmeric's anti-cancer properties, but **results are still very early**. Evidence from test tube and animal studies suggests that curcumin may help prevent or treat several types of cancers, including prostate, breast, skin, and colon cancer.

Its preventive effects may be because it is a strong antioxidant, protecting cells from damage. More research is needed. Cancer should be treated with conventional medications. Don't use alternative therapies alone to treat cancer. If you choose to use complementary therapies along with your cancer treatment, make sure you tell all your doctors.

Bacterial and Viral Infections

Test tube and animal studies suggest turmeric may kill bacteria and viruses. **But researchers don't know whether it would work in people.**

Uveitis

A preliminary study suggests curcumin may help treat uveitis, an inflammation of the eye's iris. **In one study of 32 people with chronic anterior uveitis, curcumin was effective as corticosteroids, the type of medication usually prescribed**. More research is needed.

Plant Description

A relative of ginger, turmeric is a perennial plant that grows 5 - 6 feet high in the tropical regions of Southern Asia, with trumpet-shaped, dull yellow flowers. Its roots are bulbs that also produce rhizomes, which then produce stems and roots for new plants. Turmeric is fragrant and has a bitter, somewhat sharp taste. Although it grows in many tropical locations, the majority of turmeric is grown in India, where it is used as a main ingredient in curry.

Parts Used

The roots, or rhizomes and bulbs, are used in medicine and food. They are generally boiled and then dried, turning into the familiar yellow powder. **Curcumin, the active ingredient, has antioxidant (and prooxidant) properties. Other substances in this herb have antioxidant properties as well.**

Supporting Research

(Asai, Miyazawa, 2001) (Asai A, Miyazawa T. Dietary curcuminoids prevent high-fat diet-induced lipid accumulation in rat liver and epididymal adipose tissue. *J Nutr.* 2001;131(11):2932-2935) (Baum et al, 2007) (Baum L, et al. Curcumin effects on blood lipid profile in a 6-month human study. *Pharmacol Res.* 2007;56(6):509-14) (Blumenthal et al, 2000) (Blumenthal M, Goldberg A, Brinckmann J. *Herbal Medicine: Expanded Commission E Monographs.* Newton, MA: Integrative Medicine Communications; 2000:379-384) () (Turmeric monograph, 2001Curcuma longa (turmeric). Monograph. *Altern Med Rev.* 2001;6 Suppl:S62-S66) (Darvesh et al, 2011) (Darvesh AS, Aggarwal BB, Bishayee A. Curcumin and Liver Cancer: A Review. *Curr Pharm Biotechnol.* 2011 Apr 5. [Epub ahead of print]) (Davis et al, 2007) (Davis JM, Murphy EA, Carmichael MD, Zielinski MR, Groschwitz CM, Brown AS, Ghaffar A, Mayer EP. Curcumin effects on inflammation and performance recovery following eccentric exercise-induced muscle damage. *Am J Physiol Regul Integr Comp Physiol.* 2007 Mar 1 [Epub ahead of print]) (Dorai et al, 2001) (Dorai T, Cao YC, Dorai B, Buttyan R, Katz AE. Therapeutic potential of curcumin in human prostate cancer. III. Curcumin inhibits proliferation, induces apoptosis, and inhibits angiogenesis of LNCaP prostate cancer cells in vivo. *Prostate.* 2001;47(4):293-303) (Dorai, Gehani, Katz, 2000) (Dorai T, Gehani N, Katz A. Therapeutic potential of curcumin in human prostate cancer. II. Curcumin inhibits tyrosine kinase activity of epidermal growth factor receptor and depletes the protein. *Mol Urol.* 2000;4(1):1-6) (Gautam et al, 2007) (Gautam SC, Gao X, Dulchavsky S. Immunodilation by curcumin. *Adv Exp Med Biol.* 2007;595:321-41) (Gesher et al, 2001) (Gescher A J, Sharma R A, Steward W P. Cancer chemoprevention by dietary constituents: a tale of failure and promise. *Lancet Oncol.* 2001;2(6):371-379) (Goel et al, 2008) (Goel A, Kunnumakkara AB, Aggarwal BB. Curcumin as "Curecumin": from kitchen to clinic. *Biochem Pharmacol.* 2008;75(4):787-809) (Hanni et al, 2006) (Hanai H, Iida T, Takeuchi K, Watanabe F, Maruyama Y, Andoh A, et al. Curcumin maintenance therapy for ulcerative colitis: randomized, multicenter, double-blind, placebo-controlled trial. *Clin Gastroenterol Hepatol.* 2006 Dec;4(12):1502-6) (Handler et al, 2007) (Handler N, Jaeger W, Puschacher H, Leisser K, Erker T. Synthesis of novel curcumin analogues and their evaluation as selective cyclooxygenase-1 (COX-1) inhibitors. *Chem Pharm Bull* (Tokyo). 2007 Jan;55(1):64-71) (Heck et al, 2000) (Heck AM, DeWitt BA, Lukes AL. Potential interactions between alternative therapies and warfarin. *Am J Health Syst Pharm.* 2000;57(13):1221-1227) (Jagetia, Aggarwal, 2007) (Jagetia GC, Aggarwal BB. "Spicing up" of the immune system by curcumin. *J Clin Immunol.*

2007;27(1):19-35) (Johnson, Mukhtar, 2007) (Johnson JJ, Mukhtar H. Curcumin for chemoprevention of colon cancer. Cancer Lett. 2007 Apr 18; [Epub ahead of print]) (Kim, Kang, Moon, 2001) (Kim MS, Kang HJ, Moon A. Inhibition of invasion and induction of apoptosis by curcumin in H-ras-transformed MCF10A human breast epithelial cells. *Arch Pharm Res.* 2001;24(4):349-354) (Krishnaswamy, 2008) (Krishnaswamy K. Traditional Indian spices and their health significance. *Asia Pac J Clin Nutr.* 2008;17 Suppl 1:265-8) (Pari, Tewas, Eckel, 2008) (Pari L, Tewas D, Eckel J. Role of curcumin in health and disease. *Arch Physiol Biochem.* 2008;114(2):127-49) (Phan et al, 2001) (Phan TT, See P, Lee ST, Chan SY. Protective effects of curcumin against oxidative damage on skin cells in vitro: its implication for wound healing. *J Trauma* 2001;51(5):927-931) (Rakel, 2008) (Rakel D. *Rakel: Integrative Medicine, 2nd ed.* Philadelphia, PA: Saunders; 2008;80) (Rao, 2007) (Rao CV. Regulation of COX and LOX by curcumin. *Adv Exp Med Biol.* 2007;595:213-26) (Sharma et al, 2001) (Sharma RA, Ireson CR, Verschoyle RD. Effects of dietary curcumin on glutathione S-Transferase and Malondialdehyde-DNA adducts in rat liver and colon mucosa: relationship with drug levels. *Clin Cancer Res.* 2001;7:1452-1458) (Sharma et al, 2007) (Sharma RA, Steward WP, Gescher AJ. Pharmacokinetics and pharmacodynamics of curcumin. *Adv Exp Med Biol.* 2007;595:453-70) (Shehzad et al, 2010) (Shehzad A, Khan S, Shehzad O, Lee YS. Curcumin therapeutic promises and bioavailability in colorectal cancer. *Drugs Today (Barc).* 2010 Jul;46(7):523-32. Review) (Shishoda et al, 2007) (Shishodia S, Singh T, Chaturvedi MM. Modulation of transcription factors by curcumin. *Adv Exp Med Biol.* 2007;595:127-48) (Su et al, 2006) (Su CC, Lin JG, Li TM, Chung JG, Yang JS, Ip SW, et al. Curcumin-induced apoptosis of human colon cancer colo 205 cells through the production of ROS, Ca2+ and the activation of caspase-3. *Anticancer Res.* 2006 Nov-Dec;26(6B):4379-89) (Suryanarayana et al, 2007) (Suryanarayana P, Satyanarayana A, Balakrishna N, Kumar PU, Reddy GB. Effect of turmeric and curcumin on oxidative stress and antioxidant enzymes in streptozotocin-induced diabetic rat. *Med Sci Monit.* 2007;13(12):BR286-92) (White, Judkins, 2011) (White B, Judkins DZ. Clinical Inquiry. Does turmeric relieve inflammatory conditions? *J Fam Pract.* 2011 Mar;60(3):155-6. Review) (Zafir, Banu, 2007) (Zafir A, Banu N. Antioxidant potential of fluoxetine in comparison to Curcuma longa in restraint-stressed rats. *Eur J Pharmacol.* 2007;572(1):23-31)

Alternative Names

Curcuma longa

Version Info

- Last Reviewed on 05/04/2011

Prof Randolph M. Howes MD, PhD

- Steven D. Ehrlich, NMD, Solutions Acupuncture, a private practice specializing in complementary and alternative medicine, Phoenix, AZ. Review provided by VeriMed Healthcare Network. This page was last updated: May 7, 2013

Source: Turmeric | University of Maryland Medical Center http://umm.edu/health/medical/altmed/herb/turmeric#ixzz3NrhE8JOt

University of Maryland Medical Center

The following was adapted from the excellent article by Epstein et al:

Curcumin as a therapeutic agent

Curcumin as a therapeutic agent: the evidence from *in vitro*, animal and human studies
(Epstein, Sanderson, MacDonald, 2010)

There is no explicit evidence that correlates the molecular or stoichiometric properties of curcumin or its analogues with their biological effects. While several groups have studied the differential bioactivities of these different analogues, no single curcuminoid shows overall highest potency.

Differential efficacy varies widely according to the cell type, function, disease system and organism in question. (Anand et al, 2008)

Thus, there is no consensus as to the most effective preparation for human use.

Some data suggest that a mixture of curcuminoids have synergistically greater activity than any of their individual elements. (Sandur et al, 2007)

The safety, tolerability and non-toxicity of curcumin at high doses are well established. **Oral doses up to 12 g/d are well tolerated in human subjects**, although dosing diet regimen above 8 g may be difficult to achieve due to the bulky nature of this quantity of compound. (Lao et al, 2006) (Cheng et al, 2001)

However, **drug delivery is a problem and the bioavailability of oral curcumin is low due to a combination of efficient first pass metabolism, poor gastrointestinal absorption, rapid elimination and poor aqueous solubility**. (Anand et al, 2007) (Sharma, Steward et al, 2007)

Other, potentially active, metabolites have been identified, perhaps the most important and intensively studied of which is tetrahydrocurcumin, a reduction metabolite. It lacks the yellow color and hydrophobicity of curcumin and does not occur in natural curcumin sources. While it has less anti-inflammatory activity than curcumin in terms of its ability to inhibit NF-κB, **it exhibits greater antioxidant potency than curcumin in a number of different models.** (Sandur et al, 2007) (Pan et al, 2000)

It has been reported that heat treatment improves the water solubility of curcumin. (Kurien et al, 2007)

In human trials, only minor side effects of curcumin, namely diarrhea, have been reported, and it is considered safe and well tolerated.

As a caveat, however, these trials have usually examined short-term outcomes. **There is some evidence that long-term, high-dose curcumin administration in rodents can be tumorigenic**. (NTP, 1993) (Somassundaram et al, 2002)

It has also been shown that **curcumin's predominant activity switches from antioxidant to pro-oxidant with increasing concentration**, which may provide an explanation for its seemingly opposing biological effects *in vivo*. (Sandur, Ichikawa et al, 2007)

These apparent contradictory roles of curcumin, as both anti-cancer and pro-carcinogenic agent, are as yet unexplained, and epitomize the complexity and paradoxical nature of the compound. Nevertheless, **there is good evidence from India, at a population level, about the safety of lifelong curcumin ingestion up to about 100 mg/d, and it is classified 'Generally Recognised As Safe' by the United States Food and Drug Administration**. (Chainani-Wu et al, 2003)

A wide variety of cellular properties of curcumin have been demonstrated, including antioxidant, anti-inflammatory, anti-proliferative, pro-apoptotic, anti-bacterial and anti-cancer activities.

NF-κB

NF-κB is one of the key transcription factors responsive to curcumin. In human myeloid ML-1a cells, curcumin suppresses NF-κB activation induced by TNF-α, phorbol ester and hydrogen peroxide. (Singh, Aggarwal, 1995)

The mechanism appears to be via reduced IκBα phosphorylation and degradation, suggesting that curcumin acts at a step above IκB kinase (IKK) in the NF-κB activation pathway. **Many of the observed biological effects of curcumin involve processes that are NF-κB-dependent.** (Aggarwal et al, 2006)

Signal transducer and activator of transcription

Signal transducer and activator of transcription (STAT)3 is a transcriptional activator with a ubiquitous role in tumorigenesis. It is involved in dysregulation of cell growth, invasion, angiogenesis, metastasis and resistance to apoptosis. (Aggarwal, BB, Sethi, G, Ahn, KS, et al. 2006)

Tumor suppressor p53

Mutation of the tumor suppressor p53 plays an important role in the evolution of many different human cancers. Once again, the role of curcumin is complex. In an early study of the effects of curcumin on BKS-2 and WEHI-231 cells (both immature B cell lymphoma mouse cell lines), proliferation was inhibited. (Han et al, 1999)

The finding of reduced p53 activity was confirmed in RKO cells (a colon cancer cell line), where curcumin impairs the post-translational folding of p53 required for its function and in myeloid leukaemic cells, where it induces p53 degradation. (Moos et al, 2004) (Tsvetkov et al, 2005)

Other experiments show induction of p53 by curcumin, for example in human epithelial breast cancer, prostate cancer

and B cell lymphoma cell lines and in HT-29 cells (a human colon adenocarcinoma cell line), where it induced apoptosis. (Choudhuri et al, 2005) (Song et al, 2005)

In the former work, once again the authors show differential sensitivity of cancer cells compared with healthy cells to curcumin. While some investigators have shown anti-proliferative effects despite inhibition of the tumor suppressor p53, established precedents exist where an agent that is cancer-preventative in one system can be carcinogenic in another, for example tamoxifen (therapeutic in breast; pro-neoplastic in uterus). (Fisher et al, 1998)

These cautions must be borne in mind when considering its human use.

While curcumin has shown benefits in a number of different models of inflammatory disease, particular interest has focused on its use in the gut. IBD (Crohn's disease (CD) and ulcerative colitis (UC)) is a source of considerable morbidity, and its incidence is increasing worldwide. Currently available treatments such as steroids, 5-aminosalicylic acids and immunomodulators do not offer cure, but CD responds well to polymeric or elemental feed that brings about remission in 80 % of pediatric patients. (Heuschkel et al, 2000) (Bannerjee et al, 2004)

IBD (irritable bowel disease) is less common in developing countries than in the industrialized world, and individuals emigrating from East to West take on the Western disease risk. (Goh et al, 2009)

This holds further relevance to the importance of diet in IBD, and there is keen interest to develop nutritional therapies.

These data raise once again the suggestion that curcumin can have paradoxically opposing effects at different concentrations, and when clinical studies take place, a wide range of dosages are warranted.

The molecular targets of curcumin include many pathways and processes involved in the generation and propagation of cancer. The observation that many common cancers (including colon, breast, prostate and lung) are commoner in the Western world than in countries such as India, where there is high natural dietary curcumin consumption, while not indicative of cause and effect, is intriguing.

Chemoprevention

Curcumin has been investigated as both chemotherapeutic and chemopreventive agent in many different animal (largely rodent) models of carcinogenesis. Its chemopreventive efficacy for colon cancer is particularly well established. (Rao et al, 1993) (Kim et al, 1998)

Other gastrointestinal cancers against which curcumin has shown protective effects include esophageal, stomach, liver and oral; all in rodent models.

Curcumin also shows chemopreventive properties in rodent models of various extra-intestinal cancers, including breast, lung, kidney, bladder, blood and skin.

Chemotherapy

Curcumin inhibits tumor growth and metastasis, and has chemosensitising and radiosensitizing properties. One of the earliest examples of the ability of curcumin to inhibit tumor growth is that of lymphoma cells in a mouse ascites model, when it was administered intraperitoneally at 50 mg/kg. (Kuttan et al, 1985)

Curcumin also has anti-tumor efficacy against human melanoma cell xenografts if given intraperitoneally. (Odot et al, 2004)

Also, **in xenograft models, sub-cutaneous delivery of curcumin suppresses growth of head and neck squamous carcinoma cells, and when given orally it inhibits proliferation and angiogenesis and induces apoptosis in prostate cancer cells**. (Lotempio et al, 2005)

Curcumin also suppresses proliferation and angiogenesis and enhances apoptosis in pancreatic cancer; both when given orally in combination with gemcitabine in an orthotopic model, and in a xenograft model when given intravenously in a liposomal formulation. (Kunnumakkara et al, 2007) (Li et al, 2005)

The same group have also used an intravenous liposomal curcumin preparation in luminal gastrointestinal cancers, where it has chemosensitising properties against colorectal cancer in a mouse xenograft model. (Li et al, 2007)

In this work, tumor growth and angiogenesis **were inhibited and apoptosis enhanced** in combination with oxaliplatin. In an ortho-topic implantation model of hepatocellular carcinoma, curcumin also prevented intrahepatic metastasis.

Finally, in recent work, oral curcumin has shown efficacy in preventing breast cancer metastasis to lung in orthotopic models, both as chemo-sensitizer in conjunction with paclitaxel and in the prevention of its he-matogenous spread in immuno-deficient mice. (Aggarwal, BB, Shishodia, S, Takada, Y, et al, 2005) (Bachmeier et al, 2007)

Curcumin given intraperitoneally in combination with docetaxel inhib-its tumor growth and angiogenesis in an orthotopic nude mouse model of ovarian cancer. (Lin et al, 2007)

The wealth of *in vitro* and pre-clinical data has provided a strong basis from which to progress to the trialing of curcumin in human subjects. Many of the molecular efficacies of curcumin demonstrated in cell cul-ture systems and animal models are comparable to those seen in hu-man subjects.

The anti-inflammatory targets of curcumin including reduction of NF-κB, COX2 and pro-inflammatory cytokines such as IL-1, IL-6 and TNF-α, translate into clinical anti-inflammatory efficacy **with im-provement of rheumatoid arthritis, psoriasis, post-operative inflammation, chronic anterior uveitis and orbital inflamma-tory pseudo-tumors**.

Concordant with the finding that high concentrations of curcumin are achievable in gastrointestinal tissue, **curcumin shows clinical benefit in irritable bowel syndrome, tropical pancreatitis, gall bladder and biliary motility, gastric ulceration and familial adenoma-tous polyposis coli**.

Further encouraging results came from a larger multicenter, randomized, double-blind, controlled trial of eighty-nine ulcerative colitis patients with quiescent UC, in which **two out of forty-three patients (5 %) taking oral curcumin had relapsed by 6 months compared with eight out of thirty-nine (21 %) in the placebo group**. (Hanai et al, 2006)

The investigators also **showed significant clinical and endoscopic improvements in the curcumin-treated group**.

In Summary

There is a strong foundation of evidence from both *in vitro* and animal models that **curcumin has anti-cancer actions, including its pro-apoptotic and anti-angiogenic effects** and its modulation of the cell cycle, growth factor expression and signal transduction pathways. Building upon this foundation, **curcumin appears to prevent and treat cancer in human subjects**.

These preliminary data hold promise, and interest in curcumin as a therapeutic agent continues to grow.

Since ancient times, curcumin has been used in a wide range of inflammatory, neoplastic and other conditions. In recent years, the molecular basis for its efficacy has been extensively investigated.

Many cellular and molecular targets have been identified and many questions still remain.

In complex multifactorial illnesses such as systemic inflammatory diseases and cancer, an agent that acts at a number of different cellular levels offers perhaps a better chance of effective prophylaxis or treatment.

Its non-toxicity and good tolerability in human subjects, in combination with strong promising results from cell line, animal and early human clinical studies, support the ongoing research and development of curcumin as a preventive and disease-modifying agent.

Enhancing curcumin bioavailability

Curcumin and turmeric: improving the therapeutic benefits by enhancing absorption and bioavailability

August 13, 2015

Few natural products have demonstrated the range of protective and therapeutic promise as have turmeric and its principal bioactive components, the curcuminoids.

Success in translating this potential into tangible benefits has been limited by inherently poor intestinal absorption, rapid metabolism, and limited systemic bioavailability.

Seeking to overcome these limitations, food ingredient formulators have begun to employ a variety of approaches to enhance absorption and bioavailability.

Open access article, Beyond Yellow Curry: Assessing Commercial Curcumin Absorption Technologies, is now available from the *Journal of the American College of Nutrition*, official publication of the American College of Nutrition.

Turmeric and its main bioactive components - curcumin, desmethoxycurcumin and bisdemethoxycurcumin - have many biological effects including anti-inflammatory, antioxidant, antitumor, antibacterial, and antiviral activities. Turmeric traditionally has been consumed in fat-based sauces, such as in a fat-rich yellow curry. More recently, intake of concentrated extracts of curcuminoids has become common in the form of health supplements.

This review introduces needed order to the curcumin marketplace by examining bioavailability studies on a number of commercial curcumin ingredients and evaluating them on a level playing field.

The article presented the following results:

- **A hydrophilic carrier dispersed curcuminoid formula exhibits 45.9 times the bioavailability of the standard purified 95 percent curcuminoid preparation and, based on relative mass efficiency**, 1.5 times the bioavailability of the next best commercial ingredient, a cyclodextrin complex.

Curcumin is currently being actively researched. When asked about the future of this field of research, author Dallas Clouatre said, "I would like to see and perhaps be involved in research on improving bioavailability. Also, it would be useful to test whether curcumin's benefits can be improved or even directed through use of combination products.

The "silver bullet" research model for nutritional and pharmaceutical compounds long has been questioned. Alternatives, such as an examination of what is sometimes termed the "entourage effect," need to be explored."

The article authors conclude, "**Delivery strategies can significantly improve the bioavailability of curcuminoids**. Total formula mass is important for making practical formulation decisions about dosing, cost and space." (Financial support was provided by OmniActive Health Technologies, Inc.)

My conclusions on turmeric (curcumin) are as follows:

CURCUMIN

Contradictory to the commonly-mentioned antioxidant effect, curcumin has significant prooxidant activity. Studies indicate a role of **ROS (EMODs)** in curcumin-induced cell death.

Some promising effects have been observed in patients with various pro-inflammatory diseases including cancer, cardiovascular disease, arthritis, uveitis, ulcerative proctitis, Crohn's disease, ulcerative colitis, irritable bowel disease, tropical pancreatitis, peptic ulcer, gastric ulcer, idiopathic orbital inflammatory pseudotumor, oral lichen planus, gastric inflammation, vitiligo, psoriasis, acute coronary syndrome, atherosclerosis, diabetes, diabetic nephropathy, diabetic microangiopathy, lupus nephritis, renal conditions, acquired immunodeficiency syndrome, ß-thalassemia, biliary dyskinesia, Dejerine-Sottas disease, cholecystitis, and chronic bacterial prostatitis.

Although curcumin has shown efficacy against numerous human ailments, **poor bioavailability due to poor absorption, rapid metabolism, and rapid systemic elimination have been shown to limit its therapeutic efficacy.**

The United States Food and Drug Administration has approved curcumin as being GRAS (generally recognized as safe), and the polyphenol is now being used as a supplement in several countries.

I believe that data on a wide spectrum of diseases indicate a positive potential for the clinical use of curcumin, especially for cancer treatment or as an adjunct and in the treatment of arthritis. Still, further studies are necessary.

References

(Adams et al, 2006) (Adams LS, Seeram NP, Aggarwal BB, Takada Y, Sand D, Heber D. Pomegranate juice, total pomegranate ellagitannins, and punicalagin suppress inflammatory cell signaling in colon cancer cells. J Agric Food Chem. 2006;54:980–5)

(Afaq et al, 2009) (Afaq F, Zaid MA, Khan N, Dreher M, Mukhtar H. Protective effect of pomegranate-derived products on UVB-mediated damage in human reconstituted skin. Exp Dermatol. 2009;18:553–61)

(Aggarwal, BB, Shishodia, S, Takada, Y, et al, 2005) (Aggarwal, BB, Shishodia, S, Takada, Y, et al. (2005) Curcumin suppresses the paclitaxel-induced nuclear factor-kappaB pathway in breast cancer cells and inhibits lung metastasis of human breast cancer in nude mice. Clin Cancer Res 11, 7490–7498)

(Aggarwal et al, 2006) (Aggarwal, S, Ichikawa, H, Takada, Y, et al. (2006) Curcumin (diferuloylmethane) down-regulates expression of cell pro-liferation and antiapoptotic and metastatic gene products through sup-pression of IkappaBalpha kinase and Akt activation. Mol Pharmacol 69, 195–206)

(Aggarwal et al, 2007) (Aggarwal BB, Sundaram C, Malani N, Ichikawa H. Curcumin: the Indian solid gold. *Adv Exp Med Biol.* 2007;595:1-75)

(Aggarwal, Haikumar, 2009) (Aggarwal BB, Harikumar KB. Potential therapeutic effects of curcumin, the anti-inflammatory agent, against neurodegenerative, cardiovascular, pulmonary, metabolic, autoimmune and neoplastic diseases. Int J Biochem Cell Biol. 2009;41(1):40–59)

(Aggarwal, BB, Sethi, G, Ahn, KS, et al. 2006) (Aggarwal, BB, Sethi, G, Ahn, KS, et al. (2006) Targeting signal-transducer-and-activator-of-transcrip-tion-3 for prevention and therapy of cancer: modern target but ancient solution. Ann N Y Acad Sci 1091, 151–169)

(Aggarwal, Sung, 2009) (Aggarwal BB, Sung B. Pharmacological basis for the role of curcumin in chronic diseases: an age-old spice with modern targets. Trends Pharmacol Sci. 2009;30(2):85–94)

(Albrecht et al, 2004) (Albrecht M, Jiang W, Kumi-Diaka J, Lansky EP, Gommersall LM, Patel A, et al. Pomegranate extracts potently suppress proliferation, xenograft growth, and invasion of human prostate cancer cells. J Med Food. 2004;7:274–83)

(Albright et al, 2003) (Albright, C. D., Salganik, R. I., Craciunescu, C. N., Mar, M. H. & Zeisel, S. H. (2003) Mitochondrial and microsomal derived reactive oxygen species mediate apoptosis induced by transforming growth factor-beta1 in immortalized rat hepatocytes. J. Cell Biochem. 89: 254–261)

(Albright et al, 2004) (Albright, C. D., Salganik, R. I. & Van Dyke, T. (2004) Dietary depletion of vitamin E and vitamin A inhibits mammary tumor growth and metastasis in transgenic mice. J. Nutr. 134: 1139–1144)

(Al-Jarallah et al, 2013) (Al-Jarallah A, Igdoura F, Zhang Y, et al. The effect of pomegranate extract on coronary artery atherosclerosis in SR-BI/APOE double knockout mice. Atherosclerosis. 2013 May;228(1):80-9)

(Allegri et al, 2010) (Allegri P, Mastromarino A, Neri P. Management of chronic anterior uveitis relapses: efficacy of oral phospholipidic curcumin treatment. Long-term follow-up. Clin Ophthalmol. 2010;4:1201–1206)

(Alwi et al, 2008) (Alwi I, Santoso T, Suyono S, Sutrisna B, Suyatna FD, Kresno SB, et al. The effect of curcumin on lipid level in patients with acute coronary syndrome. Acta Med Indones. 2008;40(4):201–21)

(Ames, 1983) (Ames B.N. Dietary carcinogens and anticarcinogens. Oxygen radicals and degenerative diseases. Science. 1983;221(4617):1256–1263)

(Ames, 1989) (Ames BN. Endogenous oxidative DNA damage, aging, and cancer. Free Radic Res Commun. 1989;7:121–28)

(Anand et al, 2007) (Anand P, Kunnumakkara AB, Newman RA, Aggarwal BB. Bioavailability of curcumin: problems and promises. Mol Pharm. 2007;4(6):807–818)

(Anand et al, 2008) (Anand P, Thomas, SG, Kunnumakkara, AB et al, (2008) Biological activities of curcumin and its analogues (cogeners) made by man and mother nature. Biochem Pharmacol 76, 1590-1611)

(Anisimov, 2003) (Anisimov VN. Effects of exogenous melatonin – A review. Toxicol Pathol. 2003;31:589–603)

(Antony et al, 2008) (Antony B, Merina B, Iyer VS, Judy N, Lennertz K, Joyal S. A pilot cross-over study to evaluate human oral bioavailability of BCM-95CG (Biocurcumax), a novel bioenhanced preparation of curcumin. Indian J Pharm Sci. 2008;70(4):445–449)

(Appendino et al, 2011) (Appendino G, Belcaro G, Cornelli U, Luzzi R, Togni S, Dugall M, et al. Potential role of curcumin phytosome (Meriva) in controlling the evolution of diabetic microangiopathy. A pilot study. Panminerva Med. 2011;53(3 Suppl 1):43–49)

(Araujo et al, 1999) (Araujo, M. C., Dias, F. L. and Takahashi, C. S., Potentiation by turmeric and curcumin of gamma-radiation-induced chromosome aberrations in Chinese hamster ovary cells. Teratogen. Carcinogen. Mutagen, 1999, 19, 9–18)

(AREDS report no. 9, 2001) (Age-Related Eye Disease Study Research Group. "A randomized, placebo-controlled, clinical trial of high-dose supplementation with vitamins C and E and beta carotene for age-related cataract and vision loss: AREDS report no. 9."*Archives of ophthalmology* 119.10 (2001): 1439)

(Asgary et al, 2014) (Asgary S, Sahebkar A, Afshani MR, Keshvari M, Haghjooyjavanmard S, Rafieian-Kopaei M. Clinical evaluation of blood pressure lowering, endothelial function improving, hypolipidemic and anti-Inflammatory effects of pomegranate juice in hypertensive subjects. *Phytother Res.* 2014 Feb;28)2)193-9)

(Avery et al, 2003) (Avery NG, Kaiser JL, Sharman MJ, et al. Effects of vitamin E supplementation on recovery from repeated bouts of resistance exercise. J Strength Cond Res. 2003;17(4):801–9)

(Aviram et al, 2000) (Aviram M, Dornfeld L, Rosenblat M, Volkova N, Kaplan M, Coleman R, et al. Pomegranate juice consumption reduces oxidative stress, atherogenic modifications to LDL, and platelet aggregation: Studies in humans and in atherosclerotic apolipoprotein E-deficient mice. Am J Clin Nutr. 2000;71:1062–76)

(Aviram et al, 2004) (Aviram M, Rosenblat M, Gaitini D, Nitecki S, Hoffman A, Dornfeld L, et al. Pomegranate juice consumption for 3 years by patients with carotid artery stenosis reduces common carotid intima-media thickness, blood pressure and LDL oxidation. Clin Nutr. 2004;23:423–33)

(Aviram, Rosenblat, 2012) (Aviram M, Rosenblat M. Pomegranate protection against cardiovascular diseases. *Evid Based Complement Alternat Med.* 2012;2012:382763)

(Aviram, Rosenblat, 2013) (Aviram M, Rosenblat M. Pomegranate for your cardiovascular health. *Rambam Maimonides Med J.* 2013 Apr;4(2):e0013)

(Aydogan et al, 2006) (Aydogan S, Yerer MB, Goktas A. Melatonin and nitric oxide. J Endocrinol Invest.2006;29(3):281–7)

(Bachmeier et al, 2007) (Bachmeier, B, Nerlich, AG, Iancu, CM, et al. (2007) The chemopreventive polyphenol curcumin prevents hematogenous breast cancer metastases in immunodeficient mice. Cell Physiol Biochem 19, 137–152)

(Bae et al, 2010) (Bae JY, Choi JS, Kang SW, Lee YJ, Park J, Kang YH. Dietary compound ellagic acid alleviates skin wrinkle and inflammation induced by UV-B irradiation. Exp Dermatol. 2010;19:e182–90)

(Bagri et al, 2009) (Bagri P, Ali M, Aeri V, Bhowmik M, Sultana S. Antidiabetic effect of *Punica granatum* flowers: Effect on hyperlipidemia, pancreatic cells lipid peroxidation and antioxidant enzymes in experimental diabetes. Food Chem Toxicol. 2009;47:50–4)

(Balakrishnan and Anuradha, 1998) (Balakrishnan SD, Anuradha CV. Exercise, depletion of antioxidants and antioxidant manipulation. Cell Biochem Funct. 1998;16(4):269–75)

(Bandyopadhyay et al, 1999) (Bandyopadhyay, U., Das, D. and Banerjee, R. K., Reactive oxygen species: oxidative damage and pathogenesis. Curr Sci., 1999, 77, 658–666)

(Banihani et al, 2013) (Banihani S, Swedan S, Alguraan Z. Pomegranate and type 2 diabetes. Nutr Res. 2013 May;33(5):341-8. doi: 10.1016/j. nutres.2013.03.003. Epub 2013 Apr 15)

(Bannerjee et al, 2004) (Bannerjee, K, Camacho-Hubner, C, Babinska, K, et al. (2004) Anti-inflammatory and growth-stimulating effects precede nutritional restitution during enteral feeding in Crohn disease. J Pediatr Gastroenterol Nutr 38, 270–275)

(Barja 2002) (Barja G. Rate of generation of oxidative stress-related damage and animal longevity. Free Radic Biol Med. 2002;33(9):1167–72)

(Barnett and Conlee, 2003) (Barnett DW, Conlee RK. The effects of a commercial dietary supplement on human performance. Am J Clin Nutr. 2003;40(3):287–93)

(Basak et al, 2015) (Saroj K. Basak, Alborz Zinabadi, Arthur W. Wu, Natarajan Venkatesan, Victor M. Duarte, James J. Kang, Clifton L. Dalgard, Meera Srivastava, Fazlul H. Sarkar, Marilene B. Wang and Eri S. Srivatsan. Liposome encapsulated curcumin-difluorinated (CDF) inhibits the growth of cisplatin resistant head and neck cancer stem cells, , *Oncotarget*, published 19 May 2015)

(Basu et al, 2013) (Basu A, Newman ED, Bryant AL, Lyons TJ, Betts NM. Pomegranate polyphenols lower lipid peroxidation in adults with type 2 diabetes but have no effects in healthy volunteers: a pilot study. J Nutr Metab. 2013;2013:708381. Epub 2013 Jul 10)

(Bauet-Robert et al, 2010) (Bayet-Robert M, Kwiatkowski F, Leheurteur M, Gachon F, Planchat E, Abrial C, et al. Phase I dose escalation trial of docetaxel plus curcumin in patients with advanced and metastatic breast cancer. Cancer Biol Ther. 2010;9(1):8–14)

(Baum et al, 2008) (Baum L, Lam CW, Cheung SK, Kwok T, Lui V, Tsoh J, et al. Six-month randomized, placebo-controlled, double-blind, pilot clinical trial of curcumin in patients with Alzheimer disease. J Clin Psychopharmacol. 2008;28(1):110–113)

(Belcaro et al, 2010) (Belcaro G, Cesarone MR, Dugall M, Pellegrini L, Ledda A, Grossi MG, et al. Product-evaluation registry of Meriva(R), a curcumin-phosphatidylcholine complex, for the complementary management of osteoarthritis. Panminerva Med. 2010;52(2 Suppl 1):55–62)

(Belcaro, Cesarone et al, 2010) (Belcaro G, Cesarone MR, Dugall M, Pellegrini L, Ledda A, Grossi MG, et al. Efficacy and safety of Meriva(R), a curcumin-phosphatidylcholine complex, during extended administration in osteoarthritis patients. Altern Med Rev. 2010;15(4):337–344)

(Berger, 2005) (Berger MM. Can oxidative damage be treated nutritionally? Clin Nutr. 2005;24:172–83)

(Betteridge, 2000) (Betteridge, D. John. "What is oxidative stress?." Metabolism 49.2 (2000): 3-8)

(Bhadbhade et al, 2011) (Bhadbhade SJ, Acharya AB, Rodrigues SV, Thakur SL. The antiplaque efficacy of pomegranate mouth rinse. Quintessence Int. 2011;42:29–36)

(Biswas et al, 2010) (Biswas J, Sinha D, Mukherjee S, Roy S, Siddiqi M, Roy M. Curcumin protects DNA damage in a chronically arsenic-exposed population of West Bengal. Hum Exp Toxicol. 2010;29(6):513–524)

(Bjelakovic et al, 2004) (Bjelakovic G, Nikolova D, Simonetti RG, et al. Antioxidant supplements for prevention of gastrointestinal cancers: a systematic review and meta-analysis. Lancet. 2004;364:1219–28)

(Blasiak et al, 1999) (Blasiak, J., Trzeciak, A., Malecka-Panas, E., Drzewoski, J., Iwamienko, T., Szumiel, I. and Wojewodzka, M., DNA damage and repair in human lymphocytes and gastric mucosa cells exposed to chromium and curcumin. Teratogen. Carcinogen. Mutagen, 1999, 19, 19–31)

(Boddupalli et al, 2012) (Sekhar Boddupalli, Jonathan R. Mein, Shantala Lakkanna, and Don R. James. Induction of Phase 2 Antioxidant Enzymes by Broccoli Sulforaphane: Perspectives in Maintaining the Antioxidant Activity of Vitamins A, C, and E. Front Genet. 2012; 3:7)

(Bonnesen et al, 2001) (Bonnesen et al, Dietary Indoles and Isothiocyanates That Are Generated from Cruciferous Vegetables Can Both Stimulate Apoptosis and Confer Protection against DNA Damage in Human Colon Cell Lines. CANCER RESEARCH 61, 6120–6130, August 15, 2001])

(Boussetta et al, 2009) (Boussetta T, Raad H, Lettéron P, Gougerot-Pocidalo MA, Marie JC, Driss F, et al. Punicic acid a conjugated linolenic acid inhibits TNFalpha-induced neutrophil hyperactivation and protects from experimental colon inflammation in rats. PLoS One. 2009;4:e6458)

(Bowles et al, 1991) (Bowles D, Torgan C, Ebner S, et al. Effects of acute, submaximal exercise on skeletal muscle vitamin E. Free Radic Res Commun. 1991;14:139–43)

(Brooks, Paton, Vidanes, 2001) (Brooks JD, Paton VG, Vidanes G. Potent induction of phase 2 enzymes in human prostate cells by sulforaphane. *Cancer Epidemiol Biomarkers Prev.* 2001;10:949–54)

(Bundy et al, 2004) (Bundy R, Walker AF, Middleton RW, Booth J. Turmeric extract may improve irritable bowel syndrome symptomology in otherwise healthy adults: a pilot study. J Altern Complement Med. 2004;10(6):1015–1018)

(Butler et al 2002) (Butler RN, Fossel M, Harman SM, et al. Is there an anti-aging medicine? J Gerontol A Biol Sci Med Sci. 2002;57A(9):B333–B8)

(Calabrese et al, 2003) (Calabrese V, Butterfield DA, Stella AM. Nutritional antioxidants and the heme oxygenase pathway of stress tolerance: novel targets for neuroprotection in Alzheimer's disease. Ital J Biochem. 2003;52(4):177–81)

(Cantoni, Guidarelli, 2008) (Cantoni O., Guidarelli A. Peroxynitrite damages U937 cell DNA via the intermediate formation of mitochondrial oxidants. *IUBMB Life*. 2008;60(11):753–756)

(Carroll et al, 2011) (Carroll RE, Benya RV, Turgeon DK, Vareed S, Neuman M, Rodriguez L, et al. Phase IIa clinical trial of curcumin for the prevention of colorectal neoplasia. Cancer Prev Res (Phila)2011;4(3):354–364)

(Cerda et al, 2003) (Cerdá B, Cerón JJ, Tomás-Barberán FA, Espín JC. Repeated oral administration of high doses of the pomegranate ellagitannin punicalagin to rats for 37 days is not toxic. J Agric Food. 2003;51:3493–501)

(Cesari et al, 2005) (Cesari M, Kritchevsky SB, Leeuwenburgh C, et al. Oxidative damage and platelet activation as new predictors of mobility disability and mortality in elders. Antioxid Redox Signal. 2005;8(3–4):609–19)

(Chainani-Wu et al, 2003) (Chainani-Wu, N (2003) Safety and anti-inflammatory activity of curcumin: a component of turmeric (*Curcuma longa*). J Altern Complement Med 9, 161–168)

(Chainani-Wu et al, 2007) (Chainani-Wu N, Silverman S, Jr, Reingold A, Bostrom A, Mc Culloch C, Lozada-Nur F, et al. A randomized, placebo-controlled, double-blind clinical trial of curcuminoids in oral lichen planus. Phytomedicine. 2007;14(7–8):437–446)

(Chandra and McBean, 1994) (Chandra RK, McBean LD. Zinc and immunity. Nutrition. 1994;10:79–80)

(Chattopadhyay et al, 2004) (Ishita Chattopadhyay, Kaushik Biswas, Uday Bandyopadhyay and Ranajit K. Banerjee. Current Science, VOL. 87, NO. 1, 10 JULY 2004 pg 44-53)

(Cheng et al, 2001) (Cheng AL, Hsu CH, Lin JK, Hsu MM, Ho YF, Shen TS, et al. Phase I clinical trial of curcumin, a chemopreventive agent, in patients with high-risk or pre-malignant lesions. Anticancer Res. 2001;21(4B):2895–2900)

(Chiao et al, 2002) (Chiao JW, Chung FL, Kancherla R, Ahmed T, Mittelman A, Conaway CC. Sulforaphane and its metabolite mediate growth arrest and apoptosis in human prostate cancer cells. *Int J Oncol.* 2002;20:631–6)

(Choi et al, 2008) (Choi W.Y., Choi B.T., Lee W. H., Choi Y. H. Sulforaphane generates reactive oxygen species leading to mitochondrial pertur-bation for apoptosis in human leukemia U937 cells. *Biomedicine and Pharmacotherapy.* 2008;62(9):637–644)

(Choi et al, 2009) (Choi, Kyungsun, et al. "Oxidative stress-induced ne-crotic cell death via mitochondira-dependent burst of reactive oxygen species." Current neurovascular research 6.4 (2009): 213-222)

(Christopher et al, 2010) (Christopher D. Hapner, Patricia Deuster, Yifan Chen. Inhibition of oxidative hemolysis by quercetin, but not oth-er antioxidants. Chemico-Biological Interactions. Volume 186, Issue 3, 5 August 2010, Pages 275–279)

(Chrubasik et al, 2014) (Chrubasik-Hausmann S, Vlachojannis C, Zimmermann B. Pomegranate juice and prostate cancer: importance of the characterisation of the active principle. Phytother Res. 2014 Nov;28(11):1676-8)

(Chuengsmarn et al, 2012) (Chuengsamarn S, Rattanamongkolgul S, Luechapudiporn R, Phisalaphong C, Jirawatnotai S. Curcumin extract for prevention of type 2 diabetes. Diabetes Care. 2012;35(11):2121–7)

(Cichon, Radisky, 2014) (Cichon M.A., Radisky D.C. ROS-induced epithe-lial-mesenchymal transition in mammary epithelial cells is mediated by NF-κB-dependent activation of Snail. *Oncotarget.* 2014;5(9):2827–2838)

(Chandran, Goel, 2012) (Chandran B, Goel A.A randomized, pilot study to assess the efficacy and safety of curcumin in patients with active rheumatoid arthritis. Phytother Res. 2012;26(11):1719–25)

(Chen et al, 2010) (Chen Y, Li WH et al, Plant polyphenol curcumin sig-nificantly affects CYP1A2 and CyP2A6 activity in healthy, male Chinese volunteers. Ann Pharmacother. 2010;1038-1045)

(Choudhuri et al, 2005) (Choudhuri, T, Pal, S, Das, T, et al. (2005) Curcumin selectively induces apoptosis in deregulated cyclin D1-expressed cells at G2 phase of cell cycle in a p53-dependent manner. J Biol Chem 280, 20059–20068)

(Clapp-Lilly et al, 2001) (Clapp-Lilly KL, Smith MA, Perry G, et al. Melatonin acts as antioxidant and pro-oxidant in an organotypic slice culture model of Alzheimer's disease. Neuroreport. 2001;12:1277–80)

(Clarke et al, 2011) (Clarke J. D., Hsu A., Yu Z., Dashwood R. H., Ho E. Differential effects of sulforaphane on histone deacetylases, cell cycle arrest and apoptosis in normal prostate cells versus hyperplastic and cancerous prostate cells. Molecular Nutrition and Food Research. 2011;55(7):999–1009)

(Clarkson, 1995) (Clarkson, Priscilla M. "Antioxidants and physical performance." Critical Reviews in Food Science & Nutrition 35.1-2 (1995):131-141)

(Conaway et al, 2001) (Conaway CC, Getahun SM, Liebes LL, et al. Disposition of glucosinolates and sulforaphane in humans after ingestion of steamed and fresh broccoli. Nutr Cancer. 2000;38:168–78. Erratum in: Nutr Cancer. 2001;41:196)

(Conaway et al., 2002) (Conaway CC, Yang YM, Chung FL (2002). Isothiocyanates as cancer chemopreventive agents: their biological activities and metabolism in rodents and humans. Curr. Drug Metab., 3: 233-255)

(Cook et al, 2007) (Cook, Nancy R., et al. "A randomized factorial trial of vitamins C and E and beta carotene in the secondary prevention of cardiovascular events in women: results from the Women's Antioxidant Cardiovascular Study." Archives of internal medicine 167.15 (2007): 1610-1618)

(Cruz-Correa et al, 2006) (Cruz-Correa M, Shoskes DA, Sanchez P, Zhao R, Hylind LM, Wexner SD, et al. Combination treatment with curcumin and quercetin of adenomas in familial adenomatous polyposis. Clin Gastroenterol Hepatol. 2006;4(8):1035–1038)

(Cuomo et al, 2011) (Cuomo J, Appendino G, Dern AS, Schneider E, McKinnon TP, Brown MJ, et al. Comparative absorption of a standardized curcuminoid mixture and its lecithin formulation. J Nat Prod.2011;74(4):664–669)

(Danesi et al, 2014) (Danesi F, Kroon PA, Saha S, de Biase D, D'Antuono LF, Bordoni A. Mixed pro- and anti-oxidative effects of pomegranate polyphenols in cultured cells. Int J Mol Sci. 2014 Oct 27;15(11):19458-71)

(Davidson et al, 2009) (Davidson MH, Maki KC, Dicklin MR, et al. Effects of consumption of pomegranate juice on carotid intima-media thickness in men and women at moderate risk for coronary heart disease. *Am J Cardiol.* 2009 Oct 1;104(7):936-42)

(De La Fuente 2002) (De La Fuente M. Effects of antioxidants on immune system ageing. Eur J Clin Nutr.2002;56(3):S5–S8)

(Dell'Agli et al, 2009) (Dell'Agli M, Galli GV, Corbett Y, Taramelli D, Lucantoni L, Habluetzel A, et al. Antiplasmodial activity of *Punica granatum* L. fruit rind. J Ethnopharmacol. 2009;125:279–85)

(Dell'agli et al, 2010) (Dell'agli M, Galli GV, Bulgari M, Basilico N, Romeo S, Bhattacharya D, et al. Ellagitannins of the fruit rind of pomegranate (*Punica granatum*) antagonize*in vitro* the host inflammatory response mechanisms involved in the onset of malaria. Malar J. 2010;9:208)

(De Luca, Ross, 1996) (De Luca, L. M. & Ross, S.A. (1996) Beta-carotene increases lung cancer incidence in cigarette smokers. Nutr. Rev. 54: 178–180)

(de Nigris et la, 2007) (de Nigris F, Williams-Ignarro S, Sica V, Lerman LO, D'Armiento FP, Byrns RE, et al. Effects of a pomegranate fruit extract rich in punicalagin on oxidation-sensitive genes and eNOS activity at sites of perturbed shear stress and atherogenesis. Cardiovasc Res. 2007;73:414–23)

(de Nigris et al, 2007, NO) (de Nigris F, Balestrieri ML, Williams-Ignarro S, D'Armiento FP, Fiorito C, Ignarro LJ, et al.The influence of pomegranate fruit extract in comparison to regular pomegranate juice and seed oil on nitric oxide and arterial function in obese Zucker rats. Nitric Oxide. 2007;17:50–4)

(Dengel et al, 1998) (Dengel DR, Hagberg JM, Pratley RE, et al. Improvements in blood pressure, glucose metabolism, and lipoprotein lipids after aerobic exercise plus weight loss in obese, hypertensive middle-aged men. Metabolism. 1998;47:1075–82)

(Deodhar et al, 1980) (Deodhar SD, Sethi R, Srimal RC. Preliminary study on antirheumatic activity of curcumin (diferuloyl methane) Indian J Med Res. 1980;71:632–634)

(Dhillon et al, 2008) (Dhillon N, Aggarwal BB, Newman RA, Wolff RA, Kunnumakkara AB, Abbruzzese JL, et al. Phase II trial of curcumin in patients with advanced pancreatic cancer. Clin Cancer Res.2008;14(14):4491–4499)

(DHHS, 1995) (Department of Health and Human Services, Centers for Disease Control and Prevention, and National Center for Chronic Disease Prevention and Health Promotion 1996; Pate et al 1995)

(Di Mascio et al, 1991) (Di Mascio P, Murphy ME, Sies H. Antioxidant defense systems: the role of carotenoids, tocopherols, and thiols. Am J Clin Nutr. 1991;53(Suppl):194S–200S)

(Disilvestro et al, 2012) (Disilvestro RA, Joseph E, Zhao S, Joshua B. Diverse effects of a low dose supplement of lipidated curcumin in healthy middle aged people. Nutr J. 2012;11(1):79. doi: 10.1186/1475-2891-11-79)

(Dong et al, 2012) (Dong S, Tong X, Liu H, Gao Q. Protective effects of pomegranate polyphenols on cardiac function in rats with myocardial ischemia/reperfusion injury. *Nan Fang Yi Ke Da Xue Xue Bao.* 2012 Jun;32(7):924-7)

(Doudiccan et al, 2012) (Doudican N.A., Wen S.Y., Mazumder A., Orlow S. J. Sulforaphane synergistically enhances the cytotoxicity of arsenic trioxide in multiple myeloma cells via stress-mediated pathways. *Oncology Reports.* 2012;28(5):1851–1858)

(Droge, 2002) (Dröge W. Free radicals in the physiological control of cell function. *Physiological Reviews.* 2002;82(1):47–95)

(Du et al, 2012) (Du P, et al, Anticonvulsive and antioxidant effects of curcumin on pilocarpine-induced seizures in rats. Chin Med J (Engl). 2012;125:1975-1979)

(Durgaprasad et al, 2005) (Durgaprasad S, Pai CG, Vasanthkumar, Alvres JF, Namitha S. A pilot study of the antioxidant effect of curcumin in tropical pancreatitis. Indian J Med Res. 2005;122(4):315–318)

(Edsmyr et al, 1981) (Edsmyr F, Menander-Huber KB. Orgotein efficacy in ameliorating side effects due to radiation therapy. *Eur J Rheumatol Inflamm.* 1981;4(2):228-36)

(Egner et al, 2011) (Egner P.A., Chen J. G., Wang J. B., et al. Bioavailability of sulforaphane from two broccoli sprout beverages: results of a short-term, cross-over clinical trial in Qidong, China. *Cancer Prevention Research.* 2011;4(3):384–395) (el Hamss et al, 1999) (el Hamss, R., Analla, M., Campos-Sanchez, J., Alonso-Moraga, A., Munoz-Serrano, A. and Idaomar, M., A dose dependent anti-genotoxic effect of turmeric. Mutat. Res., 1999, 446, 135–139)

(Elbarbry, Elrody, 2011) (Fawzy Elbarbry and Nehad Elrody. Potential health benefits of sulforaphane: A review of the experimental, clinical and epidemiological evidences and underlying mechanisms. Journal of Medicinal Plants Research Vol. 5(4), pp. 473-484, 18 February, 2011)

(Epelbaum et al, 2010) (Epelbaum R, Schaffer M, Vizel B, Badmaev V, Bar-Sela G. Curcumin and gemcitabine in patients with advanced pancreatic cancer. Nutr Cancer. 2010;62(8):1137–1141)

(Epstein, Sanderson, MacDonald, 2010) (Jenny Epstein, Ian R. Sanderson and Thomas T. MacDonald. Curcumin as a therapeutic agent: the evidence from *in vitro*, animal and human studies. British Journal of Nutrition / Volume 103 / Issue 11 / June 2010, pp 1545-1557)

(Ercisli et al, 2011) (Ercisli S, Gadze J, Agar G, Yildirim N, Hizarci Y. Genetic relationships among wild pomegranate (*Punica granatum*) genotypes from Coruh Valley in Turkey. Genet Mol Res. 2011;10:459–64)

(Esmaillzadeh et al, 2006) (Esmaillzadeh A, Tahbaz F, Gaieni I, Alavi-Majd H, Azadbakht L. Cholesterol-lowering effect of concentrated pomegranate juice consumption in type II diabetic patients with hyperlipidemia. Int J Vitam Nutr Res. 2006;76:147–51)

(Evans, 1999) (Evans WJ. Exercise training guidelines for the elderly. Med Sci Sports Exerc. 1999;31:12–17)

(Facchini et al, 2000) (Facchini FS, Hua NW, Reaven GM, et al. Hyperinsulinemia: the missing link among oxidative stress and age-related diseases? Free Radic Biol Med. 2000;29:1302–6)

(Fahey et al., 1997) (Fahey JW, Zhang Y, Talalay P (1997). Broccoli sprouts: an exceptionally rich source of inducers of enzymes that protect against chemical carcinogens. Proc. Natl. Acad. Sci. U. S. A., 94: 10367) (Shapiro et al., 2001)

(Fahey et al., 2001) (Fahey JW, Zalcmann AT, Talalay P (2001). The chemical diversity and distribution of glucosinolates and isothiocyanates among plants. Phytochem., 56: 5-51)

(Fahey et al, 2002) (Fahey JW, Haristoy X, Dolan PM, et al. Sulforaphane inhibits extracellular, intracellular, and antibiotic-resistant strains of

Helicobacter pylori and prevents benzo[a]pyrene-induced stomach tumors. *Proc Natl Acad Sci USA.* 2002;99:7610–7615)

(Fahey, Talalay, 1999) (Fahey JW, Talalay P. Antioxidant functions of sulforaphane: a potent inducer of Phase II detoxication enzymes. *Food Chem Toxicol.* 1999;37:973–979)

(Fan, et al, 2013) (Fan X, et al. The clinical applications of curcumin: current state and the future. Curr Pharm Des. 2013;19:2011-2031)

(Fenercioglu et al, 2010) (Fenercioglu AK, Saler T, Genc E, Sabuncu H, Altuntas Y. The effects of polyphenol-containing antioxidants on oxidative stress and lipid peroxidation in Type 2 diabetes mellitus without complications. J Endocrinol Invest. 2010;33:118–24)

(Ferrara, 2007) (Ferrara AM. Treatment of hospital-acquired pneumonia caused by methicillin-resistant *Staphylococcus aureus.* Int J Antimicrob Agents. 2007;30:19–24)

(Fiatarone Singh 1998) (Fiatarone Singh MA. Combined exercise and dietary intervention to optimize body composition in aging. Ann N Y Acad Sci. 1998;854:378–93)

(Fiatarone et al, 1994) (Fiatarone MA, O'Neill EF, Ryan ND, et al. Exercise training and nutritional supplementation for physical frailty in very elderly people. N Engl J Med. 1994;330(25):1769–75)

(Fibach, Rachmilewitz, 2008) (Fibach E, Rachmilewitz E. The role of oxidative stress in hemolytic anemia. Curr Mol Med. 2008;8(7):609–619)

(Fiebig et al, 1994) (Fiebig R, Leeuwenburgh C, Li JJ. The effects of aging and training on myocardial antioxidant systems and lipid peroxidation. Med Sci Sports Exerc. 1994;26:S133)

(Fiers et al, 1999) (W Fiers, R Beyaert, W Declercq, P Vandenabeele. More than one way to die: apoptosis, necrosis and reactive oxygen damage. Oncogene (1999) 18: 7719-30)

(Fimognari et al, 2014) (Fimognari C., Turrini E., Sestili P., et al. Antileukemic activity of sulforaphane in primary blasts from patients affected by myelo- and lympho-proliferative disorders and in hypoxic conditions. *PLoS ONE.* 2014;9(7) doi: 10.1371/journal.pone.0101991.e101991)

(Fimognari et al, 2006) (Fimognari C, Nusse M, Lenzi M, Sciuscio D, Cantelli-Forti G, Hrelia P. Sulforaphane increases the efficacy of doxorubicin in mouse fibroblasts characterized by p53 mutations. Mutat Res.2006;601:92–101)

(Fimognari, Hrelia, 2007) (Fimognari C., Hrelia P. Sulforaphane as a promising molecule for fighting cancer. *Mutation Research.* 2007;635(2-3):90–104)

(Finkel and Holbrook, 2000) (Finkel T, Holbrook NJ. Oxidants, oxidative stress and the biology of ageing. Nature.2000;408:239–47)

(Finley, Davis, Feng, 2000) (Finley J.W., Davis C. D., Feng Y. Selenium from high selenium broccoli protects rats from colon cancer. *The Journal of Nutrition.* 2000;130(9):2384–2389)

(Firuzi et al, 2011) (Firuzi, O.; Miri, R.; Tavakkoli, M.; Saso, L. Antioxidant Therapy: Current Status and Future Prospects. Current Medicinal Chemistry, Volume 18, Number 25, September 2011, pp. 3871-3888(18)

(Fisher et al, 1998) (Fisher, B, Costantino, JP, Wickerham, DL, et al. (1998) Tamoxifen for prevention of breast cancer: report of the National Surgical Adjuvant Breast and Bowel Project P-1 Study. J Natl Cancer Inst 90, 1371–1388)

(Fleury et al, 2002) (Fleury C, Mignotte B, Vayssière JL. Mitochondrial reactive oxygen species in cell death signaling. Biochimie. 2002 Feb-Mar;84(2-3):131-41)

(Frank and Gupta, 2005) (Frank B, Gupta S. A Review of antioxidants and Alzheimer's disease. Ann Clin Psychiatry. 2005;17(4):269–86)

(Frydoonfar, McGrath, Spiegelman, 2003) (Frydoonfar HR, McGrath DR, Spigelman AD. The effect of indole-3-carbinol and sulforaphane on a prostate cancer cell line. *ANZ J Surg.* 2003;73:154–6)

(Fuhrman et al, 2005) (Fuhrman B, Volkova N, Aviram M. Pomegranate juice inhibits oxidized LDL uptake and cholesterol biosynthesis in macrophages. *J Nutr Biochem.* 2005 Sep;16(9):570-6)

(Fulle et al 2004) (Fulle S, Protasi F, Di Tano G, et al. The contribution of reactive oxygen species to sarcopenia and muscle ageing. Exp Gerontol. 2004;39:17–24)

(Funk et al, 2006) (Funk JL, Frye JB, Oyarzo JN, Kuscuoglu N, Wilson J, McCaffrey G, et al. Efficacy and mechanism of action of turmeric supplements in the treatment of experimental arthritis. *Arthritis Rheum.* 2006 Nov;54(11):3452-64)

(Fusco et al, 2007) (Domenico Fusco, Giuseppe Colloca, Maria Rita Lo Monaco, and Matteo Cesari. Effects of antioxidant supplementation on the aging process. Clin Interv Aging. 2007 Sep; 2(3): 377–387)

(Galan et al., 2004) (Galan MV, Kishan AA, Silverman AL (2004). Oral broccoli sprouts for the treatment of Helicobacter pylori infection: a preliminary report. Dig. Dis. Sci., 49: 1088-1090)

(Galati et al, 2002) (Galati, G., Sabzevari, O., Wilson, J. X. and O'Brien, P. J., Prooxidant activity and cellular effects of the phenoxyl radicals of dietary flavonoids and other polyphenolics. Toxicology, 2002, 177, 91–104)

(Gamet-Payrestre et al, 2000) (Gamet-Payrastre L, Li P, Lumeau S, et al. Sulforaphane, a naturally occurring isothiocyanate, induces cell cycle arrest and apoptosis in HT29 human colon cancer cells. *Cancer Res.* 2000;60:1426–1433)

(Gao et al, 2004) (Gao X, Bermudez OI, Tucker KL. Plasma C-Reactive protein and homocysteine concentrations are related to frequent fruit and vegetable intake in Hispanic and non-Hispanic White elders. J Nutr. 2004;134:913–18)

(Garcea et al, 2005) (Garcea G, Berry DP, Jones DJ, Singh R, Dennison AR, Farmer PB, et al. Consumption of the putative chemopreventive agent curcumin by cancer patients: assessment of curcumin levels in the colorectum and their pharmacodynamic consequences. Cancer Epidemiol Biomarkers Prev.2005;14(1):120–125)

(Gibbons et al, 2003) (Gibbons RJ, Abrams J, Chatterjee K, et al. American College of Cardiology/American Heart Association Task Force on Practice Guidelines – Committee on the Management of Patients with Chronic Stable Angina ACC/AHA 2002 guideline update for the management of patients with chronic stable angina – summary article: a report of the American college of cardiology/American heart association task force on practice guidelines (committee on the management of patients with chronic stable angina) Circulation. 2003;107:149–58)

(Gil et al, 2000) (Gil MI, Tomás-Barberán FA, Hess-Pierce B, Holcroft DM, Kader AA. Antioxidant activity of pomegranate juice and its relationship with phenolic composition and processing. J Agric Food Chem. 2000;48:4581–9)

(Ginsberg et al., 2010) (Ginsberg G., Guyton K., Johns D., Schimek J., Angle K., Sonawane B. (2010). Genetic polymorphism in metabolism and host defense enzymes: implications for human health risk assessment. Crit. Rev. Toxicol. 40, 575–619)

(Goel et al, 2008) (Goel A, Jhurani S, Aggarwal BB. Multi-targeted therapy by curcumin: how spicy is it? Mol Nutr Food Res. 2008;52(9):1010–1030)

(Goel et al, 2008. Bio Pharma) (Goel A, Kunnumakkara AB, Aggarwal BB. Curcumin as "Curecumin": *from kitchen to clinic*. Biochem Pharmacol 2008; 75:787–809)

(Goh et al, 2009) (Goh, K & Xiao, SD (2009) Inflammatory bowel disease: a survey of the epidemiology in Asia. J Dig Dis 10, 1–6)

(Golombick et al, 2009) (Golombick T, Diamond TH, Badmaev V, Manoharan A, Ramakrishna R. The potential role of curcumin in patients with monoclonal gammopathy of undefined significance—its effect on paraproteinemia and the urinary N-telopeptide of type I collagen bone turnover marker. Clin Cancer Res. 2009;15(18):5917–5922)

(Golombick et al, 2012) (Golombick T, Diamond TH, Manoharan A, Ramakrishna R. Monoclonal gammopathy of undetermined significance, smoldering multiple myeloma, and curcumin: a randomized, double-blind placebo-controlled cross-over 4g study and an open-label 8g extension study. Am J Hematol. 2012 May;87(5):455-60)

(Gonzalez-Sarrias et al, 2010) (González-Sarrías A, Larrosa M, Tomás-Barberán FA, Dolara P, Espín JC. NF-kappaB-dependent anti-inflammatory activity of urolithins, gut microbiota ellagic acid-derived metabolites, in human colonic fibroblasts. Br J Nutr. 2010;104:503–12)

(Gould et al, 2009) (Gould SW, Fielder MD, Kelly AF, Naughton DP. Antimicrobial activities of pomegranate rind extracts: Enhancement by cupric sulphate against clinical isolates of S. aureus, MRSA and PVL positive CA-MSSA. BMC Complement Altern Med. 2009;9:23)

(Greco et al, 2000) (Greco A, Minghetti L, Levi G. Isoprostanes, novel markers of oxidative injury, help understanding the pathogenesis of neurodegenerative diseases. Neurochem Res. 2000;25:1357–64)

(Gupta, Patchva and Aggrarwal, 2013) (Subash C. Gupta, Sridevi Patchva, and Bharat B. Aggarwal. Therapeutic Roles of Curcumin: Lessons Learned from Clinical Trials. AAPS J. 2013 Jan; 15(1): 195–218)

(Gutteridge, 1993) (Gutteridge JMC. Free radicals in disease processes – A compilation of cause and consequence. Invited review. Free Radic Res Commun. 1993;19:141–58)

(Halliwell 1990) (Halliwell, B. and Gutteridge, J. M. C., Role of free radicals and catalytic metal ions in human disease: an overview. Methods Enzymol., 1990, 186, 1–85)

(Halliwell, 1998) (Halliwell, B., In Oxidative Stress in Skeletal Muscle (eds Reznick, A. Z. et al.), Birkhauser, Verlag Basel, Switzerland, 1998, pp. 1–27)

(Han et al, 1999) (Han, SS, Chung, ST, Robertson, DA, et al. (1999) Curcumin causes the growth arrest and apoptosis of B cell lymphoma by downregulation of egr-1, c-myc, bcl-XL, NF-kappa B, and p53. Clin Immunol 93, 152–161)

(Han et al, 2003) (Han D., Canali R., Rettori D., Kaplowitz N. Effect of glutathione depletion on sites and topology of superoxide and hydrogen peroxide production in mitochondria. *Molecular Pharmacology*. 2003;64(5):1136–1144)

(Hanai et al, 2006) (Hanai H, Iida T, Takeuchi K, Watanabe F, Maruyama Y, Andoh A, et al. Curcumin maintenance therapy for ulcerative colitis: randomized, multicenter, double-blind, placebo-controlled trial. Clin Gastroenterol Hepatol. 2006;4(12):1502–1506)

(Harman, 1956) (Harman D. Aging: a theory based on free radical and radiation chemistry. J Gerontol. 1956;11:298–300)

(Harman, 1961) (Harman D. 1961. Mutation, cancer and aging. Lancet 1: 200-201)

(Harman, 1972) (Harman D. The biologic clock: the mitochondria? J Am Geriatr Soc. 1972;20:145–147)

(Harman, 1981) (Harman D. The aging process. Proc Natl Acad Sci USA 78:7124– 7128, 1981)

(Harman, 1994) (Harman D. Free-radical theory of aging. Increasing the functional life span. Ann N Y Acad Sci. 1994;717:1–15)

(Harman, 2001) (Harman, D. 2001. Aging; overview. Ann N Y Acad Sci 928: 1-21)

(Harman 2003) (Harman D. The free radical theory of aging. Antioxid Redox Signal. 2003;5:557–61)

(Hartmann et al, 2003) (Hartmann A, Agurell E, Beevers C, et al. 4th International Comet Assay Workshop Recommendations for conducting the in vivo alkaline Comet assay. 4th International Comet Assay Workshop. Mutagenesis. 2003;18(1):45–51)

(Hartman et al, 2006) (Hartman RE, Shah A, Fagan AM, Schwetye KE, Parsadanian M, Schulman RN, et al. Pomegranate juice decreases amyloid load and improves behavior in a mouse model of Alzheimer's disease. Neurobiol Dis. 2006;24:506–15)

(Hastak et al, 1997) (Hastak K, Lubri N, Jakhi SD, More C, John A, Ghaisas SD, et al. Effect of turmeric oil and turmeric oleoresin on cytogenetic damage in patients suffering from oral submucous fibrosis. Cancer Lett. 1997;116(2):265–269)

(Hauer et al, 2003) (Hauer K, Hildebrandt W, Sehl Y, et al. Improvement in muscular performance and decrease in tumor necrosis factor level in old age after antioxidant treatment. J Mol Med.2003;81:118–25)

(Hayouni et al, 2011) (Hayouni E, Miled K, Boubaker S, Bellasfar Z, Abedrabba M, Iwaski H. Hydroalcoholic extract based-ointment from *Punica granatum* L. peels with enhanced *in vivo* healing potential on dermal wounds. Phytomedicine. 2011;18:976–84)

(He et al, 2011) (He ZY, Shi CB, Wen H, Li FL, Wang BL, Wang J. Upregulation of p53 expression in patients with colorectal cancer by administration of curcumin. Cancer Investig. 2011;29(3):208–213)

(Hecht, 1999) (Hecht SS. Chemoprevention of cancer by isothiocyanates, modifiers of carcinogen metabolism. *J Nutr.* 1999;129:768S–74S)

(Heinonen et al, 1994) (Heinonen, Olli P., and Demetrius Albanes. "The effect of vitamin E and beta carotene on the incidence of lung cancer and other cancers in male smokers." *The New England journal of medicine* 330 (1994)

(Heller et al, 1998) (Heller F, Descamps O, Hondekijn JC. LDL oxidation: therapeutic perspectives. Atherosclerosis. 1998;137(Suppl 1):S25–S31)

(Hercberg et al, 2004) (Hercberg S, Galan P, Preziosi P, et al. The SU.VI.MAX Study - A randomized, placebo-controlled trial of the health effects of antioxidant vitamins and minerals. Arch Intern Med.2004;164:2335–42)

(Hercberg et al, 2004) (Hercberg S, Czernichow S, Galan P. Antioxidant vitamins and minerals in prevention of cancers: lessons from the SU.VI. MAX study. Br J Nutr. 2006;96(Suppl 1):S28–S30)

(Hercberg et al, 2006) (Hercberg S, Czernichow S, Galan P. Antioxidant vitamins and minerals in prevention of cancers: lessons from the SU.VI. MAX study. Br J Nutr. 2006;96(Suppl 1):S28–S30)

(Hercberg et al, 2007) (Hercberg, Serge, et al. "Antioxidant supplementation increases the risk of skin cancers in women but not in men." *The Journal of nutrition* 137.9 (2007): 2098-2105)

(Heuschkel et al, 2000) (Heuschkel, RB, Menache, CC, Megerian, JT, et al. (2000) Enteral nutrition and corticosteroids in the treatment of acute Crohn's disease in children. J Pediatr Gastroenterol Nutr 31, 8–15)

(Higdon, Frei, 2003) (Higdon JV, Frei B. Tea catechins and polyphenols: health effects, metabolism, and antioxidant functions. Crit Rev Food Sci Nutr 2003;43:89–143)

(Hofling et al, 2010) (Höfling JF, Anibal PC, Obando-Pereda GA, Peixoto IA, Furletti VF, Foglio MA, Goncalves RB. Antimicrobial potential of some plant extracts against Candida species. Braz J Biol. 2010;70:1065–8)

(Holt et al, 2005) (Holt PR, Katz S, Kirshoff R. Curcumin therapy in inflammatory bowel disease: a pilot study. Dig Dis Sci. 2005;50(11):2191–2193)

(Hontecillas et al, 2009) (Hontecillas R, O'Shea M, Einerhand A, Diguardo M, Bassaganya-Riera J. Activation of PPAR gamma and alpha by punicic acid ameliorates glucose tolerance and suppresses obesity-related inflammation. J Am Coll Nutr. 2009;28:184–95)

(Hora et al, 2003) (Hora JJ, Maydew ER, Lansky EP, Dwivedi C. Chemopreventive effects of pomegranate seed oil on skin tumor development in CD1 mice. J Med Food.2003;6:157–61)

(Hou et al, 2008) (Hou XL, Takahashi K, Tanaka K, Tougou K, Qiu F, Komatsu K, Takahashi K, Azuma J. Curcuma drugs and curcumin regulate the expression and function of P-gp in Caco-2 cells in completely opposite ways. Int J Pharm. 2008 Jun 24;358(1-2):224-9)

(Houston, 2014) (Houston M. The role of nutrition and nutraceutical supplements in the treatment of hypertension. *World J Cardiol.* 2014 Feb 26;6(2):38-66)

(Howes, Steele, 1971) (Howes, R. M. and Steele, R. H., Microsomal che-miluminescence induced by NADPH and its relation to lipid peroxi-dation, Res. Commun. Chem. Path. Pharmacol., July-Sept. 1971, 2; 4 & 5:619-626)

(Howes, Steele, 1972) (Howes, R.M. and Steele, R.H., Microsomal che-miluminescence induced by NADPH and its relation to aryl-hydroxyl-ations, Res Commun. Chem. Path. Pharmacol., March 1972, 3; 2:349-357)

(Howes, Steele, 1976) (Howes, R.M., Steele, R.H. and Hoopes, J.E., Peroxide induced Chemiluminescence in an in vitro proline hydroxyl-ation system, 1976, 8; 1:77-84)

(Howes et al, 1976) (Howes, R. M., Allen, R.C., Su, C.T. and Hoopes, J.E., Altered polymorphonuclear leukocyte bioenergetics in patients with thermal injury, the Surgical Forum, 1976, 27:558-560)

(Howes et al, 1977) (Howes, R.M., Steele, R.H. and Hoopes, J.E., The role of Electronic excitation states in collagen biosynthesis, Persp. In Biol. And Med., Summer 1977, 20; 4:539-544)

(Howes, 2004, UTOPIA) (Howes, R. M. U.T.O.P.I.A. - Unified Theory of Oxygen Participation in Aerobiosis. © 2004. Free Radical Publishing Co. Kentwood, LA, available at www.iwillfindthecure.org)

(Howes, 2005, Med Sci) (Howes R. M. The Medical and Scientific Significance of Oxygen Free Radical Metabolism. © 2005. Free Radical Publishing Co. Kentwood, LA. USA. available at www.iwillfindthecure. org)

(Howes, 2005) (Howes, R.M. Tumoricidal Activity of An Injectable Singlet Oxygen System Generated From Physiological Agents: The Howes Singlet Oxygen Cancer Therapy System). In The Medical and Scientific Significance of Oxygen Free Radical Metabolism. © 2005. Free Radical Publishing Co. Kentwood, LA. pp. 893-912)

(Howes, Farber, 2005) (Howes, R.M. and Farber, G. Tumoricidal Activity of the Howes Singlet Oxygen Delivery System in Human Basal Cell Carcinoma. In The Medical and Scientific Significance of Oxygen Free Radical Metabolism. © 2005. Free Radical Publishing Co. Kentwood, LA. pp. 883-892)

(Howes, 2006, Diabetes) (Howes, R. M. Diabetes and Oxygen Free Radical Sophistry, © 2006; Free Radical Publishing Co. USA. Free Radical Publishing Co. USA. 366 pages) available at www.iwillfindthecure.org)

(Howes, 2006, H2O2) (Howes, R. M. Hydrogen Peroxide Monograph 1: Scientific, Medical and Biochemical Overview. © 2006; Free Radical Publishing Co. USA. 200 pages) available at www.iwillfindthecure.org.)

(Howes, 2006, CVD) (Howes, R. M. Cardiovascular Disease and Oxygen Free Radical Mythology, © 2006; Free Radical Publishing Co. USA. 308 pages) available at www.iwillfindthecure.org)

(Howes, 2006, AOX A, C, E) (Howes, R. M. Monograph 2: Antioxidant vitamins A, C & E: Equivocal Scientific Studies, © 2006; Free Radical Publishing Co. USA. 171 pages) available at www.iwillfindthecure.org)

(Howes, 2006, Fantasy) (Howes, R.M.: "The Free Radical Fantasy," The Annals of New York Academy of Sciences, 2006, Vol. 1067, pp. 22-26)

(Howes, 2007, #75) (Howes M.D., PhD., R. (2007). The Consequent Downfall of the Free Radical Theory. PHILICA.COM Article number 75)

(Howes, 2008, ROSI) (Howes, R. M. Reactive Oxygen Species Insufficiency (ROSI)as the Basis for Disease Allowance and Coexistence: Extraordinary Support for an Extraordinary Theory. Vol I, II & III. © 2008; 1564 pages) available at www.iwillfindthecure.org)

(Howes R.M. 2009, Am J Cosm Surg) (Howes, RM. Antioxidant Vitamins: A Review of Policy Statements and Recommendations. The American Journal of Cosmetic Surgery. 2009;26(2):63-78)

(Howes, Book 1, 2010) (Death in Small Doses? Antioxidant Vitamins A, C and E in the Twenty-first Century: A Heath Impact Statement for the Layman. Book One, Trafford Publishing, © 2010 Death in Small Doses?)

(Howes R : Hydrogen Peroxide: 2010) (R. Howes : Hydrogen Peroxide: A review of a scientifically verifiable omnipresent ubiquitous essentiality of obligate, aerobic, carbon-based life forms. The Internet Journal of Plastic Surgery. 2010 Volume 7 Number 1)

(Howes R : Cancer Therapy, 2010) (Howes R : Cancer Therapy: A Review with Scientific Validation for the Role of Electronically Modified Oxygen Derivatives in Oncologic Treatment Modalities. The Internet Journal of Alternative Medicine. 2010 Volume 8 Number 1)

(Howes, Book 2, 2011) (Antioxidant Vitamins A, C and E are Making a Killing. A Health Impact Statement for the Medical Scientist. Book Two, Trafford Publishing, © 2010, Death in Small Doses?)

(Howes, 2011,AOX Scams) (Anti-aging Anti-oxidant Scams, CreateSpace and Free Radical Publishing Co, USA, © 2011)

(Howes, 2011, AOX Failures) (Antioxidant Failures and Dangers: The Consequent Downfall of the Free Radical Theory, CreateSpace and Free Radical Publishing Co, USA, © 2011)

(Howes, 2011, Overkill) (Antioxidant Overkill. CreateSpace and Free Radical Publishing Co, USA, © 2011)

(Howes, 2011,AOX failures) (Antioxidant Failures and Dangers,The fall of the free radical theory. CreateSpace and Free Radical Publishing Co, USA, © 2011)

(Howes, 2011, Dangers) (Dangers of Excessive Antioxidants in Cancer Patients. CreateSpace and Free Radical Publishing Co, USA, © 2012)

(Howes, 2011, Heart Disease) (Heart Disease and Antioxidant Failures. CreateSpace and Free Radical Publishing Co, USA,© 2011)

(Howes, 2011, Sports) (Sports,Athletes, Exercise Facts and Antioxidant Myths. CreateSpace and Free Radical Publishing Co, USA, © 2011)

(Howes, 2012) (Antioxidant Links To Deadly Unintended Consequences. CreateSpace and Free Radical Publishing Co, USA, © 2012)

(Howes, 2012, Sex) (Sex, Performance, Naked Radicals And Antioxidants. CreateSpace and Free Radical Publishing Co, USA, © 2012)

(Howes, 2012, Alzheimer's) (Alzheimer's Disease: Forget Antioxidants and Supplements. CreateSpace and Free Radical Publishing Co, USA, © 2012)

(Howes, 2014, ROS) (Reactive Oxygen Species vs. Antioxidants: The Oxypocalypse or The War That Never Was. CreateSpace and Free Radical Publishing Co, USA, © 2014)

(Howes, 2014, Diabetes) (Diabetes and Oxygen Free Radical Sophistry, CreateSpace and Free Radical Publishing Co, USA, © 2014)

(Howes, 2014, UTOPIA) (Unified Theory of Oxygen Participation In Aerobiosis, © 2014, revised. CreateSpace and Free Radical Publishing Co, USA, © 2014)

(Howes, 2014, H2O2) (Hydrogen Peroxide: A Health, Homeostatic and Protective Essentiality, © 2014. CreateSpace and Free Radical Publishing Co, USA, © 2014)

(Howes, 2014, Fish oil) (Fish Oil (Omega3 fatty acids): Facts, Fantasies & Failures, © 2014, revised. CreateSpace and Free Radical Publishing Co, USA, © 2014)

(Howes, 2014, Vit D) (Vitamin D: Benefits & False Claims. © 2014. CreateSpace and Free Radical Publishing Co, USA, © 2014)

(Howes, 2015, Chocolate) (Chocolate & Red Wine Antioxidants (Polyphenols, Flavonoids & resveratrol): Facts vs. Falsehoods. © 2015. CreateSpace and Free Radical Publishing Co, USA, © 2015)

(Howes, 2015, Exercise) (Exercise and Reactive Oxygen Species: Likely the only health miracle out there. © 2015. CreateSpace and Free Radical Publishing Co, USA, © 2015)

(Howes, 2015, HBOT) (Hyperbaric oxygen, Hypoxia, Hyperoxia & EMODs (ROS): Separating Fact From Factitious. © 2015. CreateSpace and Free Radical Publishing Co, USA, © 2015)

(Howes, 2015, Blueberry) (Blueberry, Tomato & CoQ10 Antioxidants (Anthocyanin, Lycopene & Ubiquinone): Claims vs. Facts., © 2015. CreateSpace and Free Radical Publishing Co, USA, © 2015)

(Howes, 2015, Cancer) (Cancer and Longevity Answers: Naked mole rats, Exercise & EMODs (ROS), © 2015. CreateSpace and Free Radical Publishing Co, USA, © 2015)

(Hu et al, 2004) (Hu P, Reuben DB, Crimmins EM, et al. The effects of serum beta-carotene concentration and burden of inflammation on all-cause mortality risk in high-functioning older persons: MacArthur Studies of Successful Aging. J Gerontol A Biol Sci Med Sci.2004;59A(8):849–54)

(Hu, Hebbar et al, 2004) (Hu R., Hebbar V., Kim B.-R., et al. In vivo pharmacokinetics and regulation of gene expression profiles by isothiocyanate sulforaphane in the rat. *Journal of Pharmacology and Experimental Therapeutics*. 2004;310(1):263–271)

(Huang et al, 2005) (Huang TH, Yang Q, Harada M, Li GQ, Yamahara J, Roufogalis BD, et al. Pomegranate flower extract diminishes cardiac fibrosis in Zucker diabetic fatty rats: Modulation of cardiac endothelin-1 and nuclear factor-kappaB pathways. J Cardiovasc Pharmacol. 2005;46:856–62)

(Huang et al, 2005, BJP) (Huang TH, Peng G, Kota BP, Li GQ, Yamahara J, Roufogalis BD, et al. Pomegranate flower improves cardiac lipid metabolism in a diabetic rat model: Role of lowering circulating lipids. Br J Pharmacol. 2005;145:767–74)

(Hughes et al, 1995) (Hughes VA, Fiatarone MA, Fielding RA, et al. Long term effects of a high carbohydrate diet and exercise on insulin action in older subjects with impaired glucose tolerance. Am J Clin Nutr. 1995;62:426–33)

(Iannelli et al, 2006) (Iannelli P, Zarrilli V, Varricchio E, Tramontano D, Mancini FP. The dietary antioxidant resveratrol affects redox changes of PPARalpha activity. Nutr Metab Cardiovasc Dis.2007;17:247–256)

(Ide et al, 2010) (Ide H, Tokiwa S, Sakamaki K, Nishio K, Isotani S, Muto S, et al. Combined inhibitory effects of soy isoflavones and curcumin on the production of prostate-specific antigen. Prostate.2010;70(10):1127–1133)

(Imaida et al, 2001) (Imaida K, et al, Lack of chemopreventative effects of lycopene and curcumin on experimental rat prostate carcinogenesis. Oxford Journals. Life Sciences and medicine. Carcinogenesis. 2001. vol. 22, Issue 3. Pp. 467-472)

(Jacobs et al, 2003) (Jacobs EJ, Connell CJ, Chao A, et al. Multivitamin use and colorectal cancer incidence in a US cohort: does timing matter? Am J Epidemiol. 2003;158(7):621–8)

(Jaiswal et al, 2002) (Jaiswal AS, Marlow BP, Gupta N, Narayan S. Beta-catenin-mediated transactivation and cell-cell adhesion pathways are important in curcumin (diferuylmethane)-induced growth arrest and apoptosis in colon cancer cells. Oncogene. 2002;21:8414–27)

(James, 1996) (James JS. Curcumin: clinical trial finds no antiviral effect. AIDS Treat News. 1996;(no 242):1–2)

(Ji et al, 1991) (Ji LL, Wu E, Thomas DP. Effects of exercise training on antioxidant and metabolic functions in senescent and rat skeletal muscle. Gerontology. 1991;37:317–25)

(Ji, 1996) (Ji LL. Exercise, oxidative stress, and antioxidants. Am J Sports Med. 1996;24:S20–S24)

(Jiang et al, 2001) (Jiang Q, Christen S, Shigenaga MK, et al. Gamma-tocopherol, the major form of vitamin E in the U.S. diet, deserves more attention. Am J Clin Nutr. 2001;74:714–22)

(Jo et al, 2014) (Jo G. H., Kim G. Y., Kim W. J., Park K. Y., Choi Y. H. Sulforaphane induces apoptosis in T24 human urinary bladder cancer cells through a reactive oxygen species-mediated mitochondrial pathway: the involvement of endoplasmic reticulum stress and the Nrf2 signaling pathway. *International Journal of Oncology*. 2014;45(4):1497–1506)

(Joe et al, 1994) (Joe, B. and Lokesh, B. R., Role of capsaicin, curcumin and dietary n-3 fatty acids in lowering the generation of reactive oxygen species in rat peritoneal macrophages. Biochim. Biophys. Acta, 1994, 1224, 255–263)

(Johnston, 2004) (Johnston N. Sulforaphane halts breast cancer cell growth. *Drug Discov Today*. 2004;9:908)

(Joseph et al, 2004) (Joseph MA, Moysich KB, Freudenheim JL, et al. Cruciferous vegetables, genetic polymorphisms in glutathione S-transferases M1 and T1, and prostate cancer risk. *Nutr Cancer*. 2004;50:206–13)

(Juge et al., 2007) (Juge N, Mithen RF, Traka M (2007). Molecular basis for chemoprevention by sulforaphane: a comprehensive review. Cell Mol. Life Sci., 64: 1105-1127)

(Jung et al., 2002) (Jung Park E, Pezzuto JM (2002). Botanicals in cancer chemoprevention. Cancer Metastasis Rev., 21: 231-255)

(Jurenka, 2010) (Jurenka JS. Therapeutic applications of pomegranate (*Punica granatum* L.): A review. [Accessed September 2010];Altern Med Rev. 2008 13:128–44. USDA 2010)

(Kahya et al, 2011) (Kahya V, Meric A, Yazici M, Yuksel M, Midi A, Gedikli O. Antioxidant effect of pomegranate extract in reducing acute inflammation due to myringotomy. J Laryngol Otol. 2011;1:370–5)

(Kall, Vang, Clausen, 1997) (Kall MA, Vang O, Clausen J. Effects of dietary broccoli on human drug metabolising activity. *Cancer Lett*. 1997;114:169–70)

(Kalpravidh et al, 2010) (Kalpravidh RW, Siritanaratkul N, Insain P, Charoensakdi R, Panichkul N, Hatairaktham S, et al. Improvement in oxidative stress and antioxidant parameters in beta-thalassemia/Hb E patients treated with curcuminoids. Clin Biochem. 2010;43(4–5):424–429)

(Kanai et al, 2011) (Kanai M, Yoshimura K, Asada M, Imaizumi A, Suzuki C, Matsumoto S, et al. A phase I/II study of gemcitabine-based chemotherapy plus curcumin for patients with gemcitabine-resistant pancreatic cancer. Cancer Chemother Pharmacol. 2011;68(1):157–164

(Kaplan et al, 2001) (Kaplan M, Hayek T, Raz A, Coleman R, Dornfeld L, Vaya J, et al. Pomegranate juice supplementation to atherosclerotic mice reduces macrophage lipid peroxidation, cellular cholesterol accumulation and development of atherosclerosis. J Nutr. 2001;131:2082–9)

(Karasovskaya, 2012) (Karasovskaya V. Antioxidant Properties of Berries. Review of human studies andtheir relevance in the context of the European Food Safety Authority. Number thesis: 2012228. June 2012 Hogeschool van Amsterdam)

(Katz et al, 2007) (Katz SR, Newman RA, Lansky EP. *Punica granatum*: Heuristic treatment for diabetes mellitus. J Med Food. 2007;10:213–7)

(Kaur et al, 2014) (Kaur H, Bal A, Sandhir R. Curcumin supplementation improves mitochondrial and behavioral deficits in experimental model of chronic epilepsy. Pharmacol Biochem Behav. 2014;51:1572-1578)

(Kelloff et al, 2000) (Kelloff GJ, Crowell JA, Steele VE, et al. Progress in cancer chemoprevention: development of diet-derived chemopreventive agents. *J Nutr.* 2000;130(2S Suppl):467S–471S)

(Kelly et al, 2001) (Kelly, M. R., Xu, J., Alexander, K. E. and Loo, G., Disparate effects of similar phenolic phytochemicals as inhibitors of oxidative damage to cellular DNA. Mutat. Res., 2001, 485, 309–318)

(Khan et al, 2007) (Khan N, Hadi N, Afaq F, Syed DN, Kweon MH, Mukhtar H. Pomegranate fruit extract inhibits prosurvival pathways in human A549 lung carcinoma cells and tumor growth in athymic nude mice. Carcinogenesis. 2007;28:163–73)

(Kim et al, 1998) (Kim, JM, Araki, S, Kim, DJ, et al. (1998) Chemopreventive effects of carotenoids and curcumins on mouse colon carcinogenesis after 1,2-dimethylhydrazine initiation. Carcinogenesis 19, 81–85)

(Kim et al, 2002) (Kim ND, Mehta R, Yu W, Neeman I, Livney T, Amichay A, et al. Chemopreventive and adjuvant therapeutic potential of pomegranate (*Punica granatum*) for human breast cancer. Breast Cancer Res Treat. 2002;71:203–17)

(Kim et al, 2003) (Kim B. R., Hu R., Keum Y. S., et al. Effects of of glutathione on antioxidant response element-mediated gene expression and apoptosis elicited by sulforaphane. *Cancer Research*. 2003;63(21):7520–7525)

(Kim et al, 2011) (Kim SG, Veena MS, Basak SK, Han E, Tajima T, Gjertson DW, et al. Curcumin treatment suppresses IKKbeta kinase activity of salivary cells of patients with head and neck cancer: a pilot study. Clin Cancer Res. 2011;17(18):5953–5961)

(Kishore et al, 2009) (Kishore RK, Sudhakar D, Parthasarathy PR. Embryo protective effect of pomegranate (*Punica granatum* L.) fruit extract in adriamycin-induced oxidative stress. Indian J Biochem Biophys. 2009;46:106–11)

(Konig et al, 2001) (Konig D, Wagner KH, Elmadfa I, et al. Exercise and oxidative stress: significance of antioxidants with reference to inflammatory, muscular, and systemic stress. Exerc Immunol Rev. 2001;7:108–33)

(Kositchaiwat et al, 1993) (Kositchaiwat C, Kositchaiwat S, Havanondha J. *Curcuma longa* Linn. in the treatment of gastric ulcer comparison to liquid antacid: a controlled clinical trial. J Med Assoc Thail. 1993;76(11):601–605)

(Kramer, 2004) (Kramer MS. Randomized trials and public health interventions: time to end the scientific double standard. *ClinPerinatol*. 2003;30:351–61)

(Krauss et al, 2000) (Krauss RM, Eckel R, Howard BV, et al. AHA dietary guidelines: revision 2000: a statement for healthcare professionals from the Nutrition Committee of the American Heart Association. Circulation. 2000;102:2284–99)

(Kris-Etherton et al, 2004) (Kris-Etherton PM, Lichtenstein AH, Howard BV, et al. for the Nutrition Committee of the American Heart Association Council on Nutrition Physical Activity and Metabolism Antioxidant vitamin supplements and cardiovascular disease. Circulation. 2004;110:637–41)

(Kritchevsky et al, 2000) (Kritchevsky SB, Bush AJ, Pahor M, et al. Serum carotenoids and markers of inflammation in nonsmokers. Am J Epidemiol. 2000;152:1065–71)

(Kumar et al, 2001) (Kumar S, Votta BJ, Rieman DJ, Badger AM, Gowen M, Lee JC. IL-1- and TNF-induced bone resorption is mediated by p38 mitogen activated protein kinase. J Cell Physiol. 2001;187:294–303)

(Kunnumakkara et al, 2007) (Kunnumakkara, AB, Guha, S, Krishnan, S, et al. (2007) Curcumin potentiates antitumor activity of gemcitabine in an orthotopic model of pancreatic cancer through suppression of proliferation, angiogenesis, and inhibition of nuclear factor-kappaB-regulated gene products. Cancer Res 67, 3853–3861)

(Kunz, Oxman, 1998) (Kunz R, Oxman AD. The unpredictability paradox: review of empirical comparisons of randomised and non-randomised clinical trials. BMJ. 1998;317:1185–90)

(Kuo et al, 1996) (Kuo, M. L., Huang, T. S. and Lin, J. K., Curcumin, an antioxidant and anti-tumor promoter, induces apoptosis in human leukemia cells. Biochim. Biophys. Acta, 1996, 1317, 95–100)

(Kurien et al, 2007) (Kurien, BT, Singh, A, Matsumoto, H, et al. (2007) Improving the solubility and pharmacological efficacy of curcumin by heat treatment. Assay Drug Dev Technol 5, 567–576)

(Kuttan et al, 1985) (Kuttan, R, Bhanumathy, P, Nirmala, K, et al. (1985) Potential anticancer activity of turmeric (Curcuma longa). Cancer Lett 29, 197–202)

(Lal et al, 1999) (Lal B, Kapoor AK, Asthana OP, Agrawal PK, Prasad R, Kumar P, et al. Efficacy of curcumin in the management of chronic anterior uveitis. Phytother Res. 1999;13(4):318–322)

(Lansky, Shubert, Neeman, 2004) (Lansky E, Shubert S, Neeman I. Pharmacological and therapeutic properties of pomegranate. Israel: CIHEAM-Options Mediterraneennes; 2004;42:231–5)

(Lao et al, 2006) (Lao CD, Ruffin MT, Normolle D, Heath DD, Murray SI, Bailey JM, et al. Dose escalation of a curcuminoid formulation. BMC Complement Altern Med. 2006;6:10. doi: 10.1186/1472-6882-6-10)

(Lawler and Powers 1998) (Lawler JM, Powers SK. Oxidative stress, antioxidant status, and the contracting diafragm. Can J Appl Physiol. 1998;23:23–55)

(Lee et al, 1994) (Lee JC, Laydon JT, McDonnell PC, Gallagher TF, Kumar S, Green D. A protein kinase involved in the regulation of inflammatory cytokine biosynthesis. Nature. 1994;372:739–46)

(Leeuwenburgh and Heinecke 2001) (Leeuwenburgh C, Heinecke JW. Oxidative stress and antioxidants in exercise. Curr Med Chem. 2001;8(7):829–38)

(Lei et al, 2007) (Lei F, Zhang XN, Wang W, Xing DM, Xie WD, Su H, DU LJ. Evidence of anti-obesity effects of the pomegranate leaf extract in high-fat diet induced obese mice. Int J Obes (Lond) 2007;31:1023–9)

(Levi et al, 2001) (Levi MS, Borne RF, Williamson JS. A review of cancer chemopreventive agents [review]. *Curr Med Chem*. 2001;8:1349–62)

(Li et al, 2005) (Li, L, Braiteh, FS & Kurzrock, R (2005) Liposome-encapsulated curcumin: *in vitro* and *in vivo* effects on proliferation, apoptosis, signaling, and angiogenesis. Cancer 104, 1322–1331)

(Li et al, 2007) (Li, L, Ahmed, B, Mehta, K, et al. (2007) Liposomal curcumin with and without oxaliplatin: effects on cell growth, apoptosis, and angiogenesis in colorectal cancer. Mol Cancer Ther 6, 1276–1282)

(Li et al, 2010) (Yanyan Li, Tao Zhang, Hasan Korkaya, Suling Liu, Hsiu-Fang Lee, Bryan Newman, Yanke Yu, Shawn G. Clouthier, Steven J. Schwartz, Max S. Wicha, and Duxin Sun. Sulforaphane, a Dietary Component of Broccoli/Broccoli Sprouts, Inhibits Breast Cancer Stem Cells. Clin Cancer Res. 2010 May 1; 16(9): 2580–2590)

(Lim et al, 2001) (Lim, G. P., Chu, T., Yang, F., Beech, W., Frantschy, S. A. and Cole, G. M., The curry spice curcumin reduces oxidative damage and amyloid pathology in an Alzheimer transgenic mouse. J. Neurosci., 2001, 21, 8370–8377)

(Lin et al, 2007) (Lin, YG, Kunnumakkara, AB, Nair, A, et al. (2007) Curcumin inhibits tumor growth and angiogenesis in ovarian carcinoma by targeting the nuclear factor-kappaB pathway. Clin Cancer Res 13, 3423–3430)

(Lipman et al, 1998) (Lipman RD, Bronson RT, Wu D, et al. Disease incidence and longevity are unaltered by dietary antioxidant supplementation initiated during middle age in C57BL/6 mice. Mech Age Dev. 1998;103(3):269–84)

(Liu et al, 2008) (Liu Y.-C., Hsieh C.-W., Weng Y.-C., Chuang S.-H., Hsieh C.-Y., Wung B.-S. Sulforaphane inhibition of monocyte adhesion via the suppression of ICAM-1 and NF-κB is dependent upon glutathione depletion in endothelial cells. *Vascular Pharmacology*. 2008;48(1):54–61)

(Loeser et al, 2008) (Loeser RF, Erickson EA, Long DL. Mitogen-activated protein kinases as therapeutic targets in osteoarthritis. Curr Opin Rheumatol. 2008;20:581–6)

(Lopaczynski et al, 2001) (Lopaczynski, Wlodek, and Steven H. Zeisel. "Antioxidants, programmed cell death, and cancer." Nutrition Research 21.1 (2001): 295-307)

(Lorenz et al, 2007) (Lorenz MW, Markus HS, Bots ML, Rosvall M, Sitzer M. Prediction of clinical cardiovascular events with carotid intima-media thickness: a systematic review and meta-analysis. Circulation. 2007 Jan 30;115(4):459-67)

(Lotempio et al, 2005) (LoTempio, MM, Veena, MS, Steele, HL, et al. (2005) Curcumin suppresses growth of head and neck squamous cell carcinoma. Clin Cancer Res 11, (19 Pt 1), 6994–7002)

(Lynn et al, 2012) (Lynn A, Hamadeh H, Leung WC, Russell JM, Barker ME. Effects of pomegranate juice supplementation on pulse wave velocity and blood pressure in healthy young and middle-aged men and women. Plant Foods Hum Nutr. 2012 Sep;67(3):309-14)

(Mahakunakorn et al, 2003) (Mahakunakorn, P., Tohda, M., Murakami, Y., Matsumoto, K., Watanabe, H. and Vajragupta, O., Cytoprotective and cytotoxic effects of curcumin: dual action on H2O2 induced oxidative cell damage in NG108-15 cells. Biol. Pharm. Bull., 2003, 26, 725–728)

(Malik et al, 2005) (Malik A, Afaq F, Sarfaraz S, Adhami VM, Syed DN, Mukhtar H. Pomegranate fruit juice for chemoprevention and chemotherapy of prostate cancer. Proc Natl Acad Sci U S A. 2005;102:14813–8)

(Mandel, 2005) (S. Mandel et al. Journal of Nutritional Biochemistry. 16 (2005) 513–520)

(Mathew et al, 2012) (Mathew AS, Capel-Williams GM, Berry SE, Hall WL. Acute effects of pomegranate extract on postprandial lipaemia, vascular function and blood pressure. Plant Foods Hum Nutr. 2012 Dec;67(4):351-7)

(Matusheski et al., 2001) (Matusheski NV, Jeffery EH (2001). Comparison of the bioactivity of two glucoraphanin hydrolysis products found in broccoli, sulforaphane and sulforaphane nitrile. J. Agric. Food Chem., 49: 5743-5749)

(Mayne, 2003) (Mayne ST. Antioxidant nutrients and chronic disease: use of biomarkers of exposure and oxidative stress status in epidemiologic research. J Nutr. 2003;133(Suppl 3):933S–40S)

(McCall and Frei, 1999) (McCall MR, Frei B. Can antioxidant vitamins materially reduce oxidative damage in humans? Free Radic Biol Med. 1999;26:1034–53)

(Medjakovic, Jungbauer, 2013) (Medjakovic S, Jungbauer A. Pomegranate: a fruit that ameliorates metabolic syndrome. Food Funct. 2013 Jan;4(1):19-39)

(Medvedev, 1990) (Medvedev ZA. An attempt at a rational classification of theories of ageing. Biol Rev Camb Philos Soc. 1990 Aug;65(3):375-98)

(Mehta, Lansky, 2004) (Mehta R, Lansky EP. Breast cancer chemopreventive properties of pomegranate (*Punica granatum*) fruit extracts in a mouse mammary organ culture. Eur J Cancer Prev. 2004;13:345–8)

(Mena et al, 2011) (Mena P, Girones-Vilaplana A, Moreno Diego A, García-Viguera C. Pomegranate fruit for health promotion: Myths and realities. Funct Plant Sci Biotechnol.2011;5:33–42)

(Menezes et al, 2006) (Menezes SM, Cordeiro LN, Viana GS. *Punica granatum* (pomegranate) extract is active against dental plaque. J Herb Pharmacother. 2006;6:79–92)

(Meydani et al, 1993) (Meydani M, Evans WJ, Handelman G, et al. Protective effect of vitamin E on exercise-induced oxidative damage in young and older adults. Am J Physiol. 1993;264:R992–R8)

(Mirmiran et al, 2010) (Mirmiran P, Fazeli MR, Asghari G, Shafiee A, Azizi F. Effect of pomegranate seed oil on hyperlipidaemic subjects: A double-blind placebo-controlled clinical trial. Br J Nutr. 2010;104:402–6)

(Misaka et al, 2011) (Misaka S, Nakamura R, Uchida S, Takeuchi K, Takahashi N, Inui N, et al. Effect of 2 weeks' consumption of pomegranate juice on the pharmacokinetics of a single dose of midazolam: An open-label, randomized, single-center, 2-period crossover study in healthy Japanese volunteers. Clin Ther. 2011;33:246–52)

(Mithun et al, 2010) (Mithun P, Prashant G, Murlikrishna K, Shivakumar K, Chandu G. Antifungal efficacy of *Punica granatum*, *Acacia nilotica*, *Cuminum cyminum* and *Foeniculum vulgare* on Candida albicans: An *in vitro* study. Indian J Dent Res. 2010;21:334–6)

(Mohan, Waghulde, Kasture, 2010) (Mohan M, Waghulde H, Kasture S. Effect of pomegranate juice on Angiotensin II-induced hypertension in diabetic Wistar rats. Phytother Res.2010;24:S196–203)

(Moos et al, 2004) (Moos, PJ, Edes, K, Mullally, JE, et al. (2004) Curcumin impairs tumor suppressor p53 function in colon cancer cells. Carcinogenesis 25, 1611–1617)

(Mosca et al, 2004) (Mosca L, Appel LJ, Benjamin EJ, et al. American heart association. Evidence-based guidelines for cardiovascular disease prevention in women. Circulation. 2004;109:672–93)

(Mukherjee et al., 2007) (Mukherjee PK, Kumar V, Mal M, Houghton PJ (2007). Acetylcholinesterase inhibitors from plants. Phytomed., 14: 289-300)

(Myzak et al, 2004) (Myzak MC, Karplus PA, Chung FL, et al. A novel mechanism of chemoprotection by sulforaphane: inhibition of histone deacetylase. *Cancer Res.* 2004;64:5767–74)

(Myzak and Dashwood, 2006) (Myzak MC, Dashwood RH (2006). Chemoprotection by sulforaphane: keep one eye beyond Keap1. Cancer Lett., 233: 208-218)

(Nagata et al, 2007) (Nagata M, Hidaka M, Sekiya H, Kawano Y, Yamasaki K, Okumura M, et al. Effects of pomegranate juice on human cytochrome P450 2C9 and tolbutamide pharmacokinetics in rats. Drug Metab Dispos. 2007;35:302–5)

(Naumann et al, 2011) (Naumann P., Fortunato F., Zentgraf H., Büchler M. W., Herr I., Werner J. Autophagy and cell death signaling following dietary sulforaphane act independently of each other and require oxidative stress in pancreatic cancer. *International Journal of Oncology.* 2011;39(1):101–109)

(NCI, 1996) (NCI. Clinical development plan: *curcumin.* J Cell Biochem 1996; 26S: 72–85)

(Nestle, 1997) (Nestle M. Broccoli sprouts as inducers of carcinogen-detoxifying enzyme systems: clinical, dietary, and policy implications. *Proc Natl Acad Sci.*1997;94:11149–51)

(Nestle, 1998) (Nestle M. Broccoli sprouts in cancer prevention. *Nutr Rev.* 1998;56:127–30)

(Neurath et al, 2005) (Neurath AR, Strick N, Li YY, Debnath AK. *Punica granatum* (pomegranate) juice provides an HIV-1 entry inhibitor and candidate topical microbicide. Ann N Y Acad Sci. 2005;1056:311–27)

(Neuzil et al 1995) (Neuzil J, Darlow BA, Inder TE, Sluis KB, Winterbourn CC, Stocker R. Oxidation of parental lipid emulsions by ambient and phototherapy lights: potential toxicity of routine parenteral feeding. J Pediatr. 1995;126:785–90**)**

(Newman, 2007) (Newman RA, Lansky EP, Block ML. Pomegranate: The Most Medicinal Fruit. Laguna Beach, California: Basic Health Publications; 2007. -A Wealth of Phytochemicals; p. 120)

(Newman, 2011) (Newman R. Sydney, Australia: Readhowyouwant; 2011. A wealth of phtochemicals. Pomegranate: The Most Medicinal Fruit. p. 184)

(Nishida, 2005) (Nishida S. Metabolic effects of melatonin on oxidative stress and diabetes mellitus. Endocrine. 2005;27(2):131–6)

(Noorfshan, Ashkani-Esfahani et al, 2013) (Noorfshan, Ashkani-Esfahani, A review of therapeutic effects of curcumin. Curr Pharm Des. 2013;19:2032-2046)

(NTP, 1993) (National Toxicology Program (1993) NTP Toxicology and Carcinogenesis Studies of Turmeric Oleoresin (CAS No. 8024-37-1) (Major Component 79 %–85 % Curcumin, CAS No. 458-37-7) in F344/N Rats and B6C3F1 Mice (Feed Studies). Natl Toxicol Program Tech Rep Ser 427, 1–275)

(Obrenovich et al, 2011) (Obrenovich M, et al. Antioxidants in Health, Disease and Aging. CNS & Neurological Disorders - Drug Targets (Formerly Current Drug Targets - CNS & Neurological Disorders), Volume 10, Number 2, March 2011, pp. 192-207(16))

(Odot et al, 2004) (Odot, J, Albert, P, Carlier, A, et al. (2004) *In vitro* and *in vivo* anti-tumoral effect of curcumin against melanoma cells. Int J Cancer 111, 381–387)

(Okada et al, 2012) (NORIHISA OKADA, EITOKU MURAOKA, SEIICHIRO FUJISAWA and MAMORU MACHINO. In Vivo September-October 2012 vol. 26 no. 5. 759-764)

(Olinski et al, 2003) (Olinski R, Gackowski D, Rozalski R, Foksinski M, Bialkowski K. Oxidative DNA damage in cancer patients: a cause or a consequence of the disease development? Mutat Res. 2003;531:177–90)

(Onyango and Khan 2006) (Onyango IG, Khan SM. Oxidative stress, mitochondrial dysfunction, and stress signaling in Alzheimer's disease. Curr Alzheimer Res. 2006;3(4):339–49)

(Oppenheimer, 1937) (Oppenheimer A. Turmeric (curcumin) in biliary diseases. Lancet. 1937;229:619–621)

(Oostenbrug et al, 1997) (Oostenbrug GS, Mensink RP, Hardeman MR, et al. Exercise performance, red blood cell deformability, and lipid peroxidation: effects of fish oil and vitamin E. J Appl Physiol. 1997;83(3):746–52)

(Osseni et al, 2000) (Osseni RA, Rat P, Bogdan A, et al. Evidence of prooxidant and antioxidant action of melatonin on human liver cell line HepG2. Life Sci. 2000;68:387–99)

(Pacheco-Palencia et al, 2008) (Pacheco-Palencia LA, Noratto G, Hingorani L, Talcott ST, Mertens-Talcott SU. Protective effects of standardized pomegranate (*Punica granatum* L.) polyphenolic extract in ultraviolet-irradiated human skin fibroblasts. J Agric Food Chem. 2008;56:8434–41)

(Packer et al, 2004) (Packer L, Rosen P, Tritschler H, King GL, Azzi A, editors. Antioxidants in diabetes management. New York (NY) 7 Marcell Dekker; 2004. p. 1–349)

(Pahlke et al, 2006) (Pahlke G, Ngiewih Y, Kern M, Jakobs S, Marko D, Eisenbrand G. Impact of quercetin and EGCG on key elements of the Wnt pathway in human colon carcinoma cells. J Agric Food Chem.2006;54:7075–82)

(Pai et al, 2010) (Pai MB, Prashant GM, Murlikrishna KS, Shivakumar KM, Chandu GN. Antifungal efficacy of *Punica granatum*, *Acacia nilotica*, *Cuminum cyminum* and *Foeniculum vulgare* on *Candida albicans*: An *in vitro* study. Indian J Dent Res. 2010;21:334–6)

(Pan et al, 2000) (Pan, M-H, Lin-Shiau, S-Y & Lin, J-K (2000) Comparative studies on the suppression of nitric oxide synthase by curcumin and its hydrogenated metabolites through down-regulation of IκB kinase and NF-κB activation in macrophages. Biochem Pharmacol 60, 1665–1676)

(Park et al, 2014) (Park H. S., Han M. H., Kim G.-Y., et al. Sulforaphane induces reactive oxygen species-mediated mitotic arrest and subsequent apoptosis in human bladder cancer 5637 cells. *Food and Chemical Toxicology.* 2014;64:157–165)

(Pham et al, 2004) (Pham NA, Jacobberger JW, Schimmer AD, et al. The dietary isothiocyanate sulforaphane targets pathways of apoptosis, cell cycle arrest, and oxidative stress in human pancreatic cancer cells and inhibits tumor growth in severe combined immunodeficient mice. *Mol Cancer Ther.* 2004;3:1239–48)

(Pham and Plakogiannis 2005) (Pham DQ, Plakogiannis R. Vitamin E supplementation in cardiovascular disease and cancer prevention: Part 1. Ann Pharmacother. 2005;39(11):1870–8)

(Pieri et al, 1995) (Pieri C, Moroni F, Marra M, et al. Melatonin is an efficient antioxidant. Arch Gerontol Geriatr. 1995;20(2):159–65)

(Piralouti et al, 2010) (Pirbalouti AG, Azizi S, Koohpayeh A, Hamedi B. Wound healing activity of Malva sylvestris and *Punica granatum* in alloxan-induced diabetic rats. Acta Pol Pharm. 2010;67:511–6)

(Pirbalouti et al, 2010) (Pirbalouti AG, Koohpayeh A, Karimi I. The wound healing activity of flower extracts of *Punica granatum* and Achillea kellalensis in Wistar rats. Acta Pol Pharm. 2010;67:107–10)

(Polidori et al, 2000) (Polidori MC, Mecocci P, Cherubini A, et al. Physical activity and oxidative stress during aging. Int J Sports Med. 2000;21:154–7)

(Polasa et al, 1992) (Polasa K, Raghuram TC, Krishna TP, Krishnaswamy K. Effect of turmeric on urinary mutagens in smokers. Mutagenesis. 1992;7(2):107–109)

(Potter, 1997) (Potter JD. Beta-carotene and the role of intervention studies. Cancer Lett. 1997;114:329–31)

(Prescott,Fitzpatrick,2000) (Prescott SM, Fitzpatrick FA. Cyclooxygenase-2 and carcinogenesis. Biochim Biophys Acta. 2000;1470:69–78)

(Promprom et al, 2010) (Promprom W, Kupittayanant P, Indrapichate K, Wray S, Kupittayanant S. The effects of pomegranate seed extract and beta-sitosterol on rat uterine contractions. Reprod Sci. 2010;17:288–96)

(Proteggente et al, 2002) (Proteggente A. R., Pannala A. S., Paganga G., et al. The antioxidant activity of regularly consumed fruit and vegetables reflects their phenolic and vitamin C composition. *Free Radical Research*. 2002;36(2):217–233)

(Prucksunand et al, 2001) (Prucksunand C, Indrasukhsri B, Leethochawalit M, Hungspreugs K. Phase II clinical trial on effect of the long turmeric (*Curcuma longa* Linn) on healing of peptic ulcer. Southeast Asian J Trop Med Public Health. 2001;32(1):208–215)

(Pulla, Reddy, 1992) (Pulla Reddy, Ach. and Lokesh, B. R., Studies on spice principles as antioxidant in the inhibition of lipid peroxidation of rat liver microsomes. Mol. Cell. Biochem., 1992, 111, 117–124)

(Quindry et al, 2003) (Quindry JC, Stone WL, King J, et al. The effects of acute exercise on neutrophils and plasma oxidative stress. Med Sci Sports Exerc. 2003;35(7):1139–45)

(Rao et al, 1993) (Rao, CV, Simi, B & Reddy, BS (1993) Inhibition by dietary curcumin of azoxymethane-induced ornithine decarboxylase, tyrosine protein kinase, arachidonic acid metabolism and aberrant crypt foci formation in the rat colon. Carcinogenesis 14, 2219–2225)

(Rasheed, Akhtar, Haqqi, 2010) (Rasheed Z, Akhtar N, Haqqi TM. Pomegranate extract inhibits the interleukin-1b-induced activation of MKK-3, p38a-MAPK and transcription factor RUNX-2 in human osteoarthritis chondrocytes -Arthritis Res Ther. 2010;12:195)

(Rasyid, Lelo, 1999) (Rasyid A, Lelo A. The effect of curcumin and placebo on human gall-bladder function: an ultrasound study. Aliment Pharmacol Ther. 1999;13(2):245–249)

(Reid et al, 2002) (Reid ME, Duffield-Lillico AJ, Garland L, et al. Selenium supplementation and lung cancer incidence: an update of the nutritional prevention of cancer trial. Cancer Epidemiol Biomarkers Prev. 2002;11:1285–91)

(Renaud and de Lorgeril, 1992) (Renaud S, de Lorgeril M. Wine, alcohol, platelets, and the French paradox for coronary heart disease. Lancet. 1992;339(8808):1523–6)

(Rettig et al, 2008) (Rettig MB, Heber D, An J, Seeram NP, Rao JY, Liu H, et al. Pomegranate extract inhibits androgen-independent prostate cancer growth through a nuclear factor-kappaB-dependent mechanism. Mol Cancer Ther. 2008;7:2662–71)

(Ringman et al, 2005) (Ringman JM, Frautschy SA, Cole GM, Masterman DL, Cummings JL. A potential role of the curry spice curcumin in Alzheimer's disease. Curr Alzheimer Res. 2005;2(2):131–136)

(Rivera-Espinoza, Muriel, 2009) (Yadira Rivera-Espinoza and Pablo Muriel. Pharmacological actions of curcumin in liver diseases or damage. Liver International. Vol. 29, Issue 10, Pages 1457-1488. Nov. 2009)

(Rock et al, 2008) (Rock W, Rosenblat M, Miller-Lotan R, Levy AP, Elias M, Aviram M. Consumption of wonderful variety pomegranate juice and extract by diabetic patients increases paraoxonase 1 association with high-density lipoprotein and stimulates its catalytic activities. J Agric Food Chem. 2008;56:8704–13)

(Rose et al, 2003) (Rose et al, beta-Phenylethyl isothiocyanate-mediated apoptosis in hepatoma HepG2 cells. Cell Mol Life Sci. 2003 Jul;60(7):1489-503)

(Rosenblat, Volkova, Aviram, 2010) (Rosenblat M, Volkova N, Aviram M. Pomegranate juice (PJ) consumption antioxidative properties on mouse macrophages, but not PJ beneficial effects on macrophage cholesterol and triglyceride metabolism, are mediated via PJ-induced stimulation of macrophage PON2. *Atherosclerosis*. 2010 Sep;212(1):86-92)

(Rosenblat et al, 2013) (Rosenblat M, Volkova N, Aviram M. Addition of pomegranate juice to statin inhibits cholesterol accumulation in macrophages: protective role for the phytosterol beta-sitosterol and for the polyphenolic antioxidant punicalagin. *Harefuah*. 2013 Sep;152(9):513-5, 565)

(Sakamoto et al 2002) (Sakamoto H, Corcoran TB, Laffey JG, et al. Isoprostanes – Markers of ischemia reperfusion injury. Eur J Anaesthesiol. 2002;19:550–9)

(Salganik et al, 2000) (Salganik, R. I., Albright, C. D., Rodgers, J., Kim, J., Zeisel, S. H., Sivashinskiy, M. S. & Van Dyke, T. A. (2000) Dietary antioxidant depletion: enhancement of tumor apoptosis and inhibition of brain tumor growth in transgenic mice. Carcinogenesis 21: 909–914)

(Sandur et al, 2007) (Sandur, SK, Pandey, MK, Sung, B, et al. (2007) Curcumin, demethoxycurcumin, bisdemethoxycurcumin, tetrahydrocurcumin and tumerones differentially regulate anti-inflammatory and anti-proliferative responses through a ROS-independent mechanism. Carcinogenesis, 1765–1773)

(Sandur, Ichikawa et al, 2007) (Sandur, SK, Ichikawa, H, Pandey, MK, et al. (2007) Role of pro-oxidants and antioxidants in the anti-inflammatory and apoptotic effects of curcumin (diferuloylmethane). Free Radic Biol Med 43, 568–580)

(Satish et al, 2007) (Satish S, Mohana D, Ranhavendra M, Raveesha K. Antifungal activity of some plant extracts against important seed borne pathogens of Aspergillus sp. J Agric Sci Technol. 2007;3:109–19)

(Satoskar et al, 1986) (Satoskar RR, Shah SJ, Shenoy SG. Evaluation of anti-inflammatory property of curcumin (diferuloyl methane) in patients with postoperative inflammation. Int J Clin Pharmacol Ther Toxicol. 1986;24(12):651–654)

(Schraufstatter, Bernt, 1949) (Schraufstatter E, Bernt H. Antibacterial action of curcumin and related compounds. Nature. 1949;164(4167):456)

(Sekine-Suzuki et al, 2008) (Sekine-Suzuki E., Yu D., Kubota N., Okayasu R., Anzai K. Sulforaphane induces DNA double strand breaks predominantly repaired by homologous recombination pathway in human cancer cells. *Biochemical and Biophysical Research Communications.* 2008;377(2):341–345)

(Sesso et al, 2008) (Sesso, Howard D., et al. "Vitamins E and C in the prevention of cardiovascular disease in men: the Physicians' Health Study II randomized controlled trial." *Jama* 300.18 (2008): 2123-2133)

(Sestili et al, 1986) (Sestili P., Piedimonte G., Cattabeni F., Cantoni O. Induction of DNA breakage and suppression of DNA synthesis by the OH radical generated in a fenton-like reaction. *Biochemistry International.* 1986;12(3):493–501)

(Sestili et al, 2010) (Sestili P., Paolillo M., Lenzi M., et al. Sulforaphane induces DNA single strand breaks in cultured human cells. *Mutation Research/Fundamental and Molecular Mechanisms of Mutagenesis.* 2010;689(1-2):65–73)

(Sestili, Fimognari, 2015) (Sestili P, Fimognari C. Cytotoxic and Antitumor Activity of Sulforaphane: The Role of Reactive Oxygen Species. Biomed Res Int. 2015;2015:402386)

(Sevov et al, 2006) (Sevov M, Elfineh L, Cavelier LB. Resveratrol regulates the expression of LXR-alpha in human macrophages. Biochem Biophys Res, Comm. 2006;348(3):1047–54)

(Shaban et al, 2013) (Shaban NZ, El-Kersh MA, El-Rashidy FH, Habashy NH. Protective role of Punica granatum (pomegranate) peel and seed oil extracts on diethylnitrosamine and phenobarbital-induced hepatic injury in male rats. *Food Chem.* 2013 Dec 1;141(3):1587-96)

(Shankar et al, 2008) (Shankar et al, Sulforaphane enhances the therapeutic potential of TRAIL in prostate cancer orthotopic model through regulation of apoptosis, metastasis, and angiogenesis. Clin Cancer Res. 2008 Nov 1;14(21):6855-66)

(Shapiro et al., 2001) (Shapiro TA, Fahey JW, Wade KL, Stephenson KK, Talalay P (2001). Chemoprotective glucosinolates and isothiocyanates of broccoli sprouts: metabolism and excretion in humans. Cancer Epidemiol Biomarkers Prev., 10: 501-508)

(Sharma, 1976) (Sharma, O. P., Antioxidant activity of curcumin and related compounds. Biochem. Pharmacol., 1976, 25, 1811–1812)

(Sharma et al, 2007) (Sharma RA, McLelland HR, Hill KA, Ireson CR, Euden SA, Manson MM, et al. Pharmacodynamic and pharmacokinetic study of oral Curcuma extract in patients with colorectal cancer. Clin Cancer Res. 2001;7(7):1894–1900)

(Sharma, Steward et al, 2007) (Sharma, RA, Steward, WP & Gescher, AJ (2007) Pharmacokinetics and pharmacodynamics of curcumin. Adv Exp Med Biol 595, 453–470)

(Sharma et al, 2010) (Sharma M, Li L, Celver J, Killian C, Kovoor A, Seeram NP. Effects of fruit ellagitannin extracts, ellagic acid, and their colonic metabolite, urolithin A, on Wnt signaling. J Agric Food Chem. 2010;58:3965–9)

(Sharma, Sharma et al, 2010) (Sharma R., Sharma A., Chaudhary P., et al. Role of lipid peroxidation in cellular responses to d, l -sulforaphane, a promising cancer chemopreventive agent. *Biochemistry.* 2010;49(14):3191–3202)

(Shen, Ji, 2012) (Shen L, Ji H-F. The pharmacology of curcumin: is it the degradation products?. Trends in Molecular Medicine. Vol. 18, Issue 3, March 2012. Pages 136-144) http://www.sciencedirect.com/science/article/pii/S147149141200007X)

(Shimouchi et al, 2009) (Shimouchi A, Nose K, Takaoka M, Hayashi H, Kondo T. Effect of dietary turmeric on breath hydrogen. Dig Dis Sci. 2009;54(8):1725–1729)

(Shin et al, 2013) (Shin DM, et al, New Perspectives of Curcumin in Cancer Prevention. Cancer Prevention Research. Mar 8, 2013; doi: 10. 1158/1940. 6207. CAPR-12-0410)

(Shoba et al, 1998) (Shoba G, Joy D, Joseph T, Majeed M, Rajendran R, Srinivas PS. Influence of piperine on the pharmacokinetics of curcumin in animals and human volunteers. Planta Med. 1998;64(4):353–356)

(Shoskes et al, 2005) (Shoskes D, Lapierre C, Cruz-Correa M, Muruve N, Rosario R, Fromkin B, et al. Beneficial effects of the bioflavonoids curcumin and quercetin on early function in cadaveric renal transplantation: a randomized placebo controlled trial. Transplantation. 2005;80(11):1556–1559)

(Shukla et al, 2002) (Shukla, Y., Arora, A. and Taneja, P., Antimutagenic potential of curcumin on chromosomal aberrations in Wistar rats. Mutat. Res., 2002, 515, 197–202)

(Shukla et al, 2008) (Shukla M, Gupta K, Rasheed Z, Khan KA, Haqqi TM. Bioavailable constituents/metabolites of pomegranate (*Punica granatum* L) preferentially inhibit COX2 activity *ex vivo* and IL-1beta-induced PGE2 production in human chondrocytes *in vitro*. J Inflamm (Lond) 2008;5:9)

(Shravan et al, 2011) (Shravan Kumar Y, Adukondalu D, Bhargavi Latha A, Vamshi Vishnu Y, Ramesh G, Shiva Kumar R, et al. Effect of pomegranate pretreatment on the oral bioavailability of buspirone in male albino rabbits. Daru. 2011;19:266–9)

(Sies, 1997) (Sies, Helmut. "Oxidative stress: oxidants and antioxidants." Experimental physiology 82.2 (1997): 291-295)

(Sikka, 2003) (Sikka S. C. Role of oxidative stress response elements and antioxidants in prostate cancer pathobiology and chemoprevention—a mechanistic approach. *Current Medicinal Chemistry*. 2003;10(24):2679–2692)

(Singh, Aggarwal, 1995) (Singh, S & Aggarwal, BB (1995) Activation of transcription factor NF-kappa B is suppressed by curcumin (diferuloylmethane) [corrected]. J Biol Chem 270, 24995–25000)

(Singh et al, 2004) (Singh AV, Xiao D, Lew KL, Dhir R, Singh SV. Sulforaphane induces caspase-mediated apoptosis in cultured PC-3 human prostate cancer cells and retards growth of PC-3 xenografts in vivo. Carcinogenesis. 2004;25:83–90)

(Singh et al, 2005) (Singh S. V., Srivastava S. K., Choi S., et al. Sulforaphane-induced cell death in human prostate cancer cells is initiated by reactive oxygen species. *The Journal of Biological Chemistry.* 2005;280(20):19911–19924)

(Slater et al, 1995) (Slater, A. F., Nobel, C. S. & Orrenius, S. (1995) The role of intracellular oxidants in apoptosis. Biochim. Biophys. Acta 1271: 59–62)

(Sobieszczyk, Beckman, 2006) (Sobieszczyk P, Beckman J. Carotid artery disease. *Circulation.* 2006 Aug 15;114(7):e244-7)

(Sohrab et al, 2014) (Sohrab G, Nasrollahzadeh J, Zand H, Amiri Z, Tohidi M^3, Kimiagar M. Effects of pomegranate juice consumption on inflammatory markers in patients with type 2 diabetes: A randomized, placebo-controlled trial. J Res Med Sci. 2014 Mar;19(3):215-20)

(Solowiej et al, 2003) (Solowiej E, Kasprzycka-Guttman T, Fiedor P, Rowinski W. Chemoprevention of cancerogenesis—the role of sulforaphane. *Acta Pol Pharm.* 2003;60:97–100)

(Somassundaram et al, 2002) (Somassundaram, Somasundaram, S, Edmund, NA, Moore, DT, et al. (2002) Dietary curcumin inhibits chemotherapy-induced apoptosis in models of human breast cancer. Cancer Res 62, 3868–3875)

(Song et al, 2005) (Song, G, Mao, YB, Cai, QF, et al. (2005) Curcumin induces human HT-29 colon adenocarcinoma cell apoptosis by activating p53 and regulating apoptosis-related protein expression. Braz J Med Biol Res 38, 1791–1798)

(Steinkellner et al, 2001) (Steinkellner H, Rabot S, Freywald C, et al. Effects of cruciferous vegetables and their constituents on drug metabolizing enzymes involved in the bioactivation of DNA-reactive dietary carcinogens. *Mutat Res.* 2001;480-481:285–97)

(Stowe, 2011) (Stowe CB. The effects of pomegranate juice consumption on blood pressure and cardiovascular health. Complement Ther Clin Pract. 2011;17:113–5)

(Strimpakos, Sharma, 2008) (Strimpakos AS, Sharma RA. Curcumin: *preventive and therapeutic properties in laboratory studies and clinical trials.* Antioxid Redox Signal 2008; 10: 511–45) (Goel et al, 2008) (Goel A, Jhurani S, Aggarwal BB. Multi-targeted therapy by curcumin: *how spicy is it?* Mol Nutr Food Res 2008; 52: 1010–3)

(Subramanian et al, 1994) (Subramanian, M., Sreejayan Rao, M. N. A., Devasagayam, T. P. A. and Singh, B. B., Diminution of singlet oxygen induced DNA damage by curcumin and related antioxidants. Mutat. Res., 1994, 311, 249–255)

(Sugawara et al, 2012) (Sugawara J, Akazawa N, Miyaki A, Choi Y, Tanabe Y, Imai T, Maeda S. Effect of endurance exercise training and curcumin intake on central arterial hemodynamics in postmenopausal women: pilot study. Am J Hypertens. 2012 Jun;25(6):651-6)

(Suppipat et al, 2012) (Koramit Suppipat, Chun Shik Park, Ye Shen, Xiao Zhu, and H. Daniel Lacorazza. Sulforaphane Induces Cell Cycle Arrest and Apoptosis in Acute Lymphoblastic Leukemia Cells. PLoS One. 2012; 7(12): e51251)

(Syed et al, 2006) (Syed DN, Malik A, Hadi N, Sarfaraz S, Afaq F, Mukhtar H. Photochemopreventive effect of pomegranate fruit extract on UVA-mediated activation of cellular pathways in normal human epidermal keratinocytes. Photochem Photobiol. 2006;82:398–405)

(Szatrowski, Nathan, 1991) (Szatrowski T. P., Nathan C. F. Production of large amounts of hydrogen peroxide by human tumor cells. *Cancer Research.* 1991;51(3):794–798)

(Takanami et al, 2000) (Takanami Y, Iwane H, Kawai Y, et al. Vitamin E supplementation and endurance exercise: are there benefits? Sports Med. 2000;29(2):73–83)

(Talalay, Zhang, 1996) (Talalay P, Zhang Y. Chemoprotection against cancer by isothiocyanates and glucosinolates. *Biochem Soc Trans.* 1996;24:806–10)

(Tang et al, 2010) (Tang et al, Intake of cruciferous vegetables modifies bladder cancer survival. Cancer Epidemiol Biomarkers Prev. 2010 July ; 19(7): 1806–1811)

(Tao et al, 1998) (Tao X, Schulze-Koops H, Ma L, Cai J, Mao Y, Lipsky PE. Effects of Tripterygium wilfordii hook F extracts on induction of cyclo-oxygenase 2 activity and prostaglandin E2 production. Arthritis Rheum. 1998;41:130–8)

(Terada et al, 1999) (Terada A, Yoshida M, Seko Y, et al. Active oxygen species generation and cellular damage by additives of parenteral preparations: selenium and sulfhydryl compounds. Nutrition. 1999;15(9):651–5)

(Thompson, 1995) (Thompson, C. B. 1995. Apoptosis in the pathogenesis and treatment of disease. Science 267: 1456–146)

(Tiidus and Houston, 1995) (Tiidus PM, Houston ME. Vitamin E status and response to exercise training. Sports Med.1995;20:12–23)

(Tozzi-Ciancarelli, Penco and Di Massimo, 2002) (Tozzi-Ciancarelli MG, Penco M, Di Massimo C. Influence of acute exercise on human platelet responsiveness: possible involvement of exercise-induced oxidative stress. Eur J Appl Physiol. 2002;86(3):266–72)

(Trujillo et al., 2006) (Nutrigenomics, proteomics, metabolomics, and the practice of dietetics. J. Am. Diet. Assoc. 106, 403–41310)

(Tseng et al, 2004) (Tseng E, Scott-Ramsay EA, Morris ME. Dietary organic isothiocyanates are cytotoxic in human breast cancer MCF-7 and mammary epithelial MCF-12A cell lines. Exp Biol Med (Maywood). 2004;229:835–42)

(Tsvetkov et al, 2005) (Tsvetkov, P, Asher, G, Reiss, V, et al. (2005) Inhibition of NAD(P)H:quinone oxidoreductase 1 activity and induction of p53 degradation by the natural phenolic compound curcumin. Proc Natl Acad Sci U S A 102, 5535–5540)

(Turk et al, 2008) (Türk G, Sönmez M, Aydin M, Yüce A, Gür S, Yüksel M, et al. Effects of pomegranate juice consumption on sperm quality, spermatogenic cell density, antioxidant activity and testosterone level in male rats. Clin Nutr. 2008;27:289–96)

(Tusskom et al, 2013) (Tusskom et al, Phenethyl isothiocyanate induces apoptosis of cholangiocarcinoma cells through interruption of glutathione and mitochondrial pathway. Naunyn Schmiedebergs Arch Pharmacol. 2013 Nov;386(11):1009-16)

(Upritchard et al 2003) (Upritchard JE, Schuurman CRWC, Wiersma A, et al. Spread supplemented with moderate doses of vitamin E and carotenoids reduces lipid peroxidation in healthy, nonsmoking adults. Am J Clin Nutr. 2003;78:985–92)

(Usharani et al, 2008) (Usharani P, Mateen AA, Naidu MU, Raju YS, Chandra N. Effect of NCB-02, atorvastatin and placebo on endothelial function, oxidative stress and inflammatory markers in patients with type 2 diabetes mellitus: a randomized, parallel-group, placebo-controlled, 8-week study. Drugs R D. 2008;9(4):243-50)

(Van der Beek, 1991) (Van der Beek EJ. Vitamin supplementation and physical performance. J Sports Sci.1991;9:77–90)

(van Poppel and van den Berg, 1997) (van Poppel G, van den Berg H. Vitamins and cancer. Cancer Lett. 1997;114:195–202)

(van Poppel et al, 1999) (van Poppel G, Verhoeven DT, Verhagen H, Goldbohm RA. Brassica vegetables and cancer prevention. Epidemiology and mechanisms. *Adv Exp Med Biol.* 1999;472:159–68)

(Verhoeven et al, 1997) (Verhoeven DT, Goldbohm RA, van Poppel G, et al. A review of mechanisms underlying anticarcinogenicity by brassica vegetables. *Chem Biol Interact.* 1997;103:79–129)

(Vermeulen et al., 2008) (Vermeulen M, Klopping-Ketelaars IW, Van den BR, Vaes WH (2008). Bioavailability and kinetics of sulforaphane in humans after consumption of cooked versus raw broccoli. J. Agric. Food Chem. 56: 10505-10509)

(Vidal et al, 2003) (Vidal A, Fallarero A, Peña BR, Medina ME, Gra B, Rivera F, et al. Studies on the toxicity of *Punica granatum* L. (*Punicaceae*) whole fruit extracts. J Ethnopharmacol. 2003;89:295–300)

(Vina et al, 2004) (Vina J, Lloret A, Orti R, Alonso D. 2004Molecular bases of the treatment of Alzheimer's disease with antioxidants: prevention of oxidative stress Mol Asp Med 251–2.2117–23)

(Vinceti et al, 2001) (Vinceti M, Wei ET, Malagoli C, Bergomi M, Vivoli G. Adverse health effects of selenium in humans. Rev Environ Health. 2001;16:233–51)

(Vivekananthan et al, 2003) (Vivekananthan, Deepak P., et al. "Use of antioxidant vitamins for the prevention of cardiovascular disease: meta-analysis of randomised trials." *The Lancet* 361.9374 (2003): 2017-2023)

(Vlachojannis C, Zimmermann BF, Chrubasik-Hausmann S. Efficacy and safety of pomegranate medicinal products for cancer. Evid Based ComplementAlternatMed.2015;2015:258598.doi:10.1155/2015/258598. Epub 2015 Mar 1)

(Vlahovic et al, 2007) (P.Vlahović, T. Cvetković, V. Savić, V. Stefanović. Food and Chemical Toxicology. Volume 45, Issue 9, September 2007, Pages 1777–1782)

(Vogel, Pelletier, 1815) (Vogel A, Pelletier J. Examen chimique de la racine de Curcuma. J Pharm. 1815;1:289–300) (Gupta et al, 2012) (Gupta SC, Patchva S, Koh W, Aggarwal BB. Discovery of curcumin, a component of golden spice, and its miraculous biological activities. Clin Exp Pharmacol Physiol. 2012;39(3):283–299)

(Volak et al, 2008) (Volak LP, Ghirmai S, Cashman JR, Court MH. Curcuminoids inhibit multiple human cytochromes P450, UDP-glucuronosyltransferase, and sulfotransferase enzymes, whereas piperine is a relatively selective CYP3A4 inhibitor. Drug Metab Dispos. 2008 Aug;36(8):1594-605)

(Vouldoukis et al, 2004) (Vouldoukis I, Conti M, Krauss P, et al. Supplementation with gliadin-combined plant superoxide dismutase extract promotes antioxidant defences and protects against oxidative stress. *Phytother Res.* 2004 Dec;18(12):957-62)

(Vroegrijk et al, 2011) (Vroegrijk IO, van Diepen JA, van den Berg S, Westbroek I, Keizer H, Gambelli L. Pomegranate Seed Oil, a rich source of Punicic Acid, prevents diet-induced obesity and insulin resistance in mice. Food Chem Toxicol. 2011;49:1426–30)

(Wang et al, 2006) (Wang Z, Zhang Y, Banerjee S, Li Y, Sarkar FH. Notch-1 down-regulation by curcumin is associated with the inhibition of cell growth and the induction of apoptosis in pancreatic cancer cells. Cancer. 2006;106:2503–13)

(Waris, Ahsan, 2006) (Waris G., Ahsan H. Reactive oxygen species: role in the development of cancer and various chronic conditions. *Journal of Carcinogenesis.* 2006;5, article 14 doi: 10.1186/1477-3163-5-14)

(Watson et al, 2005) (Watson TA, Callister R, Taylor RD, et al. Antioxidant restriction and oxidative stress in short-duration exhaustive exercise. Med Sci Sports Exerc. 2005;37(1):63–71)

(Wenzel, Bearman, Edmond, 2007) (Wenzel RP, Bearman G, Edmond MB. Community-acquired methicillin-resistant *staphylococcus aureus* (MRSA): New issues for infection control. Int J Antimicrob Agents. 2007;30:210–2)

(Wiczk et al, 2012) (Wiczk A., Hofman D., Konopa G., Herman-Antosiewicz A. Sulforaphane, a cruciferous vegetable-derived isothio-cyanate, inhibits protein synthesis in human prostate cancer cells. *Biochimica et Biophysica Acta.* 2012;1823(8):1295–1305)

(Wijnen et al, 2001) (Wijnen MH WA, Coolen SA J, Vader HL, et al. Antioxidants reduce oxidative stress in claudicants. J Surg Res. 2001;96:183–7)

(Williamson et al, 1996) (Williamson G., Plumb G. W., Uda Y., Price K. R., Rhodes M. J. C. Dietary quercetin glycosides: antioxidant activity and induction of the anticarcinogenic phase II marker enzyme quinone reductase in Hepalclc7 cells. Carcinogenesis. 1996;17(11):2385–2387)

(Woo et al, 2003) (Woo, J. H. et al., Molecular mechanisms of curcumin-induced cytotoxicity: induction of apoptosis through generation of reactive oxygen species, down-regulation of Bcl-XL and IAP, the release of cytochrome c and inhibition of Akt. Carcinogenesis, 2003, 24, 1199–1208)

(Xiao et al, 2006) (Xiao et al, Benzyl isothiocyanate–induced apoptosis in human breast cancer cells is initiated by reactive oxygen species and regulated by Bax and Bak. Mol cancer Ther 2006;5(11): 2931- 2945)

(Xiao et al, 2009) (Xiao D., Powolny A. A., Antosiewicz J., et al. Cellular responses to cancer chemopreventive agent D, L-sulforaphane in human prostate cancer cells are initiated by mitochondrial reactive oxygen species. Pharmaceutical Research. 2009;26(7):1729–1738)

(Xiao et al, 2010) (Xiao et al, Phenethyl Isothiocyanate Inhibits Oxidative Phosphorylation to Trigger Reactive Oxygen Species-mediated Death of Human Prostate Cancer Cells. J Biol Chem. 2010 Aug 20; 285(34): 26558–26569)

(Xu et al, 2009) (Xu KZ, Zhu C, Kim MS, Yamahara J, Li Y. Pomegranate flower ameliorates fatty liver in an animal model of type 2 diabetes and obesity. J Ethnopharmacol. 2009;123:280–7)

(Yanyan et al, 2010) (Yanyan Li, Tao Zhang, Hasan Korkaya, Suling Liu, Hsiu-Fang Lee, Bryan Newman, Yanke Yu, Shawn G. Clouthier, Steven J. Schwartz, Max S. Wicha, and Duxin Sun. Sulforaphane, a Dietary Component of Broccoli/Broccoli Sprouts, Inhibits Breast Cancer Stem Cells. Clin Cancer Res. 2010 May 1; 16(9): 2580–2590)

(Ye et al, 2002) (Ye L., Dinkova-Kostova A. T., Wade K. L., Zhang Y., Shapiro T. A., Talalay P. Quantitative determination of dithiocarbamates in human plasma, serum, erythrocytes and urine: pharmacokinetics of broccoli sprout isothiocyanates in humans. Clinica Chimica Acta. 2002;316(1-2):43–53)

(Yoshino et al, 2004) (M. Yoshino, M. Haneda, M. B. Naruse, H.H. Hytay, R. Tsubouchi, S.L. Qiao, W. H. Li, K. Murakama, T. Yokochi. Proxidant activity of curcumin: copper-dependent formation of 8-hydroxy-2-deoxyguanosine in DNA and induction of apoptotic cell death. Toxicology in Vitro. Volume 18, Issue 6, Decimber 2004, Pages 783-789)

(Zang, Tang, 2007) (Zhang Y, Tang L. Discovery and development of sulforaphane as a cancer chemopreventive phytochemical. Acta Pharmacol Sin. 2007;28:1343–54)

(Zanichelli et al, 2012) (Zanichelli F., Capasso S., Cipollaro M., et al. Dose-dependent effects of R-sulforaphane isothiocyanate on the biology of human mesenchymal stem cells, at dietary amounts, it promotes cell proliferation and reduces senescence and apoptosis, while at anti-cancer drug doses, it has a cytotoxic effect. Age. 2012;34(2):281–293)

(Zanichelli, Capasso, et al, 2012) (Zanichelli F., Capasso S., Di Bernardo G., et al. Low concentrations of isothiocyanates protect mesenchymal stem cells from oxidative injuries, while high concentrations exacerbate DNA damage. Apoptosis. 2012;17(9):964–974)

(Zarfeshany et al, 2014) (Aida Zarfeshany, Sedigheh Asgary, and Shaghayegh Haghjoo Javanmard. Potent health effects of pomegranate. Adv Biomed Res. 2014; 3: 100)

(Zerba et al, 1990) (Zerba E, Koncikowski TE, Faulkner JA. Free radical injury to skeletal muscles of young, adult, and old mice. Am J Physiol. 1990;258:C429–C35)

(Zuccotti et al, 2009) (Zuccotti GV, Trabattoni D, Morelli M, Borgonovo S, Schneider L, Clerici M. Immune modulation by lactoferrin and curcumin in children with recurrent respiratory infections. J Biol Regul Homeost Agents. 2009;23(2):119–123)

ABOUT THE AUTHOR

Dr. Randolph M. Howes M.D., Ph.D.

Biographical sketch:

As a champion of the people, Dr. Howes anticipates and hopes for the active involvement of all connected parties (patients, caregivers, healthcare professionals, etc.) as an integral approach to educating consumers and the public about the potential dangers of excessive antioxidant-containing supplements.

Some people are born with a silver spoon in their mouth but Dr. Howes had to earn his. Even as a child, Dr. Howes could think with adult clarity. He could envision his future but it would require "decades of dedication" to make it a reality.

From childhood, Dr. Howes was motivated to become a medical doctor and scientist. Assuredly, having been born on a small strawberry farm in rural Louisiana, his journey to the top has proved to be arduous and demanding.

However, he was fortunate to acquire the confidence of Sister Elizabeth at St. Joseph's school and went on to gain the support of his high school speech teacher, Mrs. Iris Brann, who also had strong beliefs in his abilities and potential. Ultimately, with the help of his guitar and his singing ability, he defeated the star quarter back of the high school football team to become the president of the student body.

With the aid of a $25 dollar legislative scholarship, he went on to Southeastern Louisiana College (SLC). At SLC, he was selected for honors chemistry, made the Dean's list, worked at the Psychology Research Lab forty hours a week, maintained a premed study load, and was elected president of the Junior Class and the Interfraternity Council.

To earn badly needed funds, he played music on weekends in a small combo, The Three Blind Mice. Next, he matriculated to Tulane University School of Medicine.

His initial dream was to try to combine both medicine and science. In that regard, he began work as a technician with Dr. Andrew Schally at the Endocrine Polypeptide Lab in the isolation of thyrotropin releasing factor. This work led to a Nobel Prize for Dr. Schally.

Dr. Howes had been highly impressed with the enthusiasm of biochemist, Dr. Richard H. Steele, who accepted him as a doctoral candidate under his tutelage. Dr. Howes graduated in the top 10 of his class, won the Louisiana Pathology Association Award, was elected to the Sigma Xi honor fraternity and was the first in the history of Tulane to become a Doctor of Medicine and a Ph.D. in biochemistry concurrently.

Next, he was selected to pursue a career in surgery at the prestigious Johns Hopkins Hospital.

Unbelievably, at Dr. Howes' urging, he was allowed to operate his own research lab during his surgical internship and residency training while at Johns Hopkins Hospital. He worked hand in hand with the greats in American medicine and surgery.

Independently, he garnered grants, trained lab techs, wrote papers, slept on the cold floor, proudly served as a Captain in the U.S. Army Reserves Medical Corp and finished with board eligibility in both general and plastic surgery in an unheard of six year period.

In another first, he was appointed as an Adjunct Assistant Professor of Plastic Surgery at Johns Hopkins Hospital.

For decades, Dr. Howes gave unselfishly to pro bono medical missions in the Philippines and he holds the Ernesto Espaldon Chair as Professor of Plastic Surgery at the University of Santo Tomas.

Upon retirement from a career in cosmetic plastic surgery, he is living his dream of trying to revolutionize the treatment of cancer, heart disease, HIV/AIDS and malaria, with his in depth knowledge of the arcane biochemistry of oxygen metabolism. He is a work in progress! Dedicated and passionate, he is on a mission for mankind.

Dr. Howes invented the triple lumen venous catheter, which has been credited with helping save the lives of over 20 million critically ill patients worldwide. His catheter is the number one venous catheter in the world today and his name is well recognized in over 100 countries. He has been recognized as a humanitarian, visionary, entrepreneur, singer, songwriter, inventor and author.

He received the Harper Award for innovative research from the American College for Advancement in Medicine, served as their keynote speaker and his peers refer to him as "a walking encyclopedia on oxygen metabolism."

He is a Dr. Norman Vincent Peale Unsung Hero award winner, which recognized his awesome versatility. Additionally, even though he is humble and does not like talking about it, he is a self made multi-millionaire.

He is currently doing extensive research on cures for cancer and heart disease and development of revolutionary treatment modalities. He has written 16 books over the past 8 years on the subject of oxygen metabolism, as it relates to protection from cancer, heart disease, diabetes, malaria, HIV/AIDS, Alzheimer's disease, aging and arthritis. He has written many scientific and medical papers and has lectured nationally and internationally. He has written over 240 medical letters to the editor on popular topics.

His research has shown that currently common antioxidant vitamins, such as vitamins A & E, (and vitamin C to a lesser extent) can be harmful and that oxygen free radicals protect us from bacterial, fungal and viral infections and they help to control cancer growth.

He has developed an effective, inexpensive singlet oxygen generating system, from orthomolecular agents, for the treatment of cancer and heart disease. He is passionate about his research and hopes to have his discoveries at the patient's bedside in his lifetime. Admittedly, this is an extremely ambitious goal.

There are over 10,000 pages in his magnum opus and at the Howes World Selective Library on Oxygen Metabolism. **Over 3,000 pages of his opus are available online in a searchable format www. iwillfindthecure.org.**

Companion Books of Prof. R. Howes, MD, PhD:

Howes, R. M. *U.T.O.P.I.A. - Unified Theory of Oxygen Participation in Aerobiosis.* © 2004. Free Radical Publishing Co. Kentwood, LA, available at www. iwillfindthecure.org.

Howes R. M. *The Medical and Scientific Significance of Oxygen Free Radical Metabolism.* © 2005. Free Radical Publishing Co. Kentwood, LA. USA. available at www.iwillfindthecure.org.

Howes, R. M. *Hydrogen Peroxide Monograph 1: Scientific, Medical and Biochemical Overview.* © 2006; Free Radical Publishing Co. USA. 200 pages. available at www.iwillfindthecure.org.

Howes, R. M. Monograph 2: *Antioxidant vitamins A, C & E: Equivocal Scientific Studies,* © 2006; Free Radical Publishing Co. USA. 171 pages. available at www.iwillfindthecure.org.

Howes, R. M. *Cardiovascular Disease and Oxygen Free Radical Mythology,* © 2006; Free Radical Publishing Co. USA. 308 pages. available at www.iwillfindthecure.org.

Howes, R. M. *Diabetes and Oxygen Free Radical Sophistry,* © 2006; Free Radical Publishing Co. USA. Free Radical Publishing Co. USA. 366 pages. available at www.iwillfindthecure.org.

Howes, R. M. *Reactive Oxygen Species Insufficiency (ROSI)*
as the Basis for Disease Allowance and Coexistence:
Extraordinary Support for an Extraordinary Theory
Vol I, II & III. © 2008; 1564 pages. available at www.iwillfindthecure.org.
Howes, R. M. Volume I 501 pages #7 © 2008. Free Radical Publishing Co. USA.
Howes, R. M. Volume II 505 pages #8 © 2008. Free Radical Publishing Co. USA.
Howes, R. M. Volume III 562 pages #9 © 2008. Free Radical Publishing Co. USA.

Howes, R. M. *THE HOWES PAPERS*
© 2009; Free Radical Publishing Co. USA. 211 pages

Howes R.M. *"COFFEE TABLE MUSINGS of the*
Da Vinci in COWBOY BOOTS"
Pithy Prose and Perspicacious Aphorisms. © 2009; 103 pages

Howes, R. M. Reactive Oxygen Species vs. Antioxidants:
"The Oxypocalypse" or
"The war that never was" © 2010; Free Radical Publishing Co. USA. 550 pages. available at www.iwillfindthecure.org.

Howes R.M. *Death in Small Doses?:*
Antioxidant Vitamins A, C & E in the 21st Century
Book One: *A Health Impact Statement For The Layman*
© 2010; Trafford Publishing. Indianapolis, USA. 90 pages

Howes R.M. *Antioxidant Vitamins are Making A Killing;*
Antioxidant Vitamins A, C & E in the 21st Century
Book Two: *A Health Impact Statement For The Medical Scientist*
© 2010; 184 pages

- Death In Small Doses? Trafford Publishing, © 2010

- Antioxidant Overkill, CreateSpace and Free Radical Publishing, © 2011

- Dangers of Excessive Antioxidants in Cancer Patients, CreateSpace and Free Radical Publishing, © 2011

- Heart Disease and Antioxidant Failures, CreateSpace and Free Radical Publishing, © 2011

- Antioxidant Failures and Dangers, CreateSpace and Free Radical Publishing, © 2011

- Anti-Aging Anti-oxidant Scams, CreateSpace and Free Radical Publishing, © 2011

- Sports, Athletes, Exercise Facts and Antioxidant Myths, CreateSpace and Free Radical Publishing, © 2011

- Alzheimer's Disease: Forget Antioxidants and Supplements, CreateSpace and Free Radical Publishing, © 2012

- Sex, Performance, Reproduction, Naked Radicals And Antioxidants, CreateSpace and Free Radical Publishing, © 2012

- Antioxidants Linked To Deadly Unintended Consequences, CreateSpace and Free Radical Publishing, © 2012

- U.T.O.P.I.A.: Unified Theory of Oxygen Participation In Aerobiosis, CreateSpace and Free Radical Publishing, © 2014, revised

- Hydrogen Peroxide: A Health, Homeostatic and Protective Essentiality, CreateSpace and Free Radical Publishing, © 2014

- Reactive Oxygen Species vs. Antioxidants: The Oxypocalypse or The War That Never Was, CreateSpace and Free Radical Publishing, © 2014

- Diabetes and Oxygen Free Radical Sophistry, CreateSpace and Free Radical Publishing, © 2014, revised

- FISH OIL (Omega3 fatty acids): Facts, Fantasies & Failures. CreateSpace and Free Radical Publishing, © 2014

-Vitamin D: Benefits & False claims. CreateSpace and Free Radical Publishing, © 2014

- Chocolate & Red Wine Antioxidants (Polyphenols, Flavonoids & Resveratrol): Facts vs. Falsehoods. CreateSpace and Free Radical Publishing, © 2015

- Blueberry, Tomato & CoQ10 Antioxidants (Anthocyanin, Lycopene & Ubiquinone): Claims vs. Facts. CreateSpace and Free Radical Publishing, © 2015

- Exercise and Reactive Oxygen Species. Likely the only health miracle out there. CreateSpace and Free Radical Publishing, © 2015

- Hyperbaric oxygen, Hypoxia, Hyperoxia & EMODs (ROS): Separating Fact From Factitious. CreateSpace and Free Radical Publishing, © 2015.

All books available at www.amazon.com; www.barnesandno-bles.com; www.booksamillion.com.

Companion Papers of Prof. R. Howes, MD, PhD:

Dr. Howes has authored over 450 medical publications in health related editorials.

Citation: R. Howes: Mythology of Antioxidant Vitamins?. *The Journal of Evidence-Based Alternative and Complimentary Medicine.* April, 2011. 16(2): 149-189.

Citation: R. Howes: Cancer Therapy: A Review with Scientific Validation for the Role of Electronically Modified Oxygen Derivatives in Oncologic Treatment Modalities. *The Internet Journal of Alternative Medicine.* 2010 Volume 8 Number 1.

Citation: R. Howes: Hydrogen Peroxide: A review of a scientifically verifiable omnipresent ubiquitous essentiality of obligate, aerobic, carbon-based life forms. *The Internet Journal of Plastic Surgery.* 2010 Volume 7 Number 1.

Howes M.D., PhD., R. (2009). Dangers of Antioxidants in Cancer Patients: A Review. *PHILICA.COM Article number 153.* Published 7th February, 2009. (20 pages)

Howes M.D., PhD., R. (2008). Aging and anti-aging claims: a review on antioxidant vitamins A, C & E. *PHILICA.COM Article number 116.* Published on 12th January, 2008. (16 pages)

Howes M.D., PhD., R. (2007). Sleep: An original "radical" proposal. *PHILICA.COM Observation number 42.* Published on 5th October, 2007. (1 page)

Howes M.D., PhD., R. (2007). Antioxidant Vitamins A, C & E; Death in Small Doses and Legal Liability? *PHILICA.COM Article number 89.* Published on 5th April, 2007. (23 pages)

Howes M.D., PhD., R. (2007). Cancer, Apoptosis and Reactive Oxygen Species: A New Paradigm. *PHILICA.COM Article number 86.* Published on 26th February, 2007. (11 pages)

Howes M.D., PhD., R. (2007). Antioxidant Vitamins A, C and E: Assessing Potential for Harm. *PHILICA.COM Article number 83.* Published on 15th February, 2007. (14 pages)

Howes M.D., PhD., R. (2007). The Consequent Downfall of the Free Radical Theory. *PHILICA.COM Article number 75.* Published on 22nd January, 2007. (9 pages)

Howes, R.M.: "The Free Radical Fantasy," The Annals of New York Academy of Sciences, 2006, Vol. 1067, pp. 22-26.

(Howes, 2005) (Howes, R.M. Tumoricidal Activity of An Injectable Singlet Oxygen System Generated From Physiological Agents: The Howes Singlet Oxygen Cancer Therapy System). In The Medical and Scientific Significance of Oxygen Free Radical Metabolism. © 2005. Free Radical Publishing Co. Kentwood, LA. pp. 893-912).

(Howes, Farber, 2005) (Howes, R.M. and Farber, G. Tumoricidal Activity of the Howes Singlet Oxygen Delivery System in Human Basal Cell Carcinoma. In The Medical and Scientific Significance of Oxygen Free

Prof Randolph M. Howes MD, PhD

Radical Metabolism. © 2005. Free Radical Publishing Co. Kentwood, LA. pp. 883-892).

(Howes et al, 1977) (Howes, R.M., Steele, R.H. and Hoopes, J.E., The role of Electronic excitation states in collagen biosynthesis, Persp. In Biol. And Med., Summer 1977, 20; 4:539-544).

(Howes, Steele, 1976) (Howes, R.M., Steele, R.H. and Hoopes, J.E., Peroxide induced Chemiluminescence in an in vitro proline hydroxylation system, 1976, 8; 1:77-84).

(Howes et al, 1976) (Howes, R. M., Allen, R.C., Su, C.T. and Hoopes, J.E., Altered polymorphonuclear leukocyte bioenergetics in patients with thermal injury, the Surgical Forum, 1976, 27:558-560).

(Howes, Steele, 1972) (Howes, R.M. and Steele, R.H., Microsomal chemiluminescence induced by NADPH and its relation to aryl-hydroxylations, Res Commun. Chem. Path. Pharmacol., March 1972, 3; 2:349-357).

(Howes, Steele, 1971) (Howes, R. M. and Steele, R. H., Microsomal chemiluminescence induced by NADPH and its relation to lipid peroxidation, Res. Commun. Chem. Path. Pharmacol., July-Sept. 1971, 2; 4 & 5:619-626).

**I despise precious time wasted,
for it alone, is the unfinished canvas
displaying the portrait of my life.
R. M. Howes, M.D., Ph.D.
9/7/09**

"We are what we repeatedly do. Excellence then, is not an act, but a habit." ~Aristotle

OTHER BOOKS

PUBLISHED: Partial list.

The Fire Eaters, Molding your own destiny more easily, Carnivore Press, © 1982

Uplift, The Answer Book to your plastic and cosmetic surgery questions, Carnivore Press, © 1986

The Pundit Speaks, vol. I. An Anthology of Neoclassical

Poetic Philosophy, Carnivore Press,© 1990

The Pundit Speaks, Volume II, An Anthology of Neoclassical Poetic Philosophy, Free Radical Press,© 1994

The Pundit Speaks, Volume III, An Anthology of Neoclassical Poetic Philosophy, Free Radical Press,© 1996

The Pundit Speaks, Volume IV, An Anthology of Neoclassical Poetic Philosophy, Free Radical Press,© 2000

The Fable of the Chocolate Covered Strawberry Coloring Book, Free Radical Press,© 2001

The Pundit Speaks, Volume IV, An Anthology of Neoclassical Poetic Philosophy, Free Radical Press,© 2003

The Pundit Speaks, Volume V, An Anthology of Neoclassical Poetic Philosophy, Trafford Publishing,© 2009

Coffee Table Musings of The DaVinci In Cowboy Boots, Trafford Publishing,© 2010

Available at: www.philica.com
www.medi.philica.com
www.iwillfindthecure.org
www.amazon.com

DOC
R_X**ANDOLPH**
HOWES

RAD!CAL

"Future's shape is sculpted by the
persistent kneading hands of
the impossible dreamer."
R. M. Howes, M.D., Ph.D.
5/2/04